TEXTBOOK
OF
BIO-IDENTICAL
HORMONES

TEXTBOOK
OF
BIO-IDENTICAL
HORMONES

Edward M. Lichten, M.D.

First Edition
Textbook of Bio-Identical Hormones

By EDWARD M. LICHTEN, M.D., F.A.C.S., F.A.C.O.G.
Fellow, American College of Surgeons
Fellow, American College of Obstetricians and Gynecologists
Former Clinical Instructor, Wayne State University College of Medicine
PO Box 0843
Birmingham, Michigan 48012-0843

Foundation for Anti-Aging Research, LLC

Library of Congress Cataloging-in-Publication Data
Lichten, Edward M.
Textbook of Bio-Identical Hormones. 1. Insomnia. 2. Fibromyalgia & Growth
Hormone. 3. Thyroid. 4. Adrenal Fatigue.

ISBN: 978-0-9658777-2-5

Printed in the United States of America

This book is intended as a reference only, not as a medical manual. The information presented in
the following pages is designed to help you make informed decisions about your health. It is not
a substitute for any treatment that may have been prescribed by your doctor. If you suspect that
you have a medical problem, please seek competent medical care. Mention of specific companies,
organizations, or authorities does not imply endorsement by the publisher, nor does mention of
specific companies, organizations, or authorities imply their endorsement of this book.

Judge not your importance by the circle of your friends;
Judge your importance by the power and number of your enemies.

But with perseverance and reverence for the Almighty,
truth will prevail.

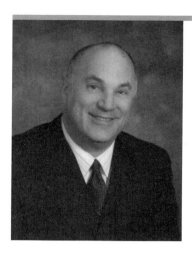

ABOUT THE AUTHOR

Edward M. Lichten, M.D., is a university-trained, board-certified obstetrician-gynecologist who has spent 30 years in private medical practice treating, researching, inventing, and rediscovering ways to use bio-identical and natural therapies to treat his patients' diseases. His philosophy is that the body can most often heal itself if supplied with the proper building blocks of vitamins, minerals, fats, and especially bio-identical hormones. A national and international lecturer, Dr. Lichten enjoys the opportunity to speak with patients and health providers alike, as they can all work together to understand better the benefits of natural and bio-identical treatments in maintaining and improving health care.

To reach the doctor:
Edward M. Lichten, M.D., F.A.C.S., F.A.C.O.G.
Fellow, American College of Surgeons
Fellow, American College of Obstetricians and Gynecologists
Birmingham, Michigan 48012-0843
Appointments: 248.593.9999
Email: drlichten@yahoo.com

ACKNOWLEDGMENTS

I would like to thank my editors, EY and CSL, for reviewing my efforts to put my thoughts together in the making of this book. To my wife, Carolynne, my daughter, Cara, and my son, Michael, thank you, for having steadfastly supported my efforts, read my text, and corrected my English.

For your efforts in loving me and caring for me through all the ups and downs that life brings, I can honestly say that you three are the essence of my continuing existence. Without you, there would have been no book and no efforts from me to continue in my quest to challenge the medical establishment to improve the lives of millions of men and women worldwide.

We all understand how important it is to care for the well-being of humanity and, on top of all that, you three unwaveringly care for me.

With respect, admiration, and a lifetime of love, thank you, my family. I dedicate my continuing medical efforts and this book to you.

DISCLAIMER

This book is written for educational purposes only.

The information contained within this book is based on the training, education, and literature references of the author and is not designated as a treatment protocol or intervention directed course for any person.

We do suggest that you have appropriate laboratory and clinical monitoring of the various endocrine systems, with the goal of finding safe and natural treatments for your medical complaints. Because there are a variety of treatments for each disorder, all medical intervention should be performed under the care of a physician.

This book is not intended to replace or displace your patient-physician relationship, only to educate and offer knowledge about alternative treatments that are based on scientific fact, clinical research, and peer-review publications.

Edward M. Lichten, M.D.

CONTENTS

FOREWORD

I have produced 40 textbooks in obstetrics and gynecology and read thousands of manuscripts as editor in chief of the *American Journal of Obstetrics and Gynecology*, but none like this book by Dr. Lichten. He was my chief resident more than 30 years ago. I would like to identify this book as the book of the future as it is not like the standard textbook of today. It will energize your thinking and will make you ask many questions about the present and the future [of health care].

The book is divided into three logical parts with many subheadings.

BOOK I: Understanding Insomnia and Fatigue. The Role of Natural Hormones, involving the Pineal, Pituitary, Thyroid, and Adrenal glands;

BOOK II: Understanding Bio-Identical Estrogen. The Role of Natural Estrogen for Women, including Menopause, Ovaries, Progesterone, Testosterone, Menstrual Migraine, and Osteoporosis; and

BOOK III: Understanding Bio-Identical Testosterone. The Role of Natural Testosterone for Men, including Male-Andropause, Heart and Cardiovascular Disease, and Diabetes.

Dr. Lichten says that the theme of this book is "The body can most often heal itself if supplied with the proper building blocks of vitamins, minerals, fats, and especially bio-identical hormones."

We live in a time of too much information to evaluate from newspapers, magazines, books, the Internet, and your health care professionals. How do you know that what you read is totally true or partially true? Your interpretation of this information makes it valuable or of no value at all. Dr. Lichten has used scientific methodology to help you understand his book. He has developed a generous scientific literature with multiple references that are both clinically and scientifically sound on each topic. This book is almost a medical autobiography of the past, as well as thought for the future. This book is not intended to be "evidence-based medicine," as this only pertains to individual publications and not textbooks.

This book also lays foundations for the future. First, people must believe that [health care] has viability [and that they are the co-pilot on their quest for good health]. The proof of the pudding can only come with time. Concepts, precepts, and understanding do not come easily. It takes cerebration, imagination, and perseverance to make things happen. May you enjoy reading this book as much as I did.

Frederick P. Zuspan, M.D.
Chairman Emeritus Department of Obstetrics and Gynecology
The Ohio State University School of Medicine and Public Health

PREFACE

Health Care Is Sacred Work

Health caring is sacred work. Health caring begins with a decision to give of one's self so that another may begin the process of healing and recovery. Health caring is a calling, a vocation. The basis of health caring is love—love for others, even for those difficult to love. Health caring is about continually improving how we care for and about others. Continually improving health caring begins with asking questions—questions about what we know and, perhaps more important, about what we do not know. This book is about asking those questions—as well as about moving all of us who provide health care back to a place of caring, which means questioning ourselves, getting to know our patients, and loving our patients.

I have known and worked with Dr. Lichten for approximately six years. During that time I have been most impressed by his absolute commitment to the health and welfare of his patients. This has caused Dr. Lichten to question constantly the traditional dogma of medicine and, at times, the traditional care provided to patients. He has been on a quest to know all that is known about health, including educating himself about traditional, complementary, and alternative forms of therapy. This has led him to collide with the medical establishment and, at times, to move toward "natural health" to support his patients as he searches for truth and patient-centered solutions.

Ernie Yoder, M.D., Ph.D., F.A.C.P.

INTRODUCTION

I am compelled to write this book because of the dangerous state of confusion that exists concerning what aging women and men should do to properly balance their hormones in order to live longer and better.

My first chapter focuses on vitamin D, which is a hormone. The majority of humans do not have adequate blood levels of vitamin D. Maladies that occur in response to less than optimal vitamin D include insomnia, hypertension, heart disease, and cancer. Vitamin D functions as a cell-regulatory brake to protect against the initiation and progression of common cancers, including those of the colon, prostate, and breast.

My second, third, and fourth chapters focus on natural occurring human growth hormone, thyroid, and adrenal hormones. As these hormones are linked to vitamin D, together they supply humans with adequate basic energy reserves. Any hormonal disruption causes an imbalance and drop in energy of the whole body as seen with fibromyalgia, fatigue, and low thyroid or adrenal function.

I am particularly concerned about women being prescribed estrogen drugs without factoring in their needs for natural progesterone, testosterone, vitamin D, and a healthy diet with supplements. Five chapters develop the role of bio-identical estrogens in treating menopause, migraine, PMS, and preventing Alzheimer's disease and osteoporosis.

Estrogen provides many desirable benefits, including stimulating cell division. Bio-identical progesterone regulates specific genes involved in aberrant cell division, thereby reducing cancer risk. Bio-identical estrogen levels should be maintained before, during, and after the onset of menopause as a mandate to healthy living.

Testosterone for both men and women provides needed energy to rebuild tissue worn-down by aging and stress. While testosterone maintains muscle, bone, and mental focus for both sexes, it is also critically necessary for the heart to function. For men, bio-identical testosterone is a key to not only maintaining normal sexual function and normal cholesterol, but also prevention, treatment, and delay of diabetes.

In my medical office, I routinely encounter a diverse group of patients suffering from serious diseases that can be effectively treated by restoring youthful hormone balance and instituting healthy lifestyle changes. To keep this accumulating wealth of knowledge within my relatively obscure private practice in Michigan would deny mankind around the world access to what I have observed, learned and documented.

I believe successful treatment of disease involves a partnership between the doctor and his patient. The doctor serves first as an educator, a mentor bringing his knowledge about health and disease in simplest terms to his patient. The patient in turn brings his experiences with the disease and the treatment outcomes back to the physician. Both do this with a deep sense of trust and humanity. Doctoring is helping your fellow man... simply, safely, and effectively.

One can find instant (and often conflicting) information by accessing the Internet. Our primary source for learning, however, still comes from books. This is because books provide information you may not realize you need to know. A Web browser, on the other hand, is limited to the "key words" you type into a search engine.

The contents of this book are aimed principally at individuals who want to take charge of their own bodies; along with progressive health care professionals who have the clear vision to see how human lives could be improved and saved by implementing this avant-garde and proven medical information into clinical practice.

This book serves as an outreach, in the broadest possible sense, to those who I will never meet, but will hopefully find effective solutions to their medical concerns via the information conveyed herein.

Thank you,

Edward Lichten, M.D., F.A.C.S.

BOOK ONE

THE ROLE *of* NATURAL HORMONES

CHAPTER 1

INSOMNIA, DAYTIME SLEEPINESS, AND LIVING A LONG AND FRUITFUL LIFE

Approximately 1 billion years ago, animal life evolved with the development of the first hormonal glands to regulate sleep. Not only was the formation of melatonin necessary as a catalyst in a number of the organelle's (primitive one-celled creatures) chemical reactions, melatonin would be involved in establishing the circadian (day-night) cycles. These approximate 12-hour cycles of bright sunlight followed by 12 hours of relative darkness established a pattern for a biological rest state, which continued to be ingrained with evolution into more effective and longer-living animalkind. When man evolved on the plains of Africa 5 million years ago, these cycles were already in place. With the migration of man from the sun-filled plains of Africa to the northern and southern latitudes, and then into the caves of industrial modern life, he gave up the sunlight and all the protection from this natural, biologically setting clock. That is why he suffers today from insomnia and its twin, midday fatigue.

At the age of 52, having given up the midnight rite of obstetrical deliveries, Dr. Lichten was faced with insomnia. Maybe because he had learned to fall asleep anywhere, anytime, he did not know that the problem of insomnia had been developing for years. Chronically sleep-deprived insomnia was not of the "Oh I can't fall asleep for an hour" variety. Rather, it was the "been up all night and it's morning and I haven't slept" kind. Being a physician, he had knowledge of the plethora of prescription sleeping medications, medications that list "sleepiness" as a side effect of treatment, and medications used to induce sleep for the worse possible hospital détentes.

Having recognized 25 years previously that women's insomnia was often due to menopausal estrogen deficiencies, he had already made sure that his testosterone level was normal and balanced. Laboratory testing had revealed no profound endocrine disease, as the thyroid levels were normal, although the adrenals were a little low, showing a generalized stress. Natural products including kava kava, valerian root, chamomile tea, and then melatonin in higher and higher dosages proved unsuccessful. So he had prescription after prescription medication offered by his family physician—all well known to the public: sleeping agents—Ambien®, Lunesta®, and Sonata®; anti-anxiety agents—Xanax®, Klonopin®, Ativan®, and Valium®; antidepressants—amitriptyline, doxepin, and trazodone; antihistamines—Benadryl® and Atarax®; narcotics—(cough medication with codeine) and even chloral hydrate. All to no avail.

The literature clearly states that, with 20 million or more Americans seeking physician intervention for insomnia every year,[1] there is great risk for addictive behavior with sleep prescriptions, especially in those over 65 years of age. Both the newer, expensive four-dollars-per-pill Lunesta®/Ambien® agents, as well as the benzodiazepines such as Valium®, are not natural and may inhibit normal slow-wave sleep (SWS).[2] In our culture, 58% of men and women do not sleep well in any given week.[3] Add the signs and symptoms of withdrawal from and potential to addiction[4] from the family of benzodiazepine derivates and this creates a major medical issue for many segments of our aging population.

Yet insomnia is no longer limited to our senior citizens. The number of younger aged adults (age 20-44) on sleeping medications doubled in the past four years. Similarly children 10-19 increased their use of sleeping aids by 85% in the same time period.[3]

Out of frustration and the knowledge that chronic insomnia is associated with a fourfold increase in mortality, Dr. Lichten, searching for a logical answer, asked for a suggestion from a natural-thinking chiropractor whom he visited twice yearly. Dr. Lichten expected to be offered a host of so-called natural cures, such as are omnipresent throughout the Internet. Some of these Internet sites do not want to just treat insomnia, but they want to treat chronic insomnia as depression at a cost of hundreds of dollars a month. Others just want to sell sleep-inducing clocks, magnetic bed pads, opaque night glasses and window shades, flashing sleep-inducing glasses, and a group of "I-don't-know-what-else" products.

The explanation Dr. Lichten received was so simple. He was asked, "How do you sleep on vacation in Florida or the Caribbean?" "Great," Lichten replied. "What is different?" "Sun," Lichten replied. And that began Dr. Lichten's study into the role of sunlight and insomnia.

Now, as a physician who never had a regular time to go to sleep, never took the warm milk, or had the time to relax with a book, this approach of re-establishing a sunlight/darkness circadian rhythm made sense. Yet, in all the literature, only six articles appear in a search of sleep disturbances with a lack of sunlight.[5]

WHY LIGHT?

In 1995, NASA scientists adjusted the circadian rhythms of workers away from the 12-hour-sun/12-hour-dark schedule to better acclimate them to the demands of their work cycles.[6] Using 10,000-lux lights, treatment subjects reported better sleep, performance, and physical and emotional well-being than control subjects, and rated the treatment as highly effective for promoting adjustment to their work schedules. There is also literature on the use of natural grow lights to treat seasonal affective disorder (SAD) and its concomitant sleep problems.[7]

But Richardson[8] notes that "practical issues sharply limit the application of artificial lighting to all shift work settings, however, and the role for a *pill to regulate sleep* (pharmacological chronobiotic agent) capable of accomplishing the same end is potentially very large." Every one wants a simple, oral, available drug.

MELATONIN

Melatonin is a neurohormone synthesized in the pineal gland deep inside the brain. Melatonin is the end product of synthesis from the naturally occurring amino acid L-tryptophan. The steps are first to 5-hydroxytryptophan (5-HTP), then to serotonin, then to *N*-acetyl-serotonin, and finally to melatonin.

Dr. Lichten's colleague, William Regelson, MD,[9] believed in melatonin and wrote the book, *Melatonin Miracle*. Although he trusted Dr. Regelson's opinion, and believed him to be a brilliant and altruistic man, Dr. Lichten never found melatonin to work that well for himself or for many of his patients. Some studies show that melatonin is effective against insomnia, while other studies do not.[10]

A study conducted by the Agency for Healthcare Research and Quality,[10] which divided individuals into (a) normal sleep, (b) primary inability to sleep, and (c) suffering from sleep restrictions, such as jet-lag disorders, concluded that "the improvement in sleep from melatonin in secondary sleep disorders was not of significant magnitude" to make a public announcement. (Other studies do, however, demonstrate efficacy at varying melatonin doses.)

VITAMIN D

"Yes, it is sunlight, not melatonin," Dr. Lichten discovered. "The answer to my insomnia problem is vitamin D."

Everyone knows about vitamin D. It is added to milk products to prevent childhood rickets, soft bones, and related teeth defects. And then the doctor's thoughts reverted to his medical school training of 25 years ago. Vitamin D is not only a vitamin; but is also a pro-hormone. And vitamin D is probably one of the most important naturally occurring pro-*hormone* substances in all of nature.

Vitamin D is a hormone produced in the skin when exposed to sunlight. The medical term is calciferol D3, to differentiate it from food substance calciferol D2. In 30 minutes of bright light exposure to the skin, the melanocytes produce approximately 10,000 IU of vitamin D. Without enough exposure to bright sunlight, especially for dark-skinned individuals and for those whose skin has thickened and become dysfunctional with age, the levels of vitamin D will be nearly universally insufficient to maintain health.

DIFFERENT TYPES OF VITAMIN D

While human cells only produce vitamin D3 naturally, there is another form, vitamin D2, that occurs in yeast, legumes, and other food sources. Vitamin D3 is present in fish and concentrated in fish oil.[11]

But they are not equal. Dr. Laura Armas[12] at Creighton, publishing in the *Journal of Clinical Endocrinology and Metabolism*, showed that 50,000 IU of vitamin D2 does not raise blood levels of vitamin D at 28 days as much as does vitamin D3. Commercially produced from plant and yeast, prescription ergocalciferol (vitamin D2) is only one-third as potent as naturally occurring vitamin D3. Her directive is that vitamin D3, naturally occurring calciferol, is more effective at treating vitamin D deficiency. And the cost difference is profound: therapy with ergocalciferol D2 is $10 a pill per week, while vitamin D3 at 2,000 IU per drop is $16 for more than six months.

ABSORPTION OF VITAMIN D

The problem with all foods, minerals, vitamins, and prescription medication is that the method by which they are delivered to the body will affect their absorption. In later chapters on vitamin supplementation, for example, we note that injectable B12 is more potent than B12 taken under the tongue (sublingual) and more potent than B12 taken orally as a capsule. When ketorolac,

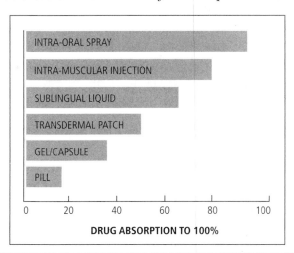

a pain-reliever drug, is taken orally, it is less potent than ketorolac injected into the muscle. The graph on the previous page shows how potency depends on route of delivery.

Now, vitamin D usually comes in a pill form. Based on an intake of a few hundred international units (IU), it is unlikely that there is adequate vitamin D in your bloodstream, let alone your children's, your family's, or your friends'. For some people over age 40, taking even 5,000 IU a day of encapsulated vitamin D does not elevate blood levels to optimal status. For those who are older, sometimes the best means to attain the higher level with many drugs is to absorb the substance directly into the bloodstream under the tongue.[13]

Secondarily, it is well known that the chemical phytic acid in grains and legumes blocks absorption of minerals. As the amounts of wheat and processed foods have increased in our diet, the effect of mineral deficiency and associated lower levels of serum vitamin D are apparent. So, if you do not want to get sick, take in more natural European grains, more body-rebuilding minerals, more essential omega-3 fats, more clean proteins, and more vitamins, including vitamin D. For without the gluten products (wheat), you may be better able to minimize inflammation, improve bones, teeth, gums, and keep your system free from disease as long as possible!

DOSAGE

The current recommended dietary allowance (RDA) for vitamin D is 400 IU. Recently, experts recommended that the RDA for vitamin D should be increased from 400 IU to 800 IU.

Previous studies have shown that the amount of vitamin D necessary to be ingested as a supplement should double recommended 1,000 IU/day during the winter months. A study of 796 Canadians showed that food sources and supplements were inadequate to maintain vitamin D serum levels during winter months.[14]

And what Dr. Lichten learned personally and what he teaches every one of his patients is that vitamin D nutritional status can only be assessed by measuring the total serum 25-hydroxyvitamin D concentration in a blood laboratory test.[15]

BLOOD LEVELS

For more than 30 years, doctors have been able to measure the metabolites of calciferol in the bloodstream. Vitamin D derivatives are measured as 25-hydroxyvitamin D, which is a summation of D3 and D2 levels. The normal range from Quest Diagnostic Laboratories is 20–100 ng/mL (or 50–250 nmol/L), while LabCorp states normal ranges of 32–100 ng/mL (or 80-250 nmol/L). Optimal values are 50+ ng/mL or 125+ nmol/L. There will be no toxicity as long as blood levels are measured at six-month intervals and kept within the normal range. In more than one year on a daily dose of 4,000 IU vitamin D3 sublingual drops, Dr. Lichten reports that his serum level is now only in the 50 ng/mL+ range. It is sound medicine to measure vitamin D levels and add back vitamin D3 supplements in sufficient enough dosages to raise the serum level to the normal range. Vitamin D drops are safe, inexpensive, and offer so many medical advantages that they should be mandatory for everyone over the age of three months. And didn't mother make every child take a teaspoon of cod liver oil at the turn of the century? Did you know that 5 g of cod liver oil, one teaspoon, contains approximately 400 IU of vitamin D3?

Mother was right. Take your vitamin D!

BENEFITS OF VITAMIN D

Although it has been recognized for hundreds of years that sunlight/vitamin D is necessary to prevent rickets, there is awareness today that vitamin D is so necessary to the normal function of at least 30 systems in the human body that not to take vitamin D supplements is outright neglectful.

- **Bone**: Not only does vitamin D affect bone mineralization, it also affects the absorption of minerals from the gastrointestinal tract. Low levels of vitamin D are consistently noted in the elderly who fall and fracture bones.[16] Treatment for osteoporosis therefore always involves additional vitamin D. Furthermore, research has shown that patients with high levels of vitamin D experience a 22% reduction in the risk of non-vertebral fracture.[15]

- **Gastrointestinal tract**: Patients with Crohn's disease and colitis are at a high risk for osteoporosis (thin bones) and fractures. Measurement of vitamin D levels as previously described[16] showed that lower levels of vitamin D were associated with worsening states of colitis and associated with extended time suffering with the disease. As the small bowel is the site for absorption of vitamin D, those who have had ulcerative colitis, distal small bowel resections, and bariatric surgery[17] are universally vitamin D deficient because of an inability to absorb adequate vitamins and minerals from an inflamed mucosa. Those who have had gallbladder surgery are also unable to absorb vitamin D, as bile is inherently necessary for its absorption. In addition, those with fatty liver and a history of alcoholism have low levels of vitamin D. Furthermore, recent genetic studies show that there is a genetic vitamin D marker that is highly associated with familial colitis.[18]

- **Chronic inflammation**: Researchers have come to understand that inflammation is associated with the increase of all maladies in man. Eating processed food, smoking, pollution, stress, and, most of all, lack of antioxidants (vitamins and hormones) contribute to our high state of disease. Not only is measurement of tumor necrosis factor (TNF) associated with major inflammatory states, but TNF correlates with lower levels of vitamin D. Increases in vitamin D through supplementation results in a lowering of TNF[19] and potentially an improvement in the medical condition.

- **Heart disease**: Heart disease is a preventable, inflammatory condition. As a later chapter will illuminate, it is not cholesterol that causes heart disease. It is oxidized LDL-cholesterol that mediates inflammatory responses, which make sticky, fluffy, plaque-forming cholesterol in the artery wall. And the use of all the natural modalities to prevent inflammation can delay and prevent the development of heart disease, thereby extending your quality of life for many years.

- **Dark skin**: 100% of immigrants were found to be vitamin D deficient even 30 years ago in England.[20] This is correlated with the preponderance of hypertension and heart disease in this racial demographic population. Furthermore, the lack of adequate sunlight may increase the risk of hypertension in blacks and other dark-skinned individuals. It is estimated that to compensate for the greater amounts of pigment in the skin, dark-skinned individuals need to increase their UV(B) exposure six-fold.

- **Myalgia, muscle pain, and low back pain**: A study of Saudi Arabian men treated with 5,000 to 10,000 IU of vitamin D daily resulted in improvement in back pain with normalization of serum vitamin D levels.[21] Patients with muscle pain have been found to have very low levels of vitamin D.[22]

- **Multiple sclerosis**: In the first large-scale, prospective study investigating the relationship between low vitamin D levels and multiple sclerosis, researchers confirmed a strong correlation. This study showed that low levels of vitamin D, confirmed before the age of 20 in the Caucasian population, carried an unacceptable risk of multiple sclerosis.[23] The explanation, not forthcoming, must be linked to the multiple aspects of normal health function that rely on vitamin D for normal myelin production.[24]

- **Cancer**: A plethora of large, multi-institutional studies from major universities here and in Europe have confirmed low levels of vitamin D in large epidemiological studies of specific cancers: breast, prostate, colon, bladder.[25-27] PubMed.com, part of the NIH national medical reference database, also notes that low vitamin D is associated with the increased incidence of esophageal, gastric, ovarian, rectal, renal, uterine, non-Hodgkin's lymphoma, cervical, gall bladder, laryngeal, oral, pancreatic, and Hodgkin's lymphoma.

  Based on the Helsinki Heart Study, researchers go so far as to state that the low circulating levels of 25-hydroxyvitamin D are associated with a "more aggressive prognosis of prostate cancer, especially before age 52" . . . "Ultraviolet light has been shown to be protective against prostate cancer." . . . "Nutrition should be maintained not only for bone health but also for the possible reduction in risk of prostate cancer and to reduce metastatic activity should prostate cancer develop."[28]

- **Protective effects of vitamin D on cancer**: Many of the newest pharmaceutical agents that are being offered as treatments for cancer are derived from naturally occurring calciferol. Calcitriol, the activated form of vitamin D, has been shown to induce cell differentiation and to control cell proliferation. People with a low vitamin D level are less able to make sufficient calcitriol to exert enough control over cell proliferation that is needed to reduce cancer.[29] Studies have shown that fatty fish oils, which offer the highest level of dietary vitamin D, protect against many types of cancer. In a study in China, use of cod liver oil was found to be protective against childhood leukemia.[30] Another study of Norwegian men and women revealed consumption of cod liver oil to protect against lung cancer.[31]

- **Pregnancy**: There is a new concern for obstetricians and pediatricians that mothers are not getting enough vitamin D and that this affects their offspring. A lack of vitamin D can lead to rickets and teeth malformation.[32,33]

- **Diabetes, heart disease, and fibromyalgia**: This will be discussed in subsequent chapters. Chronic disease states, including chronic kidney disease, rheumatoid arthritis, and psoriasis, have an association with low levels of vitamin D. It may be imperative to consider more rapid replacement and laboratory follow-up.[34-38]

- **Sunblock and skin cancer**: The problem for dermatologists is the increase in the incidence of skin cancer. Therefore, they warn their patients to "stay out of the sun" and "to wear sunscreen when they go out." But these individuals are at risk of vitamin D deficiency, which may contribute to the increased incidence of skin and other cancers.[39] Other physicians, meanwhile, tell their patients to be out in sunlight for 15 to 30 minutes every day and then apply sunscreen. What are we to do?

The solution is still the same: Take supplements of vitamin D3. Take them in sufficient amounts to raise your serum blood levels over 50 ng/mL. And if you want to follow your laboratory tests, refer to the Appendix for information on ordering your own blood profile and tracking the results.

For Dr. Lichten, the addition of vitamin D sublingual drops, one to two per night, was the magic solution. No more prescription medication to get a good night's sleep. And as stated previously, this dosage of vitamin D nightly took one full year to bring his serum laboratory tests to a normal range. Some patients have taken more, some up to four drops of sublingual vitamin D3 per day without complication. Dr. Lichten advises those using any dose over 2,000 IU per day to be cognizant of symptoms of nausea, vomiting, and malaise, which could be symptoms of vitamin D overdose. If these do occur, advise the doctor of the strength and dosage of the non-prescription vitamin D3 hormone program.

Dr. Lichten's observations are new and there have not yet been any published studies to assess the role of vitamin D in alleviating insomnia. However, given the crucial role that vitamin D plays in protecting against many disease processes, every health-conscious individual should seek to increase their serum 25-hydroxyvitamin D levels to 50-60 ng/mL. This can usually be accomplished by supplementing with 1,000 to 5,000 IU of vitamin D each night.

There are individuals for whom the above regimen just does not work to relieve insomnia. Dr. Lichten would still recommend treatment with vitamin D3, but would also advise them of the role of two other over-the-counter products for sleep. The first is L-tryptophan and the second is gamma-aminobutyric acid (GABA).

THE L-TRYPTOPHAN PATHWAY TO BETTER SLEEP

As previously described in the pathway to melatonin, L-tryptophan, an essential amino acid found in turkey, wine, and cheese, is converted to 5-HTP to cross the blood–brain barrier. There, it is converted to serotonin. The brain needs a sufficient level of serotonin to tone down or modulate the high adrenal stress hormones of daily life. In any discussion about depression, serotonin deficiencies are associated with concomitant high anxiety states.

In a recent study in Rome, 100–150 mg of 5-HTP was prescribed to a group of children aged 3-10 years who were suffering from sleep terrors. In this double-blind, randomized, controlled study, the addition of 5-HTP successfully resulted in terror-free sleep at one month in 93.5% and at six months in 83.9% of children compared with only 28.6% of children in the control group at both one and six months. The researchers concluded that 5-HTP in a dosage of 2 mg/kg/day was effective in inducing long-term improvement in sleep terrors.[40]

The dosage of 5-HTP that Dr. Lichten has added to modulate the stress of his daily life is 100 to 200 mg at bedtime, or 500 to 1,000 mg of pharmaceutical-grade L-tryptophan. Toxicity of 5-HTP has never been established,[41] although L-tryptophan might be safer in both the short and the long term. There is now tryptophan available in the United States that is certified pure before it is offered to the public.

GAMMA-AMINOBUTYRIC ACID

Gabapentin is sold as a prescription medication, Neurontin®, or as a generic, but its sleep-inducing effects can also be obtained in a supplement called GABA. It was the fifth most prescribed medication in 2003, being used for partial seizure disorders, post-herpetic neuralgias, neuropathic pain, and mood stabilization.[42,43] Because of its generic status, Pfizer has marketed Lyrica® to take its place.

This pharmaceutical agent is similar to GABA, which is a predominant neurotransmitter in the brain. It not only reduces pain perception in nerve injuries, it can also reduce the need for medication after surgery.[44] It is commonly used in dosages of up to 3,000 mg daily.

For insomnia, a small dose (125–250 mg) of GABA nightly can be taken to help induce sleep in addition to vitamin D and L-tryptophan. Dr. Lichten believes that tolerance occurs rapidly and suggests that GABA be used for only five to six nights per week.

DOSAGES USED IN DR. LICHTEN'S SLEEP-AID FORMULA

DOSAGE	FREQUENCY
Vitamin D: 4,000–5,000 IU/capsule	One capsule at bedtime; may be increased to two if blood levels remain below optimal levels
L-Tryptophan: 500 mg/capsule	One capsule at bedtime; may be increased to two
GABA: 125–250 mg sublingual lozenge	Take lozenge under tongue at bedtime

MAGNESIUM

What has not been realized, although Linus Pauling allegedly said it 50 years ago, *"You can trace every sickness, every disease, and every ailment to a mineral deficiency."* When it comes to sleep, a lack of magnesium contributes to increased states of anxiety and is probably a component of restless leg syndrome. Chronic sleep deprivation causes a decrease in intracellular magnesium.[45] Nevertheless, taking magnesium supplements of 1,000 mg daily or a couple of teaspoons, not tablespoons, of milk of magnesia at bedtime not only ensures adequate blood levels, but will also assist in a regular bowel movement so necessary in the morning.

SUCCESSFUL SLEEP MEANS NO DAYTIME SLEEPINESS

If deep sleep is a factor at night, then the resultant restful rejuvenation will prevent the mid-afternoon sleepiness that pervades our country. Adequate sleep gives one the energy to get up out of bed and go forward without *Starbuck's* or coffee in the morning. Sleep is the only effective treatment for daytime sleepiness. Add a good breakfast. *Simple, straightforward, and effective.* And there is no substitute.

In a review of Dr. Lichten's prescriptions written over the past 18 months, there were only eight patients on prescription sleep medications. They ranged in age from the late 20s to the mid 80s. Three in particular had major psychological-depression disorders and were taking significant dosages of other medications under the care of their psychiatrists. Although the Sleep-Aid Formula delineated on the previous page is not perfect, when combined with the appropriate balance of natural hormones it goes a long way to ensuring a safe, deep sleep (random eye movement [REM] sleep) for almost anyone at any age. It works well for Dr. Lichten and his patients. Almost every individual needs more vitamin D to live successful, longer, and healthier lives.

THE ROLE OF MELATONIN

With all the interest and alleged success of melatonin, Dr. Lichten was surprised that melatonin did not work to induce sleep either for him or for the patients who sought insomnia therapies. In a review of the literature, he found, among other things, that melatonin seems to work best for children:

1. Melatonin increases sleep time in ADHD children but does not change their personalities.[46,47]
2. Melatonin increases sleep patterns in children with autism.[48]
3. Sleep disorders in women outnumber men 4:1. Hormonal aspects must be considered from the initial treatment plan.[49]
4. Sleep patterns may be treated with L-tryptophan, a melatonin precursor.[49]
5. Nutritional sources are equivalent to pharmacological sources.[50]

DEPRESSION

Although depression is the second most prevalent disease in the world, Dr. Lichten believes that most endogenous (inside) depression is secondary to imbalances in the endocrine system. If one gets good nutrition, a good night's sleep, has adequate thyroid function to maintain a warm body temperature, adequate adrenal DHEA to ward off fatigue, effective glucose control, growth hormone for tissue repair, and appropriate levels of sex hormones for reproduction, then up to 75% of clinically reported depression may well be resolved. To wean off antidepressants, and only under a doctor's supervision, Dr. Lichten uses 500, 1,000, and even 1,500 mg doses of L-tryptophan (or 200 mg, 300 mg, or 400 mg of 5-HTP) daily in divided dosages. (L-tryptophan or 5-HTP naturally raises serotonin levels.) This Sleep-Aid program also incorporates a high-potency vitamin supplement taken two to three times per day. Serotonin may be one of the body's natural antidepressants, but it can only function when there are adequate levels of minerals, vitamins, amino acids (proteins), and essential fatty acids (fish oil).

CONCLUSION

Although many physicians believe it is perfectly safe to spend 20 to 30 minutes in bright sunlight without sunscreen to produce naturally up to 10,000 IU of vitamin D3, dermatologists fear that direct sun exposure will lead to an increase in skin cancers.[51] Dr. Lichten suggests that any adult can reach adequate serum levels of vitamin D3 of 50+ ng/mL by taking approximately 5,000 IU of vitamin D3 in dry-powder capsule form, or with a sublingual preparation of vitamin D3 containing 2,000 IU/drop, taking one to two drops nightly.

For those individuals with dark skins of any race or ethnicity, more vitamin D supplementation will be needed to reach adequate levels. Similarly, as individuals age, they lose their ability to manufacture vitamin D3 and are able to absorb much less from their gastrointestinal tract. That supplementation is so important.

Serum monitoring of total 25-hydroxyvitamin D can be done every six to twelve months. Toxicity should not be an issue with appropriate monitoring and oral dosages of less than 10,000 IU per day.[52]

Vitamin D replacement is not just for insomnia; it is for all aspects of general good health.

Recommended Sleep-Aid Formula

For those who wish to sample the natural, bio-identical nutraceutical, over-the-counter sleep-aid formula that Dr. Lichten uses personally and dispenses to his patients, please refer to the Appendix. Dr. Lichten makes no claim that this over-the-counter combination of products will replace prescription medication for sleep, only that it retrospectively worked for him and raised his vitamin D levels.

Caution

Vitamin D levels are monitored as total 25-hydroxyvitamin D every six months. Initial adult dosage is 1-2 drops of vitamin D in concentration of 2, 000 IU per drop. Dark skinned individuals may need twice this dosage. When the blood level reaches 60+ ng/mL, the dose may be reduced to 1,000 to 2,000 IU nightly.

1. 5- Hydroxytryptophan must be avoided if you are taking a monoamine oxidase inhibitor. It may raise blood pressure with certain medications. It is recommended that everyone have a blood pressure monitoring device and establish that the blood pressure remains normal with 5-HTP. Start with 50 mg of 5-HTP at bedtime and increase gradually over one to two weeks to the preferred dosage.

2. Gamma-aminobutyric acid is a sedative and should not be taken before driving or using any potentially dangerous equipment. Older individuals should start with just 50 mg each night. Higher dosages may induce a very deep sleep, so care must be taken to avoid slips and falls if arising in the middle of the night. Secondly, there is a tolerance to GABA that develops rapidly. Dr. Lichten recommends using GABA only five to six days per week to avoid increased tolerance.

REFERENCES:

1. Balkrishnan R, Rasu RS, Rajagopalan R. Physician and patient determinants of pharmacologic treatment of sleep difficulties in outpatient settings in the United States. *Sleep*. 2005 Jun 1;28 (6):715-9.
2. Feng Z, Gu F. Power spectral analysis of recovery sleep of sleep deprivation and hypnotic drug induced sleep. *Conf Proc IEEE Eng Med Biol Soc*. 2005 4:3593-6.
3. Available at: http://phx.corporate-ir.net/phoenix.zhtml?c=131268&p=irol-newsArticle&ID=768110&highlight=
4. Jiang Z. An epidemiological surgery on use and abuse of antianxiety drugs among Beijing residents. *Chinese Medical Journal (Engl)*. 1996 109(10):801-6.
5. Available at: pubmed.com Search: [Vitamin D and insomnia].
6. Eastman CI, Boulos Z, Terman M, Campbell SS, Dijk DJ, Lewy AJ. Light treatments for NASA shift workers. *J Biol Rhythms*. 1995 Jun;10(2):157-64.
7. Lee TM, Chan CC, Paterson JG, Janzen HL, Blashko CA. Spectral properties of phototherapy for seasonal affective disorder: a meta-analysis. *Acta Psychiatr Scand*. 1997 Aug;96(2):117-21.
8. Richardson G, Tate B. Hormonal and pharmacological manipulation of the circadian clock: recent developments and future strategies. *Sleep*. 2000 May 1;23 Suppl 3:S77-85.
9. Regelson W, Pierpaoli, W. *The Melatonin Miracle*. Pocket Books. Simon and Schuster, Inc. New York. 1995.
10. Buscemi N, Vandermeer B, Pandya R, et al. Melatonin for treatment of sleep disorders. *Evid Rep Technol Assess (Summ)*. 2004 Nov;(108):1-7.
11. Staffas A, Nyman A. Determination of cholecalciferol (vitamin D3) in selected foods by liquid chromatography: NMKL collaborative study. *J AOAC Int*. 2003 Mar-Apr;86(2):400-6.

12. Armas LA, Hollis BW, Heaney RP. Vitamin D2 is much less effective than vitamin D3 in humans. *J Clin Endocrinol Metab*. 2004 Nov;89(11):5387-91.

13. Mansur AP, Avakian SD, Paula RS, Donzella H, Santos SR, Ramires JA. Pharmacokinetics and pharmacodynamics of propranolol in hypertensive patients after sublingual administration: systemic availability. *Braz J Med Biol Res*. 1998 May;31(5):691-6.

14. Vieth R, Cole DE, Hawker GA, Trang HM, Rubin LA. Wintertime vitamin D insufficiency is common in young Canadian women, and their vitamin D intake does not prevent it. *Eur J Clin Nutr*. 2001 Dec;55(12):1091-7.

15. Bischoff HA, Stahelin HB, Dick W, et al. Effects of Vitamin D and calcium supplementation on falls: a randomized controlled trial. *J Bone Miner Res*. 2003 Feb;18(2):343–51.

16. Tajika M, Matsuura A, Nakamura T, et al. Risk factors for vitamin D deficiency in patients with Crohn's disease. *J Gastroenterol*. 2004 Jun;39(6):527-33.

17. Shah M, Simha V, Garg A. Review: long-term impact of bariatric surgery on body weight, comorbidities, and nutritional status. *J Clin Endocrinol Metab*. 2006 Nov;91(11):4223-31.

18. Dresner-Pollak R, Ackerman Z, Eliakim R, Karban A, Chowers Y, Fidder HH.The BsmI vitamin D receptor gene polymorphism is associated with ulcerative colitis in Jewish Ashkenazi patients. *Genet Test*. 2004 Winter;8(4):417-20.

19. Stio M, Martinesi M, Bruni S, et al. Interaction among vitamin D(3) analogue KH 1060, TNF-alpha, and vitamin D receptor protein in peripheral blood mononuclear cells of inflammatory bowel disease patients. *Int Immunopharmacol*. 2006 Jul;6(7):1083-92.

20. Brooke OG, Brown IR, Cleeve HJ. Vitamin D deficiency in Asian immigrants. *Br Med J*. 1979 Jul 21;2(6183):206.

21. Rostand SG. Ultraviolet light may contribute to geographic and racial blood pressure differences. *Hypertension*. 1997 Aug;30(2 Pt 1):150-6.

22. Plotnikoff GA, Quigley JM. Prevalence of severe hypovitaminosis D in patients with persistent, nonspecific musculoskeletal pain. *Mayo Clin Proc*. 2003 Dec;78(12):1463-70.

23. Munger KL, Levin LI, Hollis BW, Howard NS, Ascherio A. Serum 25-hydroxyvitamin D levels and risk of multiple sclerosis. *JAMA*. 2006 Dec 20;296(23):2832-8.

24. Kidd PM. Multiple sclerosis, an autoimmune inflammatory disease: prospects for its integrative management. *Altern Med Rev*. 2001 Dec;6(6):540-66.

25. Gorham ED, Garland CF, Garland FC, et al. Vitamin D and prevention of colorectal cancer. *J Steroid Biochem Mol Biol*. 2005 Oct;97(1–2):179-94.

26. John EM, Schwartz GG, Koo J, Van Den BD, Ingles SA. Sun exposure, Vitamin D receptor gene polymorphisms, and risk of advanced prostate cancer. *Cancer Research*. 2005 Jun 15;65(12):5470-9.

27. Cui Y, Rohan TE. Vitamin D, calcium and breast cancer risk: a review. *Cancer Epidemiol Biomarkers Prev*. 2006 Aug 15(8):1427-37.

28. Ahonen MH, Tenkanen L, Teppo L, Hakama M, Tuohimaa P. Prostate cancer risk and prediagnostic serum 25-hydroxyvitamin D levels (Finland). *Cancer Causes Control*. 2000 Oct;11(9):847-52.

29. Flynn G, Chung I, Yu WD, Romano M, et al. Calcitriol (1,25-dihydroxycholecalciferol) selectively inhibits proliferation of freshly isolated tumor-derived endothelial cells and induces apoptosis. *Oncology*. 2006 70(6): 447-57.

30. Shu XO, Gao YT, Brinton LA, et al. A population-based case-control study of childhood leukemia in Shanghai. *Cancer*. 1988 Aug 1;62(3):635-44.

31. Veierod MB, Laake P, Thelle DS. Dietary fat intake and risk of lung cancer: a prospective study of 51,452 Norwegian men and women. *Eur J Cancer Prev*. 1997 Dec;6(6):540-9.

32. Hollis BW, Wagner CL. Vitamin D deficiency during pregnancy: an ongoing epidemic. *Am J Clin Nutr*. 2006 Aug;84(2):273.

33. Walsh N. Vitamin D Deficit Affects Offspring's Bone Mass. *OB-GYN News*. Oct 1, 2006 p.1–5.

34. Hudson JQ. Secondary hyperparathyroidism in chronic kidney disease: focus on clinical consequences and vitamin D therapies. *An Pharmacother*. 2006 Sep;40(9):1584-93.

35. Qiao G, Kong J, Uskokovic M, Li YC. Analogs of 1alpha,25-dihydroxyvitamin D(3) as novel inhibitors of renin biosynthesis. *J Steroid Biochem Mol Biol*. 2005 Jun;96(1):59-66.

36. Miggiano GA, Gagliardi L. Diet, nutrition, and rheumatoid arthritis. *Clin Ter*. 2005 May–June;156(3):115–23.

37. Marniemi J, Alanen E, Impivaara O, et al. Dietary and serum vitamins and minerals as predictors of myocardial infarction and stroke in elderly subjects. *Nutr Metab Cardiovasc Dis*. 2005 Jun;15(3):188-97.

38. Woltersd M. Diet and psoriasis: experimental data and clinical evidence. *Br J Dermatol*. 2005 Oct;153(4): 706–14.

39. Zhou W, Suk R, Liu G, et al. Vitamin D is associated with improved survival in early-stage non-small cell lung cancer patients. *Cancer Epidemiol Biomarkers Prev*. 2005 Oct;14(10):2303-9.

40. Bruni O, Ferri R, Miano S, Verrillo E. L-5-Hydroxytryptophan treatment of sleep terrors in children. *Eur J Pediatr*. 2004 Jul;163(7):402-7.

41. Das YT, Bagchi M, Bagchi D, Preuss HG. Safety of 5-hydroxy-L-tryptophan. *Toxicol Lett*. 2004 Apr 15;150(1):111-22.

42. Frye MA, Ketter TA, Kimbrell TA, et al. A placebo-controlled study of lamotrigine and gabapentin monotherapy in refractory mood disorders. *J Clin Psychopharmacol*. 2000 Dec;20(6):607-14.

43. Vignatelli L, Billiard M, Clarenbach P, et al. EFNS Task Force. EFNS guidelines on management of restless legs syndrome and periodic limb movement disorder in sleep. *Eur J Neurol*. 2006 Oct;13(10):1049-65.

44. Dierking G, Duedahl TH, Rasmussen ML, et al. Effects of gabapentin on postoperative morphine consumption and pain after abdominal hysterectomy: a randomized, double-blind trial. *Acta Anaesthesiol Scand*. 2004 Mar;48(3):322-7.

45. Takase B, Akima T, Satomura K, et al. A Effects of chronic sleep deprivation on autonomic activity by examining heart rate variability, plasma catecholamine, and intracellular magnesium levels. *Biomed Pharmacother*. 2004 Oct;58 Suppl 1:S35-9.

46. Van der Heijden KB, Smits MG, Van Someren EJ, Ridderinkhof KR, Gunning WB. Effect of melatonin on sleep, behavior, and cognition in ADHD and chronic sleep-onset insomnia. *J Am Acad Child Adolesc Psychiatry*. 2007 Feb;46(2):233-41.

47. Szeinberg A, Borodkin K, Dagan Y. Melatonin treatment in adolescents with delayed sleep phase syndrome. *Clin Pediatr (Phila)*. 2006 Nov;45(9):809-18.

48. Garstang J, Wallis M. Randomized controlled trial of melatonin for children with autistic spectrum disorders and sleep problems. *Child Care Health Dev*. 2006 Sep;32(5):585-9.

49. Soares CN, Murray BJ. Sleep disorders in women: clinical evidence and treatment strategies. *Psychiatr Clin North Am*. 2006 Dec;29(4):1095-113;abstract xi.

50. Hudson C, Hudson SP, Hecht T, MacKenzie J. Protein source tryptophan versus pharmaceutical grade tryptophan as an efficacious treatment for chronic insomnia. *Nutr Neurosci*. 2005 Apr;8(2):121-7.

51. Spencer JM. Diet Not Sun Should Provide Vitamin D. *AM News*. Feb 12, 2007, p.

52. Carper J. How much vitamin D? *Parade Magazine*. Mar 25, 2007.

CHAPTER 2

FIBROMYALGIA & HUMAN GROWTH HORMONE

There existed a central controlling endocrine gland well before the emergence of mammalian animals 200 million years ago. As the size of the brain and specifically the cortex or thinking brain expanded, so did the functions of regulation by the master gland—the pituitary.[1] Today the pituitary releases four major hormones: prolactin, oxytocin, vasopressin, and growth hormone. It also releases four stimulating hormones that signal the glands of the body to release hormones: thyroid stimulating hormone (TSH); adrenal corticotropic hormone (ACTH);[15] and the sex-stimulating hormones follicle-stimulating hormone (FSH) and luteinizing hormone (LH). The ancients felt that the pituitary was the storehouse of the soul. And many modern-day physicians, including the legendary Cushing, agree.

It is important to remember that the old brain (hypothalamus) and new brain (cortex) affect release of pituitary hormones. If parts of the brain are tired, exhausted, nutritionally deprived, overstressed and suffering through chronic illnesses, neglect, or insomnia, then the pituitary will become dysfunctional. Sometimes it may produce excess hormones or excessive stimulating hormones, and other times it may just not react at all, as if it were asleep or down-regulated.[2] So when we evaluate the pituitary, we must recognize that pineal dysfunction (sleep: vitamin D, melatonin)[21] and the peripheral hormone systems (anabolic function: thyroid, adrenal, pancreatic, and sex hormones) must be concurrently evaluated. "No gland is an island" is misquoting a famous phrase, but it makes its point about the interactions of the entire endocrine system.

Biological Perspective

The master gland is divided up into the hormones it secretes and the glands it controls. Included below is a brief overview of the hormones secreted by the pituitary. It is important to note that this material illuminates the fact that no physician at this time has even the slightest idea why we mate, raise children, and stay married. But like health and disease, measuring the laboratory values gives us a rudimentary understanding of the difference between normal states and disease.

- **Oxytocin** is the hormone that causes uterine contractions. Without oxytocin, there is no onset of labor and no natural birth, nor is there milk let-down, causing a defect in maternal bonding to the newborn infant. The hormone is produced within the hypothalamus and stored in the pituitary for release. Oxytocin and vasopressin are six times higher, respectively, at climax and arousal in the male. Obviously, they play important and unexplained roles in reproduction. While the third hormone, prolactin, is directly increased by nipple stimulation.

- **Vasopressin** is the hormone that restricts urine in times of water deprivation. It is also secreted from the hypothalamus and stored in the pituitary. Studies show that higher levels of vasopressin induce a friendly approach in women to a new crowd and an aggressive facial scowl in men.[3] In lower animal life forms, vasopressin is associated with a monogamous relationship.

- **Prolactin** is a large polypeptide, similar in structure to human growth hormone. It is synthesized in the pituitary gland, but its release is regulated from the hypothalamus. Its production is increased in the presence of estrogen, and it is responsible for milk production in the female. In the male, high levels of prolactin are associated with impotence and lower levels of testosterone.

Another effect of prolactin, recently discovered by the University of Paisley and the Technische Hochschule Zürich, is to provide the body with gratification after sexual acts. Recent research suggests that the hormone prolactin may decrease the impact of dopamine, which is responsible for sexual arousal, thus causing the male's refractory period or sexual downtime.[6,30] The amount of prolactin released may be an indicator of the amount of sexual satisfaction and relaxation. Unusually high amounts are suspected to be responsible for impotence and loss of libido and can be measured in a simple laboratory test.[4]

- **Human Growth Hormone** (hGH) is produced in the anterior pituitary gland and is released in pulses approximately five times per day in adults. Baseline levels are highest in adolescent children and lowest in the aged and infirm. Growth hormone is stimulated by the emerging hormones of adolescence and in the hour before deep sleep. It is naturally responsible for growing taller and developing the muscles of adulthood.[5] Inhibition of hGH occurs naturally through the presence of somatostatin secreted from the hypothalamus and unnaturally in our environment from xenoestrogens such as DDT, plastic by-products, and biochemical estrogenic compounds fed to the livestock. Too much growth hormone results in gigantism, while too little growth hormone is the subject of the field of small-stature and anti-aging medicine.

  Measurement of hGH, or growth hormone, is difficult and unreliable except in a research setting.[7] Unless attempting to measure a chemically induced response to low blood sugar with insulin or to L-arginine, most physicians measure insulin-like growth factor-1 (IGF-1). Produced in the liver in response to hGH, IGF-1 is stable throughout the day.

Personal Perspective

When Tom T. went through his male menopause (see Book Three, chapter on "Andropause"), Dr. Lichten treated his low testosterone. Because Tom was fatigued, he would try anything over-the-counter to relieve the muscle pains in his body and the night sweats. When testosterone replacement alone did not resolve his issues of fatigue, a repeat laboratory assay confirmed that his insulin-like growth factor –1 remained very low. Dr. Lichten advised the human growth hormone itself could be replaced at a small dose of 1 IU per day. The results were dramatic: His facial frown disappeared, he grew new hair in a bald spot, his muscle tone improved, and his mental attitude cleared of depression. He noticed the difference and asked how long he could stay on hGH. Dr. Lichten suggested 3–6 months. He was fortunate, Dr. Lichten told him. Human growth hormone is usually precluded from treatment for all but the very wealthy.

Human growth hormone was first made available to children in Japan in 1980 and the United States in 1985, and the results of the Rudmans' experiments, who were leading researchers in the field of adult hGH therapy, were not published until 1991[8] and 1993.[9] All the resultant information was truly rudimentary. To review the studies is to review the association of low levels of hGH with physical and functional aspects of aging.

Donald Rudman, MD, had confirmed that aging was associated with decreasing levels of human growth hormone and questioned whether replacement would have anabolic and muscle-building effects on the volunteers. After being given doses that are now considered excessive, 22 IU per week, his subjects noted improvement in lean body mass ("muscle" up 10 pounds), reduction in adipose mass ("fat" down six pounds), improved skin thickness (20%), reversal of the shrinking of organ size (liver, spleen, kidney), and increased size of 10 muscle groups.

Now, when Rudman's wife completed a second study in 1993[9] after his death, there were so many complications of the growth hormone protocol—carpal tunnel, diabetes, and gynecomastia (breast enlargement in men)—that no one ever repeated this second study.

But the story of an "anti-aging" hormone reversing the signs of aging by 20 years (a misquote) was played to the public and a demand for anti-aging hormones and growth hormone rapidly became the cry—even though the costs of a month of hGH at half the Rudman protocol was $700. Sales in the United States of synthetic hGH reached half a billion dollars in 2004.[10]

ABUSE

There is no question that hGH has become a mainstay of bodybuilders, sports athletes, and entertainers, along with a cross section of individuals from all walks of life. They all want to achieve a more defined physique. Human growth hormone, a necessary biological hormone of life, has its own cult-like following. As physicians, we must present this information to our patients for its benefits and its disadvantages. Some would treat hGH replacement just as a prescription for plastic surgery—let the patient decide. But the information on the casual use of hGH is not positive when one considers the long-term consequences.

Personal Experience

Since Dr. Lichten established a protocol for treating adults with hGH in 1995, there has been significant knowledge derived from that database. Some men grew new hair initially, but it started to recede again 5–10 years later. Both the men and women grew significantly stronger and increased muscle mass by 5–15 pounds. With nutrition and exercise they were able to maintain their youthful weight and physique longer, but the tone of the facial muscles began to loosen again. Bone density remained the same as a young man's or woman's, but if nutritional supplements were not maintained, then mineral content started to leach away. Everyone seemed to benefit initially from a better attitude and resolve. And that, he trusts, contributed to the continuation of most in the hormonal-replacement programs and the maintenance of much of the gains. There is no shortcut to being Jack La Lanne (known as the "Godfather of fitness"), but for those not as blessed, hormonal replacement offers an improvement over programmed decline.

But what Dr. Lichten realized 15 years ago, and for which he remains eternally grateful, is that hGH and the balance of the multiple endocrine systems with replacement hormones had reversed his slide into "old age." And although many in the medical profession believe that muscle pain, strength decline, and balance deficiencies are some kind of a psychological and psychosomatic disease, Dr. Lichten knows it is in great part an endocrine disorder, and it is treatable, as many of his patients can attest.

FIBROMYALGIA

Fibromyalgia,[11] a disease recognized by the American Medical Association in 1987,[12] means "fiber"-"muscle"-"pain." It is a chronic-pain disease affecting 3% to 6% of the population, with a 9:1 predominance of females to males. More than 30% of affected individuals are unable to work. People with this disorder may qualify for long-term disability, as well as federal and state assistance. One consistent scientific finding has been the interruption of normal sleep. With a predominance of psychological explanations, almost no one had considered the disruption of hormonal endocrine systems and the resultant widespread effects such a disruption would cause.

The symptoms of fibromyalgia include widespread pain and tenderness to touch. The National Fibromyalgia Association has described 18 trigger or tender points that are usually affected, and the chart of these is usually on a female silhouette.[12] Scientists note a specific form of sleep disorder called alpha-delta sleep, in which the deep delta sleep necessary for production of human growth hormone is interrupted by bursts of alpha sleep (wakefulness). The result is that rapid eye-movement sleep stages 3 and 4 (deep REM sleep) are dramatically reduced.[13] With lack of deep REM sleep comes the muscle stiffness, the muscle pain, and the inability to concentrate, or "brain fog." As with other chronic states, there are signs of physical fatigue, irritable bowel, headaches, twitches, and temporomandibular joint pain (TMJ). Some believe this is reminiscent of, or compatible with, post-traumatic stress syndrome.

In a review of the medical literature for unbiased scientific facts, the following is noted:

With only a rudimentary understanding of the disruption of the neuroendocrine system,[20,21] one can see that the sleep disturbance is of primary concern. Whatever the causes of the endocrine disturbances listed in items #1 through #7 on the next page, their interference with quality sleep means failure for the long-term treatment of fibromyalgia.

Successful fibromyalgia treatment thus falls into broad categories listed below:

1. Normal sleep induction[17]
2. Relief of muscle pain[18]
3. Mineral replacement
4. Increased energy production with nutraceuticals & bio-identical hormones
5. Increased anabolic function
6. Tissue loading with intravenous vitamins, minerals, and antioxidants
7. Exercise
8. Anti-inflammatory agents: non-steroidal anti-inflammatory drugs (NSAIDs).[16]

NORMAL SLEEP INDUCTION

Therefore, the first step in the evaluation of fibromyalgia is to record the endocrine parameters and to treat the insomnia. The protocol begins as outlined in Chapter 1. For fibromyalgia patients, to assist with sleep disturbances, the use of vitamin D, the use of L-tryptophan or 5-hydroxytryptophan (5-HTP) to relieve depression, and the use of gamma-aminobutyric acid (GABA), or gabapentin, to decrease muscle pain are begun at once. In reference to the mineral deficiencies, such as magnesium, and liquid and intravenous vitamins are begun. One of the most important minerals Dr. Lichten uses to relieve muscle spasm is micronized silica.

THE PHYSIOLOGY OF MUSCLE PAIN

After treating the sleep disturbance, the focus is on the muscle pain. What occurs with chronic insomnia and low hGH is a buildup of lactic acid[22] in the muscles. Many patients describe the feeling as badly getting out of bed in the morning as they would the day after running a marathon. This is because the interruption of normal cellular energy, called ATP, prevents the cell from clearing the lactic acid that results from burning glucose for energy, and without lactic acid removal, the cell experiences pain.[23]

Removing lactic acid can come primarily from increasing the energy available to the cell. This is not dissimilar to those with life-threatening cardiomyopathy, described henceforth. When the mitochondria lose function, the physician can augment or increase those hormones that increase anabolic energy: hGH, testosterone, DHEA, and in special circumstances, the drug nandrolone. These hormones accelerate the amount of biochemical energy-ATP that is generated. And this additional energy, if enough, will allow the cells to clear lactic acid and slowly regenerate.

But secondarily, just as explained before, one must dramatically increase the intake and absorption of minerals. These come from the highest-grade nutraceutical products, which are necessary for cellular energy. Specifically, the supplements to add include coenzyme Q10, N-acetyl cysteine, magnesium, malic acid, and digestive enzymes. One well-respected physician has more than 131 supplements for his fibromyalgia and chronic fatigue patients. Taking these supplements weekly or intravenous mineral-vitamin therapies biweekly, and dramatically increasing tissue-repairing anabolic hormones, often result in dramatic improvement in fibromyalgia and other chronic, unexplained medical conditions in Dr. Lichten's practice.

THE ROLE OF HUMAN GROWTH HORMONE

Bennett[19] reported to Dr. Lichten in 1995 that 75% of his fibromyalgia patients showed dramatic improvement in symptoms and had returned to work after nine months of hGH replacement therapy. Dr. Lichten adopted his protocol in 1996, when hGH was made available for adult replacement. One of the first to experience a life-changing reawakening was the wife of a local physician.

Rose H. was 48 years old and had been subjected to multiple destructive courses of endocrine ablation by well-meaning specialists, leaving her with hypopituitarism. When she developed terrible headaches, they found an inflammation of her pituitary, so they added high-dose corticosteroids for eight years. When the steroids had caused osteoporosis and massive weight gain, they removed the pituitary gland. When she went through disruptive menstrual cycles, they removed her uterus and ovaries. And when she was devastated by chronic pain, insomnia, depression, and weight gain, they gave her two, not one, antidepressants. Seen by me only in desperation, she was 75 pounds overweight, almost bedridden, and in a state of true hopelessness.

Starting first with the evaluation of the six-point endocrine system, the laboratory tests showed disruption of all the following:

1. Insomnia, severe: Low levels of 25-hydroxyvitamin D[14] & melatonin[12]
2. Fibromyalgia: Low levels of IGF-1 (below 80 ng/mL)
3. Slow metabolism: Low thyroid—hypothyroidism
4. Adrenal exhaustion/fatigue: Low levels of DHEA[11,20]
5. Diabetes: Pancreatic dysfunction
6. Dysfunctional endocrines: Menopause, low testosterone, elevated FSH, elevated LH.

On the program of hormonal replacement by organ and nutritional intravenous vitamins and minerals, she made dramatic changes. No longer bedridden, she returned to work in her husband's office. So impressed by his wife's recovery, the physician basically threw his standard 25-years-in-the-making practice out the door and focused on nutritional, hormonal, and holistic medicine. The changes were so pronounced for her that she returned to her university-based endocrinologist to show him her new 60-pound lighter appearance. The doctor was aghast at the changes and so concerned about the unknown side effects of hGH that he forbade her to continue. She cried and said she would rather die than go back to feeling so destitute. And, understanding a little bit more about this disease, the university doctor became a champion for hGH for these sick and before then, hopeless individuals.

Some fibromyalgia experts believe that these people are overwhelmed by infections or viruses, Lyme disease, mycoplasma, or gastrointestinal yeast. And, to some extent, they may be correct. One doctor in my town used intravenous tetracycline for months at a cost of many thousands of dollars, but many still seemed to be afflicted even after the therapy and money had run out. It seems best that the only treatment for every one of these diseases is to improve the energy of the cell, thereby maintaining and repairing its cellular function. If this cannot be accomplished, the animal and its cells will perish. "Fix it or lose it" is so apropos.

What is not understood by most physicians who treat fibromyalgia is that the anabolic sex steroids, in Dr. Lichten's experience, are even more important than hGH. A full explanation of the role of bio-identical testosterone and its anabolic-related hormones, nandrolone and Oxandrin®, appear in the chapters on menopause, osteoporosis, and andropause. It is now confirmed that these same muscle-building hormones that propelled both men and women to world records can be immensely beneficial to those with fibromyalgia and fatigue.

Another woman in her late 30s was so afflicted with chronic pain and fibromyalgia that she was also unable to work at her family business. On the program for sleep, nutrition, intravenous bolus mineral-vitamin therapy, hGH, and anabolic testosterone, she made a dramatic recovery. She felt so good at regaining the quality of her life that she sent her husband in for his testosterone injection. At last count, the couple was living happily six years after initial therapy. Note that after recovery of normal sleep and improved nutrition, the hGH was discontinued. Sex hormone replacement, however, was not.

UNDERSTANDING THE IMPORTANCE OF HUMAN GROWTH HORMONE

In medicine, we learn from what occurs naturally. In the case of growth hormone abnormalities, there are disease states in which the body fails to produce growth hormone, cases of destruction of the pituitary gland, and cases where the body produces naturally or the individual injects unnaturally excessive amounts of growth hormone. Understanding these extremes allows the physician to modulate the abnormal back toward a normal balance.

Excessive growth hormone results in acromegaly and gigantism. Gigantism occurs when there is excessive release of hGH in a teen whose bones have not yet fused. This results in an individual growing well over six or seven feet tall. These tall individuals are at risk for hypertension and heart failure, as a normal-size heart must pump blood under more stress. Acromegaly is named because of the pronounced foreheads and thick fingers and arms of these individuals once the bones are fused. They also experience more carpal tunnel pain, more diabetes, and more gynecomastia (breast tissue in men). Just as was noted in the famous actor and TV wrestler "Andre the Giant," high levels of natural hGH are associated with a premature natural death. Andre died at age 47.

The opposite occurs in individuals with low growth hormone. These individuals are of small stature, have fine wrinkles prematurely, experience thin bones and fractures, and die early with heart failure from a lack of cellular energy. Restitution of hGH levels in teen years may offer the individual the opportunity to reach 90%–95% of expected height and to delay the onset of complications so that they live a mostly normal life.

My first patient with pituitary dwarfism was in her 40s. She was 4'6" tall. Her diagnosis was confirmed by an endocrinologist prior to recombinant hGH becoming available in the United States. She began therapy with hGH because of the association with premature heart failure. She noted renewed performance energy, reversal of unexplained heart palpitations, and a profound decrease in skin wrinkling in the first eight weeks. She attributed correctly that this life-changing event occurred because she had added nutritional supplements, hGH, and appropriate hormone replacement to her daily regimen.

MIRACLES WITH HUMAN GROWTH HORMONE

As physicians, we are still amazed at the role that our intervention can play in the recovery of quality of life. There is no greater satisfaction than knowing that your intervention saves lives. Physicians live to do their share. And with some of the dramatic cases treated with hGH, Dr. Lichten is still amazed at how resilient the human body is when given the missing key ingredients to health.

CARDIOMYOPATHY

James A. is another extreme example of what can be accomplished with nutrition, a strong faith and a good amount of anabolic therapy. He was discharged from the state university by an outstanding cardiologist, in essence to die. It seems that James contracted a viral or congenital defect in his energy-producing heart muscles. The term is cardiomyopathy for bad heart muscle. The term *mitochondrial* is added to denote that the energy-production organelles within his cells are ready to fail. So James saw Dr. Lichten in a late stage of congestive heart failure (CHF).

Just like Sam before him and Jerry after, Dr. Lichten measured James' hormones, started a replacement protocol with the anabolic hormones and began both oral and intravenous vitamin and mineral supplementation. James is still alive and active 10 years after being sent home. He helps out his parents at their business, drives his car, fixes computers, and has enough energy to enjoy sex. His workouts are strenuous for even a normal man, but James needs to work hard to maintain his body's muscle mass. James runs, not walks, seven miles every day on his treadmill. He presses weight to exhaustion. And even when his cardiac enzymes show potential cardiac damage, he completes a 12-minute Bruce hospital treadmill test without raising his heart rate over 120 beats per minute.

His doctors call him a walking miracle—Dr. Lichten calls him fortunate that his cells respond to the anabolic routine. When they don't, James too will die. But when that happens, those who treated him will have known that the university professors were wrong not to realize that the body had only wanted itself supplied with these natural substances to improve its cardiac function, and that anabolic steroids and human growth hormone do help some who would otherwise soon die.

Soon after Dr. Lichten's intervention had improved the quality of life of these two cardiomyopathy patients, Fazio[24] published the lead article in the *New England Journal of Medicine* on the use of hGH in CHF patients. Human growth hormone had increased his seven patients' ventricular mechanical (heart) efficiency from an average of 9% to 21%! His conclusions were echoed by *Le Corvoisier* in the *Journal of Clinical Endocrinology and Metabolism:* Human growth hormone improved several relevant cardiovascular parameters in patients with CHF.[25] Improvements were seen in intraventricular and posterior ventricular wall thickness, left ventricular and systemic dynamics, left ventricular ejection fraction, NY Heart Association Classification, as well as a 37.6-second increase in exercise duration.

Whether these improvements in scientific measurements are sufficient to change the quality of life of these congestive heart patients will become clearer in time. It is comforting to know, however, that when the drug therapies for congestive heart patients have reached a limit, just having the availability of human growth hormone may keep more patients alive longer and with a better quality of life instead of the obvious morbidity and death.

Jerry D.'s cardiomyopathy is different, and the entire team of university professors remains baffled. Jerry cannot walk up a flight of stairs but can bench press 180 pounds 10 times! His problem is not of "lung" origin, as his pulmonary-function tests show no obstructive disease. The regimen formulated for Jerry is similar to James' with oral supplements, 300–600 mg of coenzyme Q10, 1,500 mg of N-acetyl cysteine, and the supplementation of natural anabolic hormones. Use of testosterone, nandrolone, Oxandrin®, and hGH have allowed Jerry to leave the house and continue to work. When his muscle biopsy site failed to heal, the doctor added more intravenous minerals and vitamin C and an extra dose of nandrolone. Now, biopsy site healed, Dr. Lichten follows him closely. As already known, every patient is different, and everyone can become very ill in only a short time. Dr. Lichten's overall plan is simple: maintain sound nutrition, avoid cigarettes and bad food, and supplement the hormones into normal, approved range.

COLITIS AND CROHN'S DISEASE

When a physician is willing to listen to any patient's complaints and take that individual's concerns seriously, the word spreads within the community. So in response to these rare individuals who saw unexpected improvement on Dr. Lichten's program based on natural (bio-identical) hormonal replacement, a number of patients for whom no therapy had proved successful came to Dr. Lichten. And one of these conditions was that of an inflamed colon, called colitis. The name affixed to many of these medical diseases is Crohn's disease.

Crohn's disease is a full-wall thickness inflammation of the gastrointestinal tract. It can affect any region, from the mouth to the anus. Most cases involve the end of the small bowel and the beginning of the large bowel (ileocolonic). Most cases occur in teens, although the incidence in the elderly is increasing. The cause of the inflammation is unknown, but it is considered an autoimmune disorder. Some unknown trigger may have caused the body to start to reject its own tissues. The majority of gastrointestinal symptoms reported are abdominal pain, bloody diarrhea, and weight loss. Complications include bowel obstruction and ulcers, called fistulas, that erode the intestinal wall. Medications commonly used are anti-inflammatory agents, Asacol®, sulfasalazine, corticosteroids like prednisone, chemotherapy drugs like Imuran® or cyclosporine, and finally surgical resection. The chronic inflammation leads to pain, malabsorption, osteoporosis, muscle wasting, chronic diarrhea, and a poor quality of life. Newer medications available include Remicade®, Enbrel®, and Humira®. Limitations of these newer medications are a very high incidence of side effects, a suppression of the body's immune system, and their exorbitant costs.

Mr. H. came to Dr. Lichten on the urging of his wife. He was a tall 45-year-old Caucasian male engineer with a high-pressure job. The stress of the job and his perfectionistic personality were aggravating the Crohn's disease ulcer that was eating him up. His wife, Dr. Lichten's patient, had experienced two seemingly intractable problems that were fortunately resolved: migraine and profuse menstrual bleeding. Mr. H. had had severe bouts of ulcerative colitis for many years. Always on the brink of bowel resection, he agreed to see Dr. Lichten, though he vehemently disagreed with "alternative" medicine.

Evaluation of his endocrine parameters showed a low level of IGF-1 (for human growth hormone) and a very low level of both total and free testosterone measured as the free androgen index (FAI). With this knowledge, he began a replacement program of both nandrolone and testosterone in a 2:1 ratio. In his weekly injections were added additional B12 and B-complex vitamins. And for short-term repair, he began a program of hGH daily subcutaneous injections. Because all inflammatory diseases of the gastrointestinal tract interfere with absorption, he followed the recommended program of nutritional supplements, mixing in digestive enzymes and betaine hydrochloric acid as the enzyme activator.

"It may seem illogical to add digestive enzymes," Dr. Lichten answered when questioned. But without the ability to digest the food in the stomach, it will just "sit there" and cause heartburn, water brash (regurgitation of acid into the esophagus), and the dumping of unprocessed food from the stomach into the small bowel. As the small bowel is expecting no large particulate matter, it will cause additional inflammation and injury to the small bowel wall. "No," Dr. Lichten stated, "You should consider digestive enzymes as important to your condition with gastrointestinal dysfunction as insulin is to the diabetic."

With that, the engineer disappeared from the office to reappear every six months or so to refill his prescriptions for testosterone and anabolic steroids. For a period of six years, he avoided surgery. When last he met with Dr. Lichten, he still had not had the bowel resection that was scheduled before the first meeting.

In the medical literature, Slonim[26] reported in the *New England Journal of Medicine* that "our preliminary study suggests that growth hormone may be a beneficial treatment for patients with Crohn's disease." This reiterated what Dr. Lichten found with the engineer and others: Adding back nutritional supplements and protein and then "super-charging" the body to heal with anabolic steroids offers an opportunity to repair. And what the body can repair is truly remarkable.

Hospital patients with burns and on long-term respiratory support suffer an extreme degree of malnutrition, misery, and death. The faster these individuals can be weaned off a respirator, the sooner the burned tissue heals, keeping life-sustaining fluids from evaporating and improving the opportunities for survival. Doctors across the world have seen human growth hormone and anabolic sex steroids as a potential tool to keep these individuals alive long enough to recover and hopefully live a normal life.[27] Why should treatment of wasting surgical diseases be treated differently from the wasting AIDs disease? AIDs patients receive both anabolic steroids and hGH.

And although the cost of human growth hormone can range from $500 to $1,500 per month, the cost savings for medical expenses alone can justify the treatment for these sick and infirm individuals.[28] Whether it can assist in weaning off mechanical ventilation is in question.[29]

FIBROMYALGIA FORMULA

MEDICATION-OTC	DOSAGE/ FREQUENCY
Sleep Formula	Bedtime: A) 4,000–5,000 IU of vitamin D taken as a capsule or liquid drops B) 500–1,000 mg of L-tryptophan (500 mg of L-tryptophan can be also be taken in the daytime) C) 125–250 mg of GABA
Nutrient Formula Pack Number One	As directed in Appendix
Hormone Formula	As prescribed

HORMONAL REPLACEMENT PROTOCOL

(Range of doses based on the results of individual blood testing)

HORMONE	GENERIC	DOSAGE/FREQUENCY
Thyroid (Armour®)		30 mcg one to two times daily (if tests reveal thyroid deficiency)
DHEA		25–50 mg one to two times daily (if blood tests indicate DHEA deficiency)
Cortef®	cortisol	10 mg one to four times daily (if blood tests indicate cortisol deficiency)
Testosterone (men)	cypionate	50–200 mg weekly (if blood tests indicate testosterone deficiency)
Deca-Durabo-lin (men)	nandrolone	50–200 mg weekly (based on androgen blood test levels)
hGH: Saizen® Genotropin®	somatotropin	1 IU/day five to seven days per week (based on surrogate marker growth hormone blood levels)

Drugs Delegated to Secondary Status—No FDA drug approval exists for fibromyalgia

MEDICATION	GENERIC	DOSAGE
Neurontin®	GABA	500–1,500 mg at bedtime
Milnacipran®	SNRI	25 mg
Mirapex®	dopamine agonist/pramipexole	1 mg
Lyrica®	GABA	100 mg
Cymbalta®	SNRI	30 mg
Pamelor®	nortriptyline	50 mg
Elavil®	amitriptyline	50 mg
Paxil®	paroxetine	30 mg
Sinequan®	doxepin	25 mg
Zoloft®	sertraline	50 mg
Celexa®	citalopram	20 mg
Prozac®	fluoxetine	20 mg
Lunesta®	eszopiclone	2 mg
Rozerem®	ramelteon	8 mg
Ambien®	zolpidem	10 mg
Sonata®	pyrazolopyrimidine	10 mg
Halcion®	triazolam	0.25 mg
Restoril®	temazepam	15 mg
Valium®	diazepam	10 mg
Ultracet®	tramadol APAP	37.5 mg
Flexeril®	cyclobenzaprine	10 mg
Soma®	carisoprodol	350 mg
Klonopin®	clonazepam	1 mg
Ativan®	lorazepam	1 mg
Provigil®	modafinil	100 mg
Strattera®	atomoxetine	60 mg
Adderall-XL®	controlled substance	20 mg
Adipex®	phentermine	37.5 mg
Xyrem®	gamma-hydroxybutyrate	6 g powder
Ritalin®	methylphenidate	10 mg
amphetamine		37.5 mg

EXPLANATION OF HOW BIO-IDENTICAL HORMONES WORK

1. Sleep formula: By re-establishing normal sleep with vitamin D, L-tryptophan (or 5-HTP), and GABA (or gabapentin), the circadian rhythm is reset and brain–pituitary interaction may be normalized.
2. Pituitary dysfunction: When low levels of IGF-1 are confirmed, temporary hGH replacement may improve repair of damaged tissue.
3. Thyroid dysfunction: Active T3 is the key to the ATP-energy cycle, increased wakefulness, and the lessening of fatigue. Dosage may be increased from Armour® Thyroid 30 mcg to a maximum of Armour® Thyroid 240 mcg based on clinical symptomatology and laboratory testing.
4. Adrenal dysfunction: Two separate dysfunctions are commonly treated: The replacement of DHEA starting with 10-25 mg and as much as 100 mg daily may result in increased energy. Secondarily, short-term replacement of cortisone 2.5–5 mg one to four times daily may increase energy dramatically.
5. Sex hormone dysfunction (male): Lack of testosterone in males (and some females) is a key to the lack of energy and suppressed immune system. Replacement with bio-identical testosterone or the more potent nandrolone is of primary importance. (Females use much lower doses than males.)
6. Sex hormone dysfunction (female): Low-dose estradiol tablets, patches, or pellets, combined with oral or topical progesterone, help to establish a baseline hormone level in affected women.
7. Nutraceuticals: High-dose vitamins, minerals, amino acids, and essential fatty acids are necessary to supply the building blocks of repair. Energy is supplied to the cells with the addition of coenzyme Q10 creatine and L-carnitine, N-acetyl cysteine, and glutathione. Mineral replacement with silica in micronized form improves clearance of lactic acidosis contributing to a reduction in muscle pain. Most important is that high doses of B vitamins, betaine hydrochloric acid, and digestive enzymes are prescribed to improve absorption of nutrients and decrease inflammatory response.

8. Intravenous vitamins will be briefly mentioned here. It need not be explained that the disruption in the gastrointestinal tract by any chronic disease prevents absorption of nutrients and minerals. Loading minerals and vitamins intravenously allows for more efficient absorption.

9. Intravenous minerals were first formulated by John A. Myers, MD, in the 1930s. The preparations Dr. Lichten uses are based on maximizing the concentration that can be tolerated in a 250 ml volume of Ringer's lactate.

REFERENCES

1. MacLullich AM, Ferguson KJ, Wardlaw JM, et al. Smaller left anterior cingulate cortex volumes are associated with impaired hypothalamic-pituitary-adrenal axis regulation in healthy elderly men. *J Clin Endocrinol Metab*. 2006 Apr;91(4):1591-4.
2. Avishai-Eliner S, Eghbal-Ahmadi M, Tabachnik E, et al. Down-regulation of hypothalamic corticotropin-releasing hormone messenger ribonucleic acid (mRNA) precedes early-life experience-induced changes in hippocampal glucocorticoid receptor mRNA. *Endocrinology*. 2001 Jan;142(1):89-97.
3. Thompson RR, George K, Walton JC, et al. Sex-specific influences of vasopressin on human social communication. *Proc Natl Acad Sci U S A*. 2006 May 16;103(20):7889-94.
4. Available at: http://www.wikipedia.com [prolactin].
5. Available at: http://www.wikipedia.com [human growth hormone].
6. Brody S, Krüger TH. The post-orgasmic prolactin increase following intercourse is greater than following masturbation and suggests greater satiety. *Biol Psychol*. 2006 Mar;71(3):312-5.
7. Ranke M.B. Standardization of Growth Hormone Measurement, Evidence-Based Medicine3rd KIGS/KIMS Expert Meeting on Growth and Growth Disorder. Sorrento, Italy, November 19–20, 1998. *Hormone Research* 1999; 51(Supplement 1); page 1.
8. Rudman D, Feller AG, Cohn L, et al. Effects of human growth hormone on body composition in elderly men. *Horm Res*. 1991 36 Suppl 1:73-81.
9. Cohn L, Feller AG, Draper MW, et al. Carpal tunnel syndrome and gynaecomastia during growth hormone treatment of elderly men with low circulating IGF-I concentrations. *Clin Endocrinol (Oxf)*. 1993 Oct;39(4):417-25.
10. Barclay L. Growth Hormone Deemed Illegal for Off-Label Antiaging Use. 2005 Oct 28. Available at: http://www.medscape.com/viewarticle/515665.
11. Available at: http://www.wikipedia.com [fibromyalgia].
12. Goldenberg DL. Fibromyalgia syndrome. An emerging but controversial condition. *JAMA*. 1987 May 22-29;257(20):2782-7.
13. Branco J, Atalaia A, Paiva T. Sleep cycles and alpha-delta sleep in fibromyalgia syndrome. *J Rheumatol*. 1994 Jun;21(6):1113-7.
14. Armstrong DJ. Vitamin D deficiency is associated with anxiety and depression in fibromyalgia. *Clinical Rheumatology* 2007 Apr;26(4):551-4.

15. Adler GK, et al. Reduced hypothalamic-pituitary and sympatho-adrenal responses to hypo-glycemia in women with fibromyalgia syndrome. *Am J Med*. 1999; 106(5): 534–43.

16. Torpy DJ, et al. Responses of the sympathetic nervous system and the hypothalamic-pituitary-adrenal axis to interleukin-6: a pilot study in fibromyalgia. *Arth Rheum*. 2000; 43(4):872–80.

17. Moldofsky H. Management of sleep disorders in Fibromyalgia. *Rheumatol Dis Cl N Am*. 2002; 28(2): 353–65.

18. Bennett RM, et al. Low levels of somatomedin C in patients with the fibromyalgia syndrome. Possible links between sleep and muscle pain. *Arthritis and Rheumatism*. 1992; 35(10): 1113–6.

19. Bennett RM, et al. A randomized double blind placebo controlled study of growth hormone in the treatment of fibromyalgia. *Am J Med.*. 1998; 104(3): 227–31.

20. Dessein PH, et al. Hyposecretion of adrenal androgens and the relation of serum adrenal steroids, serotonin and insulin-like growth factor-1 to clinical features in women with fibromyalgia. *Pain*. 1999; 83(2): 313–9.

21. Korszun A, et al. Melatonin levels in women with fibromyalgia and chronic fatigue syndrome. *J Rheumatol*. 1999; 26(12): 2675–80.

22. Scroop G. CFS- Quo Vadimus? *Adelaine University Research Group-1*. November 7, 2004.

23. Available at: http://www.bowen-therapy.info/musclepain.shtml.

24. Fazio S, Sabatini D, Capaldo B, et al. A preliminary study of growth hormone in the treatment of dilated cardiomyopathy. *N Engl J Med*. 1996 Mar 28;334(13):809-14.

25. Le Corvoisier P, Hittinger L, Chanson P, et al. Cardiac effects of growth hormone treatment in chronic heart failure: A meta-analysis. *J Clin Endocrinol Metab*. 2007 Jan;92(1):180-5.

26. Slonim AE, Bulone L, Damore MB, et al. A preliminary study of growth hormone therapy for Crohn's disease. *N Engl J Med*. 2000 Jun 1;342(22):1633-7.

27. Przkora R, Herndon DN, et al. Beneficial effects of extended growth hormone treatment after hospital discharge in pediatric burn patients. *Ann Surg*. 2006 Jun;243(6):796-801.

28. Migliaccio-Walle K, Caro JJ, Möller J. Economic implications of growth hormone use in patients with short bowel syndrome. *Curr Med Res Opin*. 2006 Oct;22(10):2055-63.

29. Cook D, Meade M, Guyatt G, et al. Trials of miscellaneous interventions to wean from mechanical ventilation. *Chest*. 2001 Dec;120(6 Suppl):438S-44S.

30. Krüger TH, Hartmann U, Schedlowski M. Prolactinergic and dopaminergic mechanisms underlying sexual arousal and orgasm in humans. *World J Urol*. 2005 Jun;23(2):130-8.

CHAPTER 3

THYROID DISEASE: THE UNSUSPECTED ILLNESS

It seems that every other person seen in Dr. Lichten's office has thyroid disease or thyroid symptoms. It is routine here in Michigan and in the Midwest because of their iodine-poor soil. Eighty years ago, almost half the children of school age were diagnosed with hypothyroidism because they had visible goiters. A goiter is a swollen thyroid gland. Because the cause of goiter was inadequate iodine in the Midwestern diet, the governments of Michigan and Ohio mandated that iodine be added to salt.[1] This practice was found effective in shrinking the goiters; thereafter, iodized salt soon spread throughout the entire United States and Canada. With the use of small amounts of iodized salt, the disease is not visible; it is just hiding below the surface. The problems faced with hypothyroidism in medical practice today are even more insidious than those faced 80 years ago, when it was recognized that 40% of the population[2] was being affected and less than 10% being diagnosed.

Though thyroid dysfunction contributes to an extensive symptom list that includes cold hands, cold feet, brittle nails, hair loss, and a host of other problems, the connection to all aspects of general health makes the thyroid gland so very important. What most physicians and health professionals fail to connect is that the changes in the Western diet correlate with the proliferation of thyroid disease and its connection to various health issues. And if Broda Barnes, M.D., is correct, hypothyroidism is one of the basic deficiencies that contributes to the proliferation of coronary artery disease.[3]

The Biological Perspective

The thyroid gland is a butterfly-shaped organ that sits in the lower part of the neck and spans across the larynx. It is responsible for maintaining the metabolic rate and keeping the human body warm. Slight variations in normal thyroid function can dramatically affect health.

Every cell in the body depends on adequate levels of thyroid hormones to function. Thyroid hormones function as the "spark plugs" that trigger the Krebs cycle or ATP cycle. ATP is how the body generates energy. If there is a relatively low level of thyroid hormone, called hypothyroidism, then the body will generate less energy and less heat, and the individual will be lethargic and suffer from a lack of energy. In states of excess thyroid release, called hyperthyroidism, the body will generate more energy, and the individual will be both warm and overenergized, and will lose weight.

As described previously, in our model of the endocrine system, the pituitary is the master gland that controls the four endocrine systems, one of which is the thyroid. The pituitary releases thyroid-stimulating hormone (TSH), and the thyroid gland in turn manufactures thyroxine (T4) and triiodothyronine (T3). The thyroid production is four parts T4 to one part T3 (a ratio of 4:1). Thyroxine is thought to be more of a storage hormone, and T3 is found to be the biochemically active hormone. Under normal circumstances, T4 can be converted into T3 inside and outside the cell.

An important part of the endocrine model is that the hormones secreted by the thyroid glands feedback to the pituitary and turn down TSH. This is called a negative feedback loop. If there were no feedback, then the thyroid-stimulating hormone would push production of T4 and T3 to very high levels. The results are proper amounts of T4 and T3 produced to satisfy the body's and brain's needs.

Lastly, this thermoregulation function of the thyroid hormone may play a major role in childhood and adult obesity. In studies of body temperature, the potential to gain weight under stable caloric intake may be due to the body's inability to raise body temperature.[4]

DIAGNOSING HYPOTHYROIDISM

There are three ways of diagnosing a problem such as hypothyroidism:
1. Symptom list
2. Laboratory tests
3. Metabolic parameters: basal body temperature

Symptom List

Cold hands and feet	Inability to concentrate
Cold intolerance	Infertility
Constipation	Irritability, depression, moodiness
Difficulty in verbal expression	Menstrual pain, menstrual irregularities
Dry skin, brittle nails	Muscle weakness
Elevated cholesterol	Slow heart rate
Essential hypertension	Weight gain
Swollen eyelids, ankles	Nervousness
Fatigue	Poor memory
Hair loss	

As one can see, there are a plethora of symptoms related to hypothyroidism. The key is to recognize these symptoms as a fundamental problem with the body generating energy.

Mary S. is a 39-year-old married woman with two children and no energy. She suffers most of the symptoms listed above: cold hands and feet, low body temperature, cold intolerance, short-term memory lapses, swollen eyelids, no energy, and weight gain. She used to exercise and had even run two marathons, but now she is too tired to take care of her children. "Life is not fun," she states, "when you would rather stay in bed all day long than go out with your family."

The endocrinologist to whom she was referred recognized her complaints. The laboratory tests confirmed a borderline TSH of 7.5 mIU/L, and the physician put her on thyroxine 100 mcg for six days per week. The problem was that the patient did not feel any differently. When she returned to her endocrinologist, he looked at the blood work, and the TSH had now normalized under 5.0 mIU/L, and her T3 and T4 RIA were within normal range. He said that everything was now normal.

The patient found Dr. Lichten's website and references from other thyroid sites as well. She asked him to review the laboratory tests. He put them down and asked, "Do you feel like the laboratory tests are all right?" Mary S. said, "No." Dr. Lichten said, "Then they are not normal. We treat patients and we thoroughly monitor the correct laboratory tests." Then the complaints of cold hands, feet, fatigue, brittle nails, and memory issues were discussed. Dr. Lichten asked if she took her basal body temperature before arising in the morning. She had, and the temperature was 96.4° F. When Mary S. brought this fact up to her endocrinologist, he had made fun of her, and she was embarrassed. "Broda Barnes, M.D., the premier thyroid specialist of the 20th century, used the basal body temperature as the key parameter in judging thyroid balance. We won't ever laugh at your efforts to understand your body and feeling better," clarified Dr. Lichten.

What many people don't know is that the body functions best within a narrow basal body temperature. The catalytic and enzymatic processes, the vitamins and hormones, work best at 97.8°F–99.8°F. Being cold means being less biologically active. Being cold means that the body is not functioning well enough to raise the body's core temperature to a normal functioning level. The measurement of basal body temperature is key to finding proper thyroid activity and, when deficient, correct replacement dosing.

Physically, there is a simple test that medical students are taught to determine if the hypothyroidism affects other body functions. This is called the Achilles Reflex Test. The patient sits on a chair on their knees, with their shoes and socks off facing to the front of the chair. A reflex hammer is used to demonstrate a normal, brisk jerk when the tendon is tapped. The absence of the ankle jerk is a sign of severe, systemic hypothyroidism. The test is not very accurate but makes the point that low thyroid affects every tissue in the body.

Next, repeat laboratory tests are drawn. Instead of the antiquated T3 and T4 RIA, Dr. Lichten orders the free T3, free T4, and reverse T3. The presence of reverse T3 occurs not infrequently in individuals who are taking synthetic thyroid or have a problem with making appropriate amounts of T3 when stressed. The T3 molecule is supposed to be "left-handed," designated as L-T3. All active hormones have a "left" molecular orientation. Reverse T3 has a "right"-handed orientation and is not only worthless as a thyroid T3, but it also ties up a binding site that could be offered to L-T3. In any of the above cases, a low free T3 or high T3r are laboratory tests that confirm hypothyroidism. Secondly, Dr. Lichten orders the thyroid antibody and thyroid peroxidase antibody tests to determine if an inflammatory process is involving the thyroid. The next table shows the different thyroid blood tests, along with conventional normal ranges and what Dr. Lichten considers to be optimal ranges.

THYROID TESTS	NORMAL RANGE	OPTIMAL RANGE
Thyroid-Stimulating Hormone-TSH	0.2–5 mU/L	<2.0 mU/L
Thyroxine-T4 Free	0.8–1.8 ng/dL	>1.2 ng/dL
Triiodothyronine T3 Free	230–420 pg/ dL	<300 pg/ dL
Reverse T3	<0.25 ng/mL	<0.25 ng/mL
Thyroid Antibodies	<20 IU/ mL	<20 IU/ mL
Thyroid Peroxidase Antibodies-TPO	<35 IU/mL	<35 IU/mL
Sedimentation Rate	<20 mm/hr	<20 mm/hr

The thyroid produces both T4-thyroxine and T3-triiodo-thyronine.[5] While classically trained doctors feel that synthetic thyroid is adequate, based on the premise that the body will synthesize all the T3 that it needs, bio-identical doctors believe that the free-T3 levels may be too low, so they prescribe Armour® Thyroid, a combination of T4 and T3 from desiccated pig thyroid gland. The endocrinologist contends that if they needed to add T3, then they would add Cytomel®.

All three thyroid replacement products are bio-identical, prescription- and FDA-approved products: note that only Armour® Thyroid contains the balance of thyroid hormones.

	Synthroid® (pure T4)	Armour® Thyroid 60mg	Cytomel® (pure T3)
Dosages:	0.025–0.2 mcg	38 mcg T4	25 mcg T3
	9 mcg T3		

Based on the clinical experience of B. Siegal, M.D., in *Is Your Thyroid Making You Fat?*[6] about 70% of women will feel better on either Synthroid® or Armour® Thyroid. To them, it may not make any difference at all. For the remaining 30%, some prefer synthetic thyroid, and a number will prefer or better tolerate Armour® Thyroid. So, although on principle Dr. Lichten prefers Armour® Thyroid, he does not always take patients immediately off synthetic thyroid. What he may do next is add back low doses of Armour ® Thyroid, or replace the synthetic thyroid with Armour® Thyroid or leave the patient on synthetic thyroid and add back compounded T3. No one prescription medication fits all.

Mary S. was unhappy and she wanted a change. Dr. Lichten discontinued the synthetic thyroid. He explained that the half-life of the synthetic thyroid was about a week; that means that the thyroid medication would still be in her system when she started the Armour® Thyroid. But, the Armour® Thyroid is short-acting; hypothyroid individuals need to take the Armour® Thyroid twice daily. The compromise is to take the thyroid just once daily for the first week and increase the dosage to twice daily the second week.

Because nutritional deficiencies are an integral part of hypothyroidism, Mary S. started on two packages of vitamins with extracolloidal minerals (magnesium, zinc, selenium), iodine, and vitamins (A, B, C, and D). At this visit, Dr. Lichten did an intravenous vitamin and mineral loading with 4,000 mg of B complex, 4,000 mcg of B12, 5,000 units of vitamin A, 2,500 mg of magnesium, 10,000 mg of ascorbic acid, and 10 cc of trace minerals, including zinc, chromium, selenium, and calcium. The intravenous therapy usually gives the patients an energy boost and is offered as proof that there is something that can be done to bring natural energy back into the person's system.

Mary S. returned in two weeks to tell us she was feeling better and at six weeks from her initial visit that she was a "reinvigorated" new woman. Her basal body temperature was in the 97°F range and she was feeling much better. Dr. Lichten redrew her laboratory thyroid tests and explained that she could increase her Armour® Thyroid by another half-grain. The patient was instructed to notify the doctor if there were complaints of heart palpitations or shortness of breath. If that happened, she was to stop the thyroid medication until speaking to the doctor. The patient understood.

The patient returned after another six weeks to report that she was "cured." The doctor reviewed with her the vitamin/mineral/essential fatty acid supplements, her vitamin D intake and sleep pattern, her DHEA and vitamin C intake, and her remaining complaints. The patient was happy with the treatment and her basal body temperature was just below or at 98°F. She reported feeling warm and that her skin looked better. Moreover, when Dr. Lichten repeated her Achilles reflex, it was more brisk. Simple, safe, and FDA-approved treatment with bio-identical hormones.

Dr. Lichten explained that all three thyroid products are truly bio-identical. However, the Synthroid®-T4 and the Cytomel®-T3 are both incomplete thyroid hormones. Together, he explained, one would consider them complete, but the problem with Cytomel® is that it has such a short half-life—two hours, called blood T1/2—that to be effective one would have to take it five times per day to maintain adequate tissue T1/2 levels. The simplest treatment is Armour® Thyroid with a 4:1 balance of T4 to T3 taken twice daily.

Some, Dr. Lichten explains, may develop goiter-like symptoms on Armour® Thyroid alone. They feel their neck is swollen or the TSH values never seem to suppress adequately. For these, Dr. Lichten will add 50–100 mcg of synthetic T4 thyroid; this combination seems to work well. Again, the goals are normal thyroid parameters, a normal basal body temperature, no heart palpitations, and no trouble sleeping at night.

For some, the Armour® Thyroid does not raise the basal body temperature. Dr. Lichten prefers to keep the dosage of Armour® Thyroid under the prescribed mandate of four grains daily. However, based on biochemical studies of 25 years ago, the normal dosage of Armour® Thyroid may be as high as six grains![5] For those that still have low body temperatures, low energy, and complaints of fatigue and depression, Dr. Lichten will turn to one of the compounding pharmacies in his vicinity to make up a slow-release T3 to which is added thyroxine for twice a day dosing.

While Cytomel®, T3, comes in 25 mcg dosages and has a very short half-life, the compounding pharmacists will make up 7.5 mcg – 15 mcg of T3 in a base that retards absorption. This slow-release formula allows the capsule to disperse the dosage of T3 throughout 6-8 hours. This is important when the discussion focuses on the changing problems of thyroid disease and why supplementary T3 may be of greater significance in light of the increase in reverse T3 and thyroid antibodies.

What many doctors are seeing is the development of more and more reverse T3 even in those individuals not taking synthetic thyroid. There is really no explanation for the thyroid patient to make reverse T3.[7] What is the impetus for the body to do so? The literature does not have an answer, but the addition of supplementary T3 can make a biological difference.

Since the reverse T3 is a right-handed molecule, then L-T3 is the active hormone. Dr. Lichten's approach to elevated reverse T3 is to add more L-T3. By adding more 'good' L-T3, the L-T3 can both suppress the formation of both R-T3 and L-T3 and start to push the R-T3 out of binding sites. The process is ongoing, and the dosage may need to be increased to 15 mcg twice daily or more, but in time and medical observation, some of the debilitating signs and symptoms of this thyroid dysfunction can be partially rectified.

The other problem that is developing to a greater extent is a proliferation of Hashimoto's thyroiditis. This is an immune disorder that attacks the thyroid gland. The inflammation destroys the thyroid producing glands and the patient presents with hypothyroidism. With measurement and screening for thyroid antibodies and thyroid peroxidase antibodies, this condition may be diagnosed before full-blown thyroid disease develops.

THE "SPIN" STORY AGAINST ARMOUR® THYROID

When any person looks at the composition of synthetic thyroid and Armour® Thyroid, one can see that there is a difference: One has only T4, and the other has T3, T4, and a little T2 and T1 to be exact. For most people, it makes no difference, so why the war over synthetic or bio-identical? It seems that the pharmaceutical spin on which is best started back in 1939, with Dr. Broda Barnes' rejection of synthetic thyroid.[8] The medical schools were taught to use synthetic thyroid because its dosing was "more accurate" or, rather, the pharmaceutical companies may have offered more financial incentives. The doctors were warned that Cytomel® and T3 in Armour® Thyroid could cause heart palpitations, but so can synthetic thyroid. The unsubstantiated complaints of quality issues and alleged contamination went on and on.

What has 80 years uncovered in the medical/pharmacological literature?

First, Armour® Thyroid is FDA-approved, and the amount of thyroid contained within the formulation meets government standards, which are approximately plus or minus 10%. That means that the amount of T4 in Armour® Thyroid must be between 35 and 43 mcg, and T3 between 8 and 10 mcg. As the amount of thyroid one's body needs per day varies by more than these amounts, this degree of specificity is well within acceptable range.

Secondly, a large study at Stanford showed that the Synthroid® preparations had as much or more variation. But Boots Pharmaceuticals at that time was so distraught over the results of the study that they took legal action to block Betty Dong from the University of California, San Francisco (UCSF),[9] from releasing the results to medical peer-review journals. It took five years before the article appeared, during which time Boots sold more than $3 billion worth of Synthroid® worldwide. The federal government fined Boots $180 million, and Knoll Pharmaceuticals bought out the rights[10] to Synthroid®.

As the literature reports, Betty Dong agreed to study Synthroid® for its manufacturer, Boots, Inc. Boots designed the protocol, monitored the project, but in the end all the different forms of thyroid replacement were found to be equivalent. Dong had contracted with the company not to publish without permission, so she did not. The company published the study with a conclusion favorable to themselves. When Boots sold Synthroid® to Knoll Pharmaceuticals, a division of BASF, Knoll relented, and the article was published in the *Journal of the American Medical Association* (*JAMA*) in 1997.[11]

The conclusion of that study was that all thyroid medication had a significant degree of variation, and the policy of trying to be so exact with the dosing of synthetic thyroid remains an exercise in futility. Based on the UCSF study, the generic thyroid was just as good as the brand name.

Dr. Lichten had a further question for the experts in thyroid replacement. It seems that a number of European studies had shown that the T3 component was effective in treating or preventing depression. A study from Lithuania appeared prominently in the *New England Journal of Medicine* (*NEJM*).[12] The American Association of Clinical Endocrinologists (AACE) backed a study to disprove the *New England Journal of Medicine* article and published it in *JAMA*. When Dr. Lichten saw the study's conclusion, he wrote a letter to the editor, which was published, probably because of the simplicity of the question. Dr. Lichten wrote, "If the author is stating that natural thyroid is no better than synthetic thyroid, then we should be writing prescriptions for natural thyroid because it is cheaper." The response to that simple question was two full pages long and ended with "we have to trust what the AACE says."

SYNTHETIC THYROXINE VS. DESICCATED THYROID

Edward M. Lichten, M.D., *JAMA*. 2004; 291: 1445.[13]

To the Editor: Dr Clyde and colleagues[14] concluded that treatment of primary hypothyroidism with combination levothyroxine plus liothyronine was not superior to levothyroxine alone in terms of body weight, serum lipid levels, hypothyroid symptoms, or cognitive performance. Although Clyde, et al. recommend that patients should be treated with synthetic thyroid on the basis of cost, natural desiccated thyroid is considerably less expensive. Thus, perhaps this would be the most rational treatment choice.

There is an inherent fallacy that the clinical endocrinologists continue to restate. They state that the blood tests are *"sine qua non,"* the "whole ball of wax." But what about the thermogenic properties of thyroid—if the thyroid is truly balanced, then why are the patients still cold, fatigued, and getting fat?

The answer is that the two thyroid hormones are not balanced. Studies have now shown that a deficiency in the minerals selenium[15] and possibly zinc and magnesium affect the ability of the cells to convert T4 to T3. A significant mineral deficiency seen in the nutritionally deprived, those who are gastronomically stressed, and most older populations will prevent adequate T4 conversion, and these people will do better on Armour® Thyroid and mineral/vitamin replacement. The proof may very well be the low body temperature and fatigue that never seems to improve.

There is also an inherent fallacy that the holistic physicians continue to restate. They believe the Armour® Thyroid is the only thyroid to use. Yet some of Dr. Lichten's patients seem to have an immune reaction to Armour® Thyroid and never really feel well. Some of these individuals have a hidden gluten or corn starch allergy and will do better on a corn-free, gluten-free natural thyroid from Bio Tech.[16] And some patients just feel better or have a decrease in thyroid gland size on synthetic thyroid.

HYPERTHYROIDISM

Hyperthyroidism is a state of overt excitement. Grave's disease is the most common cause of hyperthyroidism. It is caused by the body's self-destruction of some normal thyroid regulators. This leads to thyroid cellular overgrowth and excessive production of thyroid hormone. The symptoms of hyperthyroidism are listed below:[17]

SYMPTOMS OF HYPERTHYROIDISM	
Fatigue	Weight Loss
Goiter	Tremor
Heat Intolerance	Menstrual disturbance: light flow
Hypertension	Nervousness, palpitations

A Health Center researcher has found that if autoimmune diseases were counted as a single category instead of more than 20 separate illnesses, they would move on to the federal government's list of the 10 most common causes of death for women younger than age 65.[18] Immune disorders are by nature up to 10 times more frequent in women than men. A list of potentially related autoimmune diseases include:

Crohn's disease	Polymyalgia Rheumatica
Ulcerative colitis	Arthritis- juvenile and psoriatic
Grave's disease	Rheumatoid Arthritis
Hashimoto's thyroiditis	Scleroderma
Lupus	Sjogren's
Multiple Sclerosis	

In reference to these listed autoimmune conditions, not only is there a greater risk of patients having thyroid disease, but there is also an elevated risk of patients with thyroid disease having concurrent rheumatoid factors.[19]

The treatment of inflammatory disorders by conventional medication has been unsuccessful, and the reliance on corticosteroids and chemotherapy agents such as methotrexate is disheartening. But an old treatment has been revised and rejuvenated by a number of local and national physicians. They believe that inflammation is caused by a microscopic bacterial infection. Whether it is a mycoplasma[20] or another organism, the treatment of their choice is three months of a form of tetracycline, most often with minocycline. Interestingly, minocycline will suppress both thyroxine (T4) and triiodothyronine (T3) without suppressing TSH.[21] Minocin® (or generic minocycline) 100 mg once a day is their regimen. This information is included for completeness, for there can be an unusual effect on thyroid from long-term Minocin® use, called black thyroid.[22] With black thyroid there can be deposits of pigment contained within the thyroid gland and thyroid abnormalities. Although rare, it is a side effect that should be discussed if a patient elects this unconventional treatment.

The newest genetic studies show that the allele for hypothyroidism, diabetes, and heart disease is located in close proximity on one of the autosomal linked chromosomes.[23] So, whether the human race has inborn genetic markers for these chronic diseases, or whether the human race has a susceptibility to infections that start an inflammatory response that triggers these diseases, is not well understood.

What medical science does have, however, is the ability to reduce the inflammation with natural bio-identical hormones. The anti-inflammatory effects of these hormones are documented in the following chapters:

1. Pineal hormone: Melatonin
2. Pituitary hormone   Human growth hormone
3. Thyroid hormones   Thyroxin triiodothyronine
4. Adrenal hormones   DHEA and cortisol
5. Women's hormones   Estradiol and progesterone
6. Men's hormones   Testosterone

We recognize that those chronic diseases, no matter what the origin, are inflammatory and that the body has developed (over millions of years) the ability to repair and provide humankind with the ability to prosper and reproduce. These effective and reparative forces are anabolic hormones. Humankind cannot survive without them.

THYROID RESISTANT SYNDROME

In nature, there are a few individuals who are resistant to their own thyroid.[7] Even if the numbers for the TSH, T3, and T4 are normal or even elevated, these individuals act like they have no thyroid at all. Higher and higher dosages of thyroid are prescribed, with temporary or albeit no response at all. These individuals may need six grains[24] of natural thyroid some days and less other days. Their management is difficult and time consuming.

In the practice of medicine, physicians first look at some anomaly in nature to try to understand the process exactly. For hypothyroidism, 100 years of therapy has taught doctors to replace thyroid and thereby prevent the dropsy, heart failure, elevated cholesterol, and weakened immune system. For those with hyperthyroid, the strain on the heart and body necessitate that the over-release of thyroid hormone be turned off or, more commonly, the thyroid gland surgically removed or destroyed by radiation and then supplemented back to normal. But the confusion over thyroid-resistant syndrome runs over into what Dr. Lichten sees as a new and emerging problem: a syndrome of resistance to thyroid replacement.

RESISTANCE TO THYROID REPLACEMENT

So many women and men are taking thyroid replacement yet are unable to raise their body temperatures toward normal. They still have cold hands and feet and extra weight they cannot lose, yet their thyroid replacement values for TSH, T3, and T4 free are normal to high normal. The only consistent finding is the development of thyroid antibodies, and even the addition of adequate colloidal minerals still does not change the course of the disease.

Now, if the underlying problems of the thyroid are minerals, as proposed by John Myers, M.D.,[25] 70 years ago, then the lifelong deficiency in iodine creates a physical demand by the body for iodine. A number of "goiter belts" exist throughout the world around inland areas where the iodine content is severely deficient. This would include every state west of Pennsylvania up to the Rocky Mountains. Similar areas are located in Canada.[26]

If iodine deficiency were not enough to cause hypothyroidism by itself, then the addition of large amounts of fluoride and chloride[27] in the water supply may interfere with iodine stores. To date, testing has been limited to fluoride concentrations alone. To this add bromide, which was substituted for iodine in the raising of bread 30 years ago. Reviewing the periodic chemistry table from high school, one finds that these aforementioned molecules are lighter than iodine and may easily displace iodine within the biological system. Whether significant or not, Americans are suffering from iodine deficiencies.

If this were not enough, the presence of percholate, thiocyanate and nitrate has attracted widespread attention because of the chemicals' abilities to interfere with iodine uptake by the thyroid. Cruciferous vegetables such as: cabbage, cauliflower, Brussels sprouts, kale, mustard, and turnips contain progoitrin which acts like thiocyanate. That is why walnuts, soy, Brussels sprouts, and millet can worsen thyroid problems. And the widespread use of DDT-like organophosphates in food often leaves the thyroid gland dsyfunctional.[28]

Only time will tell. In the meantime, Dr. Lichten prefers for these individuals a program that merges two FDA prescription thyroid preparations: Armour® Thyroid and small doses of synthetic thyroid. Iodine replacement is offered as topical iodine (Lugol's solution), iodine salts in the vitamin packages, and iodine contained within the compounded thyroid products. When the dosage is stabilized, small increments of sustained-release T3 are added to raise the basal body temperature.

Because of the need to balance all the hormone systems, some of Dr. Lichten's patients may need up to four grains of Armour® Thyroid[29] 100 mcg Synthroid®[30], Cortef® 5–10 mg, DHEA 25–50 mg, and replacement sex hormones before the quest for balance is at least partially met. Nutrition and environmental poisons may be major factors in contributing to low thyroid.

THYROID DISEASE AND DIABETES

The focus of every chapter is that the endocrine glands work as part of one interactive endocrine system; for example, disruptions of sleep and vitamin D deficiency affect the pituitary hormones. Disruption of the release of human growth hormone affects the adrenal release of DHEA and cortisol and, if severe enough, the sex hormones as well. Little is written to identify how interactive thyroid hormone is with all the other endocrine systems. Although it was stated that hyperthyroid and hypothyroid states can affect female fertility—and the next chapter will focus on the adrenal interaction with thyroid— there are still other unexplained interactions.

One of them is the interaction of hypothyroidism and diabetes.

THE AUTOIMMUNE ASPECTS OF DISEASE

While there is a 4:1 ratio of women to men in all cases of thyroid disease, the ratio of female to male is 9:1 for states of hyperthyroidism, and for postpartum thyroiditis, obviously 100%.[31] The question is raised as to what correlation may exist between a state of Grave's disease (hyperthyroidism), the postpartum thyroiditis, and diabetes.

The answer is that all three of these conditions are considered autoimmune diseases. But genetic evaluation research shows that type I insulin-dependent diabetes mellitus-IDDM is linked to autoimmune thyroiditis (Hashimoto's) by a dominant haplotype; they sit in close proximity on the chromosome fragment, so they tend to be genetically inherited together. Similarly, IDDM is closely associated with rheumatoid arthritis-RA.[32] Yet thyroid and RA are not related. Epidemiologic studies confirm the above. So one must screen patients with hypothyroidism for diabetes using the hemoglobin A1c, but expect little or no rheumatoid arthritis. A common screen Dr. Lichten uses for arthritis is the sedimentation rate. Only if elevated are further rheumatoid, sarcoidosis, and lupus antibodies ordered.

While only 4% of the general population is confirmed to be hypothyroid, fully 30% of type I diabetic women are afflicted with this disease. The rate of thyroid disease immediately after childbirth is triple the rate of non-pregnancy. Studies imply that this is due to the profound rebound in the immune system after suppression during pregnancy. But this accounts for only a few percentage points of thyroid disease.

It is important to follow those individuals with antithyroid peroxidase antibodies, as they predict the development of autoimmune thyroid disease and other autoimmune conditions. Thyroid disease and diabetes are linked by being in the same region on the same chromosome (and parts of genetic code).[33]

THE EFFECT OF THYROID DISEASE ON DIABETES AND CARDIOVASCULAR CONDITIONS

Hyperthyroidism is associated with an increase in insulin resistance, seen in worsening insulin requirements and worsening glycemic control. Hyperthyroidism, just like pregnancy, may unmask diabetes for the first time. Only with appropriate thyroid control will the blood sugar mechanisms return toward normal.

If fact, poorly controlled diabetes will shift the laboratory tests to a lower serum T3, as there is impaired conversion of T4–T3, a low serum T4 due to protein binding, and inappropriately low serum TSH. Hypothyroidism may affect diabetes by lowering insulin requirements as the metabolic rate declines. The most common biochemical signs of hypothyroidism are the abnormalities of plasma lipids. This includes elevated triglycerides and elevated low-density lipoprotein (LDL). Because even subclinical hypothyroidism can worsen these signs of dyslipidemia commonly found in diabetics and obese pre-diabetics, it is mandatory to address the underlying issues and try to reverse the lipid abnormalities with adequate thyroxine [thyroid] replacment. We treat subclinical hypothyroidism.

As Wu states,[32] the patients have elevated LDL-cholesterol worsened by hypothyroidism.
1. Detectible serum anti-TPO antibodies.
2. They are symptomatic.[31]

Cost of Thyroid Preparations Explaining that Natural thyroid is cheaper

PRODUCT	GENERIC	DOSAGE/FREQUENCY	100 QUANTITY
Armour® Thyroid		one grain/one to four perday	$16.76
Bio-Tech			
Synthroid®		100 mcg/one per day	$46.45
Levoxyl®	levothroid	100 mcg/one per day	$19.97
Unithroid®		100 mcg/one per day	$32.21

REFERENCES:

1. Kimball OP. Prevention of goiter in Michigan and Ohio. *Journal of the American Medical Association* 1937; 108:860–864.
2. Barnes, Broda. *Hypothyroidism: The unsuspected illness*. Harper and Row. 1939.
3. ibid.
4. Rising R, Keys A, Ravussin E, Bogardus C. Concomitant interindividual variation in body temperature and metabolic rate. *Am J Physiol*. 1992 Oct;263(4 Pt 1):E730-4.
5. Gaby AR. Sub-laboratory hypothyroidism and the empirical use of Armour Thyroid. *Alt Med Rev*. 2004 Jun;9(2): 157–179.
6. Siegal S. *Is Your Thyroid Making You Fat?* Warner Books. 2000.
7. Yen PM. Molecular basis of resistance to thyroid hormone. *Trends Endocrinol Metab*. 2003 Sept;14(7): 327–33.
8. Barnes B. Hypothyroidism: The Unsuspected Illness. Harper and Row. 1939.
9. Rennie D. Thyroid storm. *JAMA*. 1997 Apr 16;277(15):1238-43.
10. BASF financial statement. corporate.basf.com/.../publikationen/berichte/ BASF_ZB_2_1999_e.pdf?MTITEL= Second-Quarter%20Results%201999.
11. Dong BJ, Hauck WW, Gambertoglio JG, et al. Bioequivalence of generic and brand-name levothyroxine products in the treatment of hypothyroidism. *JAMA*. 1997 Apr 16;277(15):1205-13.
12. Bunevicius R, Kazanavicius G, Zalinkevicius R, Prange AJ Jr. Effects of thyroxine as compared with thyroxine plus triiodothyronine in patients with hypothyroidism. *N Engl J Med*. 1999 Feb 11;340(6):424-9.
13. Lichten EM. Synthetic Thyroxine vs. Desiccated Thyroid. *JAMA*. 2004 Mar 24;291(12):1445.
14. Clyde PW, Harari AE, Getka EJ, Shakir KM. Combined Levothyroxine Plus Liothyronine Compared with Levothyroxine Alone in Primary Hypothyroidism. *JAMA*. 2003 Dec 10;290(22):2952–2958.
15. Olivieri O, Girelli D, Stanzial AM, Rossi L, Bassi A, Corrocher R Selenium, zinc, and thyroid hormones in healthy subjects: low T3/T4 ratio in the elderly is related to impaired selenium status. *Biol Trace Elem Res*. 1996 Jan;51(1):31-41.
16. Available at: Bio Tech Thyroid. www.bio-tech-pharm.com.
17. Brownstein D. *Overcoming Thyroid Disorders. Medical Alternatives Press*. 2002

18. Available at: http://advance.uconn.edu/2000/000918/00091813.htm.
19. Soy M, Guldiken S, Arikan E, Altun BU, Tugrul A. Frequency of rheumatic diseases in patients with autoimmune thyroid disease. *Rheumatol Int*. 2007 Apr;27(6):575-7.
20. Sack J. Binding of thyrotropin to selected Mycoplasma species: detection of serum antibodies against a specific Mycoplasma membrane antigen in patients with autoimmune thyroid disease. *J Endocrinol Invest*. 1989 12(2):77-86.
21. Shigematsu T, Matsumoto F, Imai T, et al. Suppressive effects of minocycline on the pituitary-thyroid axis in humans. *J Infect Chemother*. 1995 1(2):116-121.
22. Miller BT, Lewis C, Bentz BG. Black thyroid resulting from short-term doxycycline use: case report, review of the literature, and discussion of implications. *Head Neck*. 2006 Apr;28(4):373-7.
23. Golden B, Levin L, Ban Y, Concepcion E, Greenberg DA, Tomer Y. Genetic analysis of families with autoimmune diabetes and thyroiditis: evidence for common and unique genes. *J Clin Endocrinol Metab*. 2005 Aug;90(8):4904-11.
24. LeBoff MS, Kaplan MM, Silva JE, Larsen PR. Bioavailability of thyroid hormones from oral replacement preparations. *Metabolism*. 1982 Sep;31(9):900-5.
25. Myers J. *Metabolic Aspects of Health*. 1979.
26. Langer, S. *Solved: The Riddle of Illness*. Keats. 1995.p. 18.
27. Bürgi H, Siebenhüner L, Miloni E. Fluorine and thyroid gland function: a review of the literature. *Klin Wochenschr*. 1984 Jun 15;62(12):564-9.
28. Langer P, Kocan A, Tajtaková M et al. Fish from industrially polluted freshwater as the main source of organochlorinated pollutants and increased frequency of thyroid disorders and dysglycemia. *Chemosphere*. 2007 Apr;67(9):S379-8.
29. Rees-Jones RW, Larsen PR. Triiodothyronine and thyroxine content of desiccated thyroid tablets. *Metabolism*.1977 Nov;26(11):1213-8.
30. Hennessey JV, Evaul JE, Tseng YC, Burman KD, Wartofsky L. L-thyroxine dosage: a reevaluation of therapy with contemporary preparations. *Ann Intern Med*. 1986 Jul;105(1):11-5.
31 . Carle A, Laurberg P, Pedersen IB, et al. Epidemiology of subtypes of hypothyroidism in Denmark. *Eur J Endocrinol*. 2006 Jan;154(1):21-28.
32. Wu, P. Clinical Diabetes. Thyroid Disease and Diabetes. 2000; 18(1):1- http://journal.diabetes.org/clinicaldiabetes/v18n12000/Pg38.htm
33. Torfs CP. King MC, Huey B, Malmgren J, Grumet FC. Genetic interrelationship between insulin-dependent diabetes mellitus, the autoimmune thyroid diseases, and rheumatoid arthritis. *Am J Hum Genet*. 1986 Feb;38(2):170–187.

CHAPTER 4

THE BIOLOGY OF ADRENAL EXHAUSTION

HORMONES AND FATIGUE

It seems strange that the same hormones that are needed for man's survival are belittled and seemingly considered dangerous in our modern medical world. No one thinks about taking vitamin D to sleep better, doctors who use human growth hormone to improve tissue repair are criticized, and natural thyroid is somehow considered inferior to the synthetic variety. And now the two most misaligned hormones of all—DHEA and cortisol—will be the focus of discussion. Note that DHEA is officially banned in Canada[1] as an anabolic hormone, while in Japan[2] it is used intravenously to soften the cervix of a laboring mother. And cortisol, only one-fifth as strong as prednisone, is rarely used because it allegedly causes osteoporosis and even Cushing's disease.

As Selye[3] proved 75 years ago, and as Jeffries[4] wrote 50 years ago, the problem for physicians is that they are educated on the most potent of therapeutic regimens and the most severe states of disease. When there is a life-threatening allergic reaction, physicians know to order a Medrol Dosepak® with Prednisone® and treat for five days. The same physician will be unsure how to prescribe Cortisone® in the morning and afternoon for a mild or early allergic reaction. The emphasis in physicians' medical training is on overkill: Doctors only recognize the life-threatening disease states, leaving the day-to-day practice woefully unattended. The purpose of the chapter on the history of the adrenal glands is to refocus the doctor and medical attention on the role of the natural hormones.

Natural hormones have special roles as anti-inflammatory agents and as anabolic, pro-repair functions as delineated in every chapter in this book. There are natural treatments with these natural hormones for arthritis, fatigue, and many other allergic or unexpected reactions.

Nature usually has good reasons for her choice of agents participating in the physiology of life. Hence a schedule of administration that mimics the normal production pattern of cortisol[4] and every other bio-identical hormone should be the first and last thing taught future and present doctors.

Historical Perspective

With the discovery of each natural and bio-identical hormone in the earlier parts of the 20th century came an awareness of tremendous medical power. Here, we were men with one of the magic wands of creation. Originally, only very small amounts of these hormones could be produced at great cost, so their use was discriminating and careful. But with the synthesis of each hormone came a readiness to see how far and how fast we as doctors could go to effect treatment.

After duplicating the natural hormones, it seemed that man sought to manufacture stronger and stronger hormones. Then the problems of pharmaceutical versus physiologic medications occurred from overprescribing large doses of hormonal lookalikes. Sometimes this led to catastrophic side effects and even death. Then, in their haste to protect the same public for which these super synthetic hormones were hatched, the FDA grouped natural steroids with pharmacologic concoctions by issuing the same warnings on both. A travesty and a great injustice were perpetrated again; because the government does not understand the safety and benefit of bio-identical hormones.

Before reviewing the action of natural and pharmaceutical drugs, one must review what each natural hormone was intended to treat. The understanding of the disease called "stress" started with the research of Selye before World War II.

More than 70 years ago, Hans Selye[3] described the basic work that has defined the word *stress* and what is perceived as adrenal exhaustion. It seems that Dr. Selye, although extremely bright, was not the most coordinated of individuals. Although he would publish more than 1,600 articles and write 33 books, he had trouble containing the rats in their cages. As the story goes, one day, when doing an experiment on his rats, he found that, no matter what he did to the rats, they all showed the same enlargement of the adrenal cortex, atrophy of the thymus, spleen, lymph nodes, and deep bleeding ulcers in the lining of the stomach and duodenum. Even the rats that were the control group were what Selye called "stressed." The more he processed the animals, the greater the changes in the adrenal organs. He finally realized that he was the cause of the "stress," by virtue of his dropping them out of the cages and chasing them all over the laboratory. So no matter what was done or injected into the rats, whether it was the environmental poisons or the environmental "chasing of the rats around the lab," the biological system of the rat interpreted this as stress. Stress was definitely a disease that could detrimentally affect the life of animals and, by supposition, man.

Selye came to the conclusion that there were three stages of the body's reaction to stress. He called this G.A.S.: General Adaptation Syndrome.[3] These are the three steps he hypothesized:

1. Fight or Flight (stress)
2. Adaptation (stress managed)
3. Exhaustion (worn out)

Selye noted that the initial reaction to stress was for the adrenal gland to enlarge or hypertrophy. The larger gland could manufacture more adrenal hormones. Then, as the stress factor became a stable part of the animal's environment, the size of the adrenal gland returned to normal size. But, with chronic unremitting stress, the gland shrunk in size, and the release of adrenal hormones was significantly decreased.

In our hectic and most stressed world, Selye's work is even more important than the fact that he did this work before and after WWII. The key to Selye's stress is that there is bad stress called *distress*, and good stress called *eustress*. For a maximal existence, there must be good stress. Lying around will not cause muscles to grow and lungs to expand, so one must exercise. But being at war in a life or death situation causes destructive stress. Life exists best when balanced.

Selye added another dimension to his concept of stress by identifying two levels of stress: a superficial level that is used and replenished, much like the adrenal hormones on which this chapter focuses. But on a deeper, almost metaphysical level, he speaks of the inner life force that is depleted as one ages.

Hans Selye: "It is not stress that kills us, it is our reaction to it."

The Biological Perspective

The adrenal gland has been called the second pituitary because this small 3- to 5-gram gland is seat to production of more than five separate hormones. Each endocrine hormone works by being secreted into the bloodstream and being carried to every cell in the body. There the hormone "excites" the cell into action. The hormone is carried on a protein and is bound to specific receptor sites on the cell wall. This docking occurs much as the space shuttle "docks" to the space station. Once attached, the hormone molecule is carried through the cell wall bound to a ligand and taken to the nucleus (control center). Then the hormone relays its message to the nucleus, by binding to cellular DNA genetic material. These DNA sites in the nucleus produce RNA messengers to go out from the nucleus of the cell and turn on or turn off many cellular functions, including: the manufacturing of proteins, production of energy, and, most of all, release of sugar. The adrenal gland produces hormones from the inner layer of the gland called adrenalines. The cortex layers produce a number of steroids. The first of these steroid hormones, cortisone or hydrocortisone, is from a family of glucocorticoids. They are called glucocorticoids because their first role in human existence is to release sugar for energy.[4]

In summary, the adrenal cortex produces:[5]
1. Glucocorticoids: cortisol or hydrocortisol
2. Mineralocorticoids: aldosterone
3. Androgens: DHEA and testosterone
4. Estrogens: Estrone and estradiol

Diseases of the adrenal gland include:
1. Cushing's syndrome: overproduction of cortisol
2. Conn's syndrome: underproduction of aldosterone
3. Addison's disease: lack of production of DHEA, cortisol

The source of all adrenal cortical hormones is cholesterol. The adrenal gland receives a general call to produce hormones by the pituitary hormone-stimulating factor, adrenocorticotropin hormone (ACTH). The exact mechanism by which one hormone is produced in excess of another is unknown but generally considered a selective response to Selye's concept of internal stress.

One of the primary functions of cortisol is the production of glucose from stored glycogen, protein, and fats in time of stress. The body breaks down all forms of stored energy to generate the glucose to activate all parts of the voluntary muscle system in a "fight or flight" response. The body does not need stored fat or muscle when trying to escape an enemy. Therefore, the major actions of large doses of cortisol are considered catabolic. *Catabolic* means to "eat away," versus the concept of rebuilding, called *anabolic*. These terms are most important to differentiate between a distressed individual and one who is exercising to build stronger muscles and physical fitness through anabolic actions, or eustress.

The second role for glucocorticoids is to reduce inflammation. By depressing the immune system, the stressed body does not attempt to repair damage. Biologically the body needs to escape danger before worrying about repair. As the body's normal response to tissue damage, whether it be weightlifting or cardio-pulmonary exercise, is to send in inflammatory cells to first clear the debris of damaged tissue; this process is "placed on hold" while the major stressor is resolved. The failure to end the stressor, whether it would have been a saber-tooth tiger at the mouth of a cave or an unremitting boss working you day or night, is what is important, not its cause. It is logical to assume that the majority of stress must stop for the body to start to affect its necessary repair.

An excess of production of corticosteroids is caused naturally by a medical condition called Cushing's disease. It this case, a pituitary tumor secrets excess ACTH that causes the adrenal to overproduce cortisol. Any condition that shows excess amount of cortisol in the blood without a pituitary tumor is called Cushing's disease.

Sometimes adrenal tumors are identified in Cushing's disease, but most often no operable or treatable cause is identified.

Cushing's syndrome and disease,[5] a condition of excessive cortisol, creates a condition of excess stress on the body. The high levels of circulating cortisol lead to these physical signs:

1. Moon face (puffy appearance)
2. Central obesity
3. Thinning skin with bruises
4. Purple or red striae or stretch marks
5. Hirsutism: excessive facial or body hair on women
6. Buffalo hump: deposits of fat on back behind neck
7. Increased pigmentation

The high levels of circulating cortisol lead to these physical diseases:

1. High blood pressure
2. Diabetes and insulin resistance (pre-diabetes)
3. Reproduction disturbances: infertility, impotence, no menstruation, and no libido or sex drive
4. Mood disturbances: depression, anxiety, panic, insomnia, and even frank psychosis
5. Heart disease

The key here is to understand that excessive production or intake of high potency corticosteroids leads to all the signs of aging: puffy, fat, thin skin, high blood pressure, diabetes, and heart disease. If there is one hormone integrated into the aging process it is cortisol: High levels and high response to stress ages man.

STRESS AND CORTISOL

As Selye had noted, life must have stress to maximize the body's response potential. Yet the stress must not be excessive or continuous. Note Paula's story.

Paula is a 43-year-old attorney and mother. She is significantly overweight, concerned about family, children, and getting everything done throughout the day. She is obviously stressed and unable to deal effectively with her chronic daily stressors. She is unable to sleep and unable to deal with her teenage children. She stopped working outside the home and has no energy to clean, let alone perform more than perfunctory review of legal papers. She has allergies when exposed to grass and mold. But most of all, she says she looks and feels old.

Paula reported being unable to sleep every night. The cause may well be that the high levels of cortisol and adrenaline she releases during the day may still be elevated at night, which cause her body and mind to race when they should shut down. So Paula has insomnia, and even if she does fall asleep, she wakes at 3:00 a.m. and cannot easily fall back asleep. Therefore she is exhausted but wired, starting in the wee hours of the morning.

Paula complains of weight gain and muscle weakness. She has a full, moon face, central obesity of 50 pounds, and increased body mass index with more fat than muscle and an appearance of being 20 years older than her stated age.

The stress and the caffeine trigger migraines; the low levels of growth hormones triggers fibromyalgia-like symptoms of total body aching; the thyroid disruption is noted in cold hands, brittle nails, and hair loss; and the hormonal imbalances trigger menstrual irregularities. With the increased weight and stress, she is clinically diabetic.

And confirmation is found in performing the LAB TESTS listed in the Appendix.

The pathophysiology of pineal, pituitary, and thyroid dysfunction were reviewed in detail in the previous three chapters. The pathophysiology of estrogens are the subject for all of Book Two, and testosterone in men the subject of Book Three.

The treatment Dr. Lichten offers focuses on the disrupted endocrine hormones:

Lichten Six-Step Program
1. Pineal Dysfunction:
   L-tryptophan (or 5-HTP) increases serotonin and turn down excess adrenal hormones. GABA, or gabapentin, for muscle relaxation and decreased muscle pain
2. Pituitary Dysfunction:
   Offer to cycle three months of low-dose human growth hormone to restart the anabolic processes of tissue repair
3. Thyroid Dysfunction:
   a. Armour Thyroid® starting at 1 grain and increasing incrementally until TSH is less than 2 and body temperature is approaching 98°F.
   b. Mineral supplementation with extra iodine
4. Adrenal Dysfunction:
   a. Small dosages of DHEA are supplemented twice daily. Fluid retention was treated with spironolactone, blocking excess aldosterone
   b. Vitamin C 6000 mg taken as sips of ascorbic acid in orange juice all day long
5. Pancreatic Dysfunction:
   a. Use Metformin to lower blood glucose levels, increase insulin sensitivity and reduce the risk of diabetic complications.
   b. Dietary program is offered with monitoring of glucose before and after meals.
   c. Exercise and weight loss program
6. Menstrual irregularities, no libido, and depression:
   a. Testosterone injections are added every 1–2 weeks
   b. Anabolic steroid with B vitamins are then added every 1–2 weeks

Although Paula was also treated with loading doses of intravenous vitamins for a few weeks, she felt compelled to stop treatment. Dr. Lichten next learned that Paula was admitted to the hospital with a perforated bowel and an abscess (infection). Due to Paula's weakened ability to fight infection and affect anabolic healing, this stress resulted in her spending 30 days in the hospital: She had three surgeries, including a diverting colostomy, and was discharged with an ileostomy (bowel bag) and a worsened medical status than before discontinuing her "build me back up" program. The program is outlined in the Six-Step Program. Her body looked like and was hormonally identical to a 90-year-old's, and she responded to stress like one, too. Paula proved the concept that you are as old as your hormone levels. Your biological hormone levels are the keys to a fulfilling life and whether you live long and well or are stricken by disease and premature death.

When Paula came back to the office of Dr. Lichten, she was terribly inflammatory. Even the weakest intravenous therapy was met with complaints of burning. Food caused gastric irritation, her skin was thin and bruised, and the tissue around the colostomy bag was raw and not healed. Paula had gone to the third step of the Generalized Adaptive Syndrome, Selye's G.A.S—she was burned out. There was no adrenal reserve. She was constantly inflamed and in much worse condition than three months previously.

The necessity of replacing her natural cortisol levels had been usurped by the internists who placed Paula on high doses of prednisone. Synthetic prednisone is four times more potent than cortisol, so the side effects will be four times more pronounced: 10 mg of prednisone is equivalent to 40 mg of cortisol, and the replacement dose for Paula was 20 mg of prednisone daily. Dr. Lichten would have to wean her off gradually and convert her over to 80 mg of natural cortisol divided over the entire day, with two-thirds before noon.

TOO LITTLE CORTISOL AND DISEASE

The doctors knew that Paula's inflammatory processes would consume her with pain and an inability to move around. They knew that the synthetic corticosteroids would worsen weight gain and the diabetes. But their concern was the immediate need to suppress this inflammation so that the body might heal. They just were not trained to use the less expensive and much weaker doses of natural cortisol or Cortef®.

Typical uses of hydrocortisone and natural corticosteroids in medical textbooks.

1. Rheumatoid arthritis[6]
2. Rejection of transplanted organs[7]
3. Asthma[8]

JOHN F. KENNEDY[9] AND ADDISON'S DISEASE

Addison's disease is a disease of low cortisol release and sometimes low aldosterone release as well. Before WWII, this was a more common disease, as tuberculosis could infect and destroy the adrenal gland. As most destruction of the adrenal gland now is considered to be autoimmune, it shares signs and symptoms with other like diseases. The abnormal attack by the body's immune system on its own tissues in the adrenal gland is called Addison's disease; on the tissue in the joints is called rheumatoid arthritis; and on the colon is called colitis. The process is the same. The underlying cause of why this occurs is still unknown, but there are genetic and environmental factors.

John F. Kennedy was first diagnosed and treated for low levels of cortisol in England. The European physicians first used cortisol pellets, not unlike the hormone pellets Dr. Lichten uses today. But the pellets were replaced by injections and, as the technology improved, oral medication. Kennedy learned to take the largest portion of medication in the morning and less in the afternoon. Cortisol is not taken at bedtime because it may keep certain individual awake. This pattern roughly mimics the normal circadian rhythm cycle necessary for normal wake-sleep cycles.

But when there is extra stress, pain, or infection, the dose of natural cortisol must be increased, often by 100%. Without appropriate cortisol the patient is listless, prone to infection and in almost a hibernation state. Low cortisol is destructive differently but just as importantly as excess cortisol. The body needs balance.

A recent review of JFK's medical files showed that he suffered from other endocrine dysfunction: just as Dr. Lichten has noted in so many of his patients in the chapters of this book. JFK was on testosterone injections, and because of a lack of DHEA replacement to offset his cortisol prescription, he was not in endocrine balance. He was on major pain medication, the stress of which wiped out his DHEA levels. The X-rays showed extensive osteoporosis from the excess of stress versus the body's ability to heal: He remained deficient in testosterone, thyroid, human growth hormone, and DHEA. But even the president in 1960 could not get the medical attention placed at your fingertips today. He suffered in quiet solitude with so many pain medications that it is best for us to avoid the errors of the past and use balanced hormonal therapy initially and preferably today.

Proved in JFK's case, Addison's disease can be life threatening. Fortunately, replacement therapy with glucocorticoids and mineralocorticoids can permit a normal life. Aldosterone as Florinef® is available as a nasal spray.

But more about cortisol treatments will be delineated later.

ALDOSTERONE AND MINERALOCORTICOID REPLACEMENT

The second hormone produced within the cortex of the tiny adrenal gland is aldosterone, a mineralocorticoid. A "mineral"-o-corticoid is a hormone that regulates minerals or salts in the body. Aldosterone stabilizes the blood pressure by regulating the absorption of salts, especially sodium. Lack of this hormone can present with symptoms such as weakness, low blood pressure, and exhaustion, as seen in the JFK saga. Aldosterone is released to keep the blood pressure adequate for life and survival. An increase of mineralocorticoid production is called Conn's syndrome.[10]

Conn's syndrome causes the body to retain sodium and excrete potassium. This disrupts the careful sodium-potassium balance and results in weakness and high volumes of urine, especially at night. The high blood pressure correlates with an elevated laboratory measurement of aldosterone and low levels of renin. Some endocrinologists believe that up to 10% of those with essential elevated blood pressure will show elevated aldosterone levels.[11]

There is a simple diuretic that blocks aldosterone. It is called spironolactone. Spirolactone is one of Dr. Lichten's preferred treatments in his attempts to regulate the interaction of the various hormone systems. Spirolactone is unique in that it blocks the excess natural production of aldosterone. As high levels of aldosterone affect salt, blood pressure, and energy levels, the treating physician must block these excessive and destructive processes. To do so, spironolactone competes for the receptor sites in the distal tubules of the kidney. Any site filled by spironolactone cannot take up aldosterone. Henceforth, high levels of aldactone are mitigated.

A positive and unexpected side effect of spironolactone is that it blocks the conversion of testosterone to the more potent dihydro-testosterone.[12] This is especially important in darker-complected and heavier-set women, to block their tendency to become hirsute (hairy) whenever overweight or on testosterone supplementation. It is a mainstay of Dr. Lichten's hormonal balancing program and may cause minor weight and fluid loss in both women and men. Its role in hypertension is helpful, but it is not a potent antihypertensive agent. Side effects are rare and usually limited to gastric distress. In Dr. Lichten's experience, it may decrease the taste for salt.

DHEA:
THE UNAPPRECIATED HORMONE

The third hormone secreted by the adrenal cortex is DHEA, dihydroepiandosterone. This is both the hormone in the greatest concentration in the human body and a precursor or prohormone serving as an adrenal source of both testosterone and estradiol. But modern research finds DHEA to be an important cellular trigger for energy production in every cell in the body. DHEA has now been found to be manufactured in the walls of the heart.[13]

In classical education of physicians, the only function of DHEA is that it is a precursor for testosterone in women. In men, this DHEA-to-testosterone conversion is a minor factor, but for women the adrenal is the major source of testosterone. Higher levels of DHEA and testosterone in women can produce the increased facial and body hair, male pattern baldness, male abdominal hair distribution, and a disruption of menstruation seen in the polycystic ovarian syndrome.[14] The term "Stein-Leventhal syndrome" was used to describe these afflicted women, who represented a body type morphism seen in the Mediterranean and ethic populations.

DHEA LEVELS MAY BE DIRECTLY
LINKED TO AGING

While DHEA is the most abundant active steroid, it and cortisol are the twin keys used by the body in the response to stress. In large amounts, cortisol is catabolic, breaking down stored tissue glycogen, proteins, and fats into the components necessary to feed the body's response to acute stress. DHEA, on the other hand, is anabolic, using these same building blocks to rebuild tissue and to remake the complex proteins into muscle and the lipids into the matrix that supports all the tissue. Just as Selye described two layers of stress response, Dr. Lichten sees these two adrenal hormones: one replenishable (cortisol) and one slowly consumed (DHEA). While even the most exhausted individuals can usually, with proper rest and nutrition, build back their cortisol response; the loss of DHEA production that occurs with aging, however, is usually an irreplaceable event.

The highest levels of DHEA are noted in men and women in their early 20s. Subsequently, the levels of DHEA drop by 2% per year.[15] At the age of 20, a male's level of DHEA (measured as the sulfate) may be 500 mcg/dL, while at 50 years of age the average male's level may be 150 mcg/dL. Meanwhile, cortisol secretion increases as the individual ages. So, if DHEA is the spark plug of life, the older man is running on only two cylinders instead of eight.

DHEA is secreted in a pattern that is part of the circadian rhythm of sleep and wakefulness. DHEA and cortisol levels are highest between 4 a.m. and 8 a.m., preceding or part of the waking cycle. Both hormones are lowest prior to going to sleep. When cortisol levels and stress increase, DHEA-sulfate levels decrease. Increasing levels of DHEA are seen when the stress is reduced. As the medical literature documents below, chronic stress, chronic insomnia, and chronic disease are associated with low levels of DHEA.[16-30]

A search noted below of the literature determines what disease states are recorded as being associated with low levels of DHEA. Review of the most recent 100 articles on Pubmed.org, the N.H.I.

website, for the first quarter of 2007, found the following diseases strongly correlate to low levels of DHEA measurements:

Diseases States and Low DHEA

1. Chronic infections: cutaneous leishmaniasis,[17] malaria[18]
2. Allergic reactions: chronic uticaria[19]
3. Psychiatric stress: schizophrenia,[20] posttraumatic stress[21]
4. Medication stress: opioid use[22]
5. Autoimmune stress: lupus,[23] arthritis,[24] mild adrenocortica efficiency[25]
6. Sclerosis: systemic sclerosis,[26] multiple sclerosis[27]
7. Neurological stress: Alzheimer's disease,[28] Parkinsonism[29]
8. Heart disease stress: Coronary artery wall thickening[30]
9. Immune responses: DHEA levels low in cancer[31]
10. Terminal events: Low DHEA found in dying states[32]

DHEA AND HEALTH: THE CONNECTION

The above evidence establishes an association between low levels of DHEA and several disease states. It is also a fact that menopausal women have significantly lower levels of not only DHEA but also immune function than do women of reproductive age. In a concept of inflammation and aging, it is hypothesized that, or assumed that, the hormonal deficiencies of aging have left these older women "open" or "susceptible" to the increase prevalence of autoimmune diseases: thyroiditis, Grave's disease, rheumatoid arthritis, lupus and more. This observation must be answered by clinical trials of DHEA replacement to establish whether the hypothesis can be proven.

APPLYING THE SCIENTIFIC METHOD

As discussed in other chapters in this book, true science is the application of the scientific method. This involves a five-step process to first:

1. Make the observation— LOW LEVELS of DHEA are seen in autoimmune diseases such as rheumatoid arthritis[24] and lupus erythematosis[23]
2. Form the hypothesis that DHEA DEFICIENCY is associated with this process. ABNORMALLY LOW LEVELS of T-LYMPHOCYTES ACTIVITY[33] are noted.
3. Predict a scientific fact or observation, and in this case it is that DHEA replacement can affect some aspect of the immune system.[34] The fourth and final fifth steps are to apply this third scientific theorem, and:
4. Confirm that it (DHEA replacement) has an effect on the problem seen originally. Lastly, and of most importance, is:
5. The hypothesis is left standing after everyone attacks the logic and hypothesis. That is proof—that is true science.

Peter Casson, M.D., in an elegant study out of Baylor in 1995,[33] showed that DHEA enhanced T-lymphocyte activity by up to tenfold. McGuire[34] out of Stanford showed that DHEA replacement reversed some of the protein loss from the kidney disease associated with lupus erythematosus. DHEA has shown to relieve the pain of women with rheumatoid arthritis when given in large doses. Could this be because DHEA reduces the inflammatory response of T-cells in rheumatoid arthritis? It seems so.

This is not to say that these individuals may need cortisol or even prednisone to function; but it is to state that DHEA should be one of the first drugs prescribed for these inflammatory conditions, arthritis for example. This is not to state that methotrexate,[35] Humira®[36], Remicade®, and Embrel®[37] are not applicable drugs, just to state that they are the drugs of last, not first, resort. Natural DHEA is best because it is nontoxic even in high doses. Furthermore, researchers state that the reversal of DHEA to cortisol ratio may have profound correlation with the extent and potential to recover from disease.[38]

Dr. Lichten advises his patients that there may be an increased appearance of acne, which can be easily treated with spironolactone and antibiotic face pads. But there will not be the increased cases of tuberculosis noted with Embrel®[37] nor the increase in cancer associated with immune-suppressing drugs like Humira®.[36]

McGuire,[34] chairman of medicine at Stanford, asked what was the role of DHEA when treating women with advanced lupus erythematosus. Lupus is an autoimmune connective-tissue disease in which the markers of inflammation are measured as laboratory tests of sedimentation rate and antinuclear antibody. Nuclear antibodies may be 10 to 100 times normal. The inflammation is related to joint pain and tissue destruction. One of the organs affected is the renal system. McGuire shows that the protein spilled in these individuals is reduced dramatically when DHEA was given in adequate amounts of supplementation.

Solerte[39] in an elegant study shows that the immune cells of women with Grave's disease and autoimmune thyroiditis could be reactivated with supplementary DHEA. DHEA is known to be an important regulator of normal thyroid function.[40]

And Huang showed that liver cancer turns off the enzymes to activate DHEA.[41]

If present theory holds that inflammation is the key to cell destruction and aging, then the use of DHEA to retard these inflammatory markers would be a logical step.[41] DHEA replacement seems to increase IGF-1 (growth hormone) levels in both sexes. It has an effect on increasing muscle mass in those who exercise. DHEA is associated with less depression, and increases in DHEA affect maturation and development of the brain's cortex. DHEA is simple and safe, inexpensive and efficient.

DHEA DOSAGE

The dosage Dr. Lichten uses for women is 25 mg and for men 50 mg. In a 1995 pilot office study, Dr. Lichten shows that DHEA levels were more consistent over time when the preparation was micronized, so he favors sustained-release formulations and their use in the morning and early afternoon.

THE CHANGING PICTURE OF ENDOCRINOLOGY

Labrie[42] has gone on to explain that DHEA works also within the cell. By bringing DHEA to the cell and into the cell, the cell becomes its own manufacturer of hormones. Therefore, starting from DHEA, estradiol and testosterone are actively produced for use within the cell.

Labrie reasons that it is more difficult for DHEA and other hormones to penetrate or be taken up by the cell with advanced age.[42] If this hypothesis and logic holds true, then it is imperative to increase the bio-available free portion of these active hormones to compensate, not decrease them. Note that because DHEA-sulfate measurements are relatively stable over a 24-hour period, laboratory measurements of DHEA-Sulfate are greatly preferred to measurement of DHEA.

ADRENALINE AND NOREPINEPHRINE

The center two-third of the adrenal gland is made up of tissues that produce adrenalines, which are chemically identified as epinephrine and norepinephrine. No other stressor except for surgical removal can lower the production of these epinephrine hormones. A panicking person close to death will produce as much adrenaline as he or she ever has.

CORTISOL:
SECRETS UNVEILED

The use of natural cortisol as a tool to reverse the General Adaptation Syndrome of Selye has been a goal of physicians and researchers ever since William Jefferies, M.D.,[43] lectured about this same subject more than 50 years ago. The problem with cortisol, as Dr. Lichten sees it, is that no one has figured out a means to differentiate from mildly deficient cortisol to a state of major burnout. Long-term use of cortisol may actually suppress normal adrenal function, and major dosages of DHEA may suppress cortisol as well.

The following information is gleaned from Dr. Lichten's 25 years of using small doses of cortisol, as first proposed by Jefferies and modified in his medical practice.

Everyone seems to be stressed, and more so than at any time in the past 200 years. The support of the adrenal gland cortex depends on adequate intake of vitamin C[43] and the American diet is woefully lacking in this. Therefore, it is not unusual to find these characteristics of poor adrenal reserve:

1. Fasting cortisol less than 20 mcg/dL
2. Fasting DHEA-sulfate less than 100 mcg/dL
3. Variation in fasting serum glucose and after three hours GTT

Historical Perspective

The classical testing of the adrenal gland as performed for the last 50 years focuses on the response of the adrenal gland to pituitary stimulation. The pituitary gland produces not only TSH to stimulate the thyroid and FSH and LH to stimulate the ovaries and testes but also a polypeptide protein called adrenocorticotropin hormone-ACTH. If the ACTH production is low because of injury or destruction of the pituitary gland, then an injection of .25 mg of ACTH will cause at least a doubling, often a quadrupling, of the baseline cortisol level. This is called the Cortrosyn® stimulation test.[44]

The way this test is performed is that the baseline fasting cortisol blood level is drawn and the injection is given into the deltoid muscle. Increased cortisol levels should appear in the blood sample drawn 30 minutes later.

The patient may report feeling significantly better or not in the next four days.

Consider the Cortrosyn® Stimulation test as Adrenal Test One in Dr. Lichten's office. Classically, if the blood samples show a twofold to fourfold increase in cortisol levels, the test is considered normal. Normal means that the pituitary-adrenal axis is intact. But if the patient reports any positive changes in his or her symptoms over the next 24 hours, then there is a disruption at one of three levels of the hypothalamic-pituitary-adrenal (HPA) axis. The purpose of the test is to determine at what levels there is a block:

1. A decrease in the responsiveness of the glucocorticoids receptors in the *hypothalamus* may be a normal hypothalamic response to aging. There is decreased hypothalamic secretion of CRH.
2. Low levels of ACTH may occur in individuals as they age, and this is called ACTH resistance: The down regulation or unresponsiveness does not generate the appropriate *pituitary* response. This result from chronic exposure to high levels of cortisol to the corticosteroid receptors in the hypothalamus and indirectly the pituitary: The receptors in the "old brain" burn out and are no longer receptive.[45]

There is decreased hypothalamic secretion of CRH. In cases (1) and (2), ACTH injections or increasing higher levels of cortisol should give a positive patient response.

Adrenal Test Two, as defined by Dr. Lichten, is performed at the second visit. This test is reserved for individuals who do not note improvement after the ACTH stimulation test. At this visit, the patient receives a concentrated Myer's[48] intravenous vitamin and mineral infusion over 20 minutes. Loading with 15,000 mg of vitamin C, B vitamins, trace minerals, selenium, and magnesium is followed by an intravenous injection of 10–25 mg of Solu-Cortef®. While higher doses of soluble cortisol are used for medical emergencies, this dosage will be sufficient to generate an appropriate response in those individuals who are blood tested low in cortisol and clinically unresponsive to ACTH.

Those who respond to the injection of Solu-Cortef® have "burned out" their adrenal glands and are in Selye's third stage of General Adaptation Syndrome. This is described as "adrenal problem level 3"—adrenal burnout.

Whether the patient has either low or insensitive ACTH response, or his or her adrenal cortex is completely exhausted, the treatment is exactly the same:

1. High-dose vitamin C replacement by intravenous and oral therapy
2. High-dose B vitamin replacement by intravenous and oral therapy
3. Mineral replacement by intravenous and oral therapy
4. Oral cortisol in divided dosages

As spontaneous adrenal insufficiency results from progressive destruction of adrenal tissue, symptoms appear when the process reaches 90% of the glandular tissue. Based on the work of Jefferies,[43] a maintenance dose of 20–30 mg daily of cortisol seems most applicable.

Some individuals seem to have enough cortisol upon awakening but are exhausted in mid-afternoon. It is preferred to measure cortisol levels in blood at noon with expected levels of 8–10 mg/mL. Alternatively, saliva measurements of cortisol and DHEA can be measured. The saliva measurements may be more dynamic as they record four measurements throughout the day. Relative values may not be as reproducible as serum measurements but are useful in correlating his or her symptoms to saliva hormone levels.

Dr. Lichten has reduced the dosage of Cortrosyn® from 0.250 mg to .05 mg and to 0.01mg.[46] The reason is that as little as .01 mg of Cortrosyn® given intravenously should stimulate a response at 30 minutes, comparable to higher doses.[47] Using 250 times as much will generate a response in anyone with 10% of reserve left. In using .01 mg, a normal response differentiates some of the individuals with borderline adrenal reserve.

In Dr. Lichten's experience, the majority of individuals consulting for adrenal fatigue will have Selye's stage two of the G.A.S. response. They will have normal to low morning cortisol but lose their reserve to handle additional stress. Selye called this stage "adaptation." Dr. Lichten calls this a "coffee break" and "caffeinated soda drink break" or "cigarette break" adaptation response. In a situation where the hypothalamic-pituitary-adrenal axis—HPA axis—is intact, these caffeine and nicotine products can stimulate and force the pituitary to release more ACTH.[48] This drives up the exhausted cortisol release for a short time.

In those individuals with more extreme adrenal exhaustion, Dr. Lichten routinely finds very low fasting blood glucose. As the disease becomes more advanced, the clinical symptoms that correlate to very low levels of ACTH are more pronounced. Clinical response to supplementing cortisol is Dr. Lichten's third series of tests. And the dosage of cortisol is titrated from the lowest level to give the patients the best response.

To understand more about cortisol deficiency, the following applicable information appears in the medical literature.

1. Hypopituitarism. In our patient with hypopituitarism and low levels of ACTH, the fasting glucose in routinely below 60 mg/mL. As the function of cortisol is to raise glucose, the presence of very low fasting glucose levels may be a sign of a lack of cortisol. After confirming a baseline cortisol morning level below 15–18 mcg/dL, Dr. Lichten might consider Cortef® replacement starting at 2.5–7.5 mg[49] upon arising and then perhaps repeating the smaller dose with meals. The last dose is no later than 4 p.m. to 6 p.m. For most, regular inexpensive cortisol seems to work better than sustained-release compounded forms, as the rapid absorption of cortisol seems to sensitize receptors and activate the awakening processes of cortisol. Dosages of cortisol are doubled in times of infection or severe stress.

2. Addisonian individuals have increased pigmentation. Therefore, those individuals who show increased facial pigmentation, ruddy or darker non-confluent reddened skin, are presumed to have adrenal burnout

with low levels of both DHEA-S and cortisol.[43] These individuals remain redder longer after chemical peels and skin treatments. This is to differentiate them from those individuals who have a pasty appearance and low cortisol but adequate or low DHEA-S. A drop in DHEA levels are associated with a loss of axillary hair.[50]

3. Adrenal stressed individuals may find that they get some relief from caffeine.[51] Each four ounces of coffee or two ounces of espresso has 100 mg of caffeine; red bull has 80 mg; and tea, diet Coke, and Mountain Dew have 40–55 mg of caffeine.[52] While Snapple has 12 mg, Sprite and some fruit drinks have 0 mg of caffeine. Individuals with excessive caffeine intake find that when they take cortisol replacement there is a reduction in their need for caffeine, but at the same time cortisol may be associated with insomnia.

4. Situational fatigue. With aging, two aspects of the feedback loop are affected. The first is that the secretion of ACTH is down regulated by a "sleepy" or "aged" hypothalamic-pituitary axis. Down regulation because of decreased CRH occurs normally with all the pituitary stimulatory hormones with aging. As these must feedback though corticotropin releasing hormone (CRH) to induce the ACTH release, the process of down regulation is amplified, resulting in adrenal hypoplasia. In those women with high levels of circulating androgens, the fasting glucose will be elevated. Although there are concerns about insulin resistance and diabetes, treatment may start with small doses of cortisol for another reason. The reason is that the enzymatic defect in producing cortisol increases ACTH release that raises both androgen and DHEA. In fact, to some degree, the excess of androgens contribute to some suppression of normal cortisol function.

5. Multiple endocrine dysfunctions. As adrenal insufficiency is considered to be a developing autoimmune disorder, its association with Grave's disease and amenorrhea is not uncommon. Replacement therapy with Solu-Cortef® 7.5mg 4x/day

for 12 weeks may allow regeneration of some adrenal tissue.[43] At the end of the three months, an ACTH stimulation test will show whether complete burnout has occurred.

6. Patients with the psychiatric disorders of anxiety and depression will tend to have higher baseline cortisol levels and be hyper-responsive to ACTH stimulation.[28]

7. The role of nicotine and caffeine is to cause significant rise in plasma and urinary 11-OH corticosteroid from enhanced ACTH release.[48]

8. Testosterone therapy in low dose may stimulate ACTH, but high dose will suppress it.[53]

9. Thyroid antibodies may be grounds to start Cortef®. The presence of thyroid antibodies increases the risk of future diseases including diabetes[54] and breast cancer.[55]

10. Rheumatoid arthritis patients improve on low-dose cortisol. Studies of these individuals show that they have an unexplained loss of diurnal cortisol release. They also have an abnormal response to stress, implying that an underlying genetic or environmental condition affects cortisol release and leaves the patient susceptible to rheumatoid arthritis. Similar implications are made for those who develop asthma and atopic allergic reactions.[56]

Twenty-five years ago, a 30ish-year-old heavy-set hirsute Jewish woman was seen by Dr. Lichten with complaints of infertility. Ovulation had failed to occur with Pergonal® therapy with two infertility experts. Although her DHEA-S was elevated, no one had considered the role of cortisol as a modulator of androgen activity. Two pregnancies resulted from the use of spironolactone and 7.5 mg of cortisol before breakfast and lunch and another 2.5 mg in the early afternoon. Jefferies[43] had reported the same 30 years earlier.

Frequent use of small doses of cortisol, along with mineral and vitamin supplementation, may allow for regeneration of adrenal tissue and provide for increased adrenal reserve at times of stress. Those individuals who show chronic stress and immunological deficient states will need some cortisol replacement for the rest of their lives.

The adrenal gland is more complex in its response than the thyroid or the ovary because of the role of the glucocorticoid receptors in the hypothalamus. To restate the physiology, there are three levels of response in the hypothalamic pituitary axis (HPA):

1. Hypothalamus: The old brain contains receptors for both glucocorticoids and corticotropin-releasing hormone. When the glucocorticoid receptors are burned out, they do not have the ability to stimulate the release of CRH to affect the pituitary. This is the effect of prolonged stress and aging.

2. Pituitary: The new brain, the cortex, contains storage and control of release of ACTH within the pituitary. Without CRH from hypothalamus or stimulation from the brain cortex, no release of ACTH occurs. This is documented by a positive response to ACTH stimulation testing.

3. Adrenal: This gland cortex produces cortisol and DHEA. With destruction of the adrenal gland from disease or burnout, there is lack of cortisol response to stress or testing. This is documented by a positive response to Solu-Cortef® injection.

4. Because of the continuous interaction between cortisol and DHEA, with high cortisol suppressing DHEA and high DHEA modulating and lowering cortisol, the last step is to add back 25 mg of DHEA to these patients. Two things are noted. First, there is more energy, and second there is not as many problems with mid-afternoon fatigue. Each patient learns by trial and error what dosage combination seems to work best within the parameters set by the physician.

CONCLUSION: CORTISOL

In practice, Dr. Lichten has moved from a diagnostic to a combined diagnostic-therapeutic program to evaluate adrenal reserve. After laboratory tests are drawn, the ACTH stimulation test is performed at the first visit. At the second visit with hypokalemia not present, Dr. Lichten uses an IV infusion called a concentrated Meyer's protocol to load the individual with vitamin C, trace minerals, B vitamins, and magnesium.[57] At the end of the infusion, Dr. Lichten will push 10 mg of Solu-Cortef® and ask the patient to report changes in symptoms over the next 24 to 48 hours. Replacement of DHEA and other bio-identical hormones is begun concurrently.

Clinical symptoms that are diagnostic for adrenal deficiency include extreme weakness, fatigue, dizziness, migraine, chills, hot flashes, nausea, uncontrollable shaking, body aches, low pulse (30s), vomiting, racing pulse, very disoriented, passing out, etc.

As one patient reported, "I feel awful and it comes on very suddenly." Physicians have to be concerned about low levels of potassium, because they could worsen with Solu-Cortef®. Failure to improve with higher dosages is a cause to repeat potassium levels. On the other hand, taking supplementary potassium with Cortef® may be considered, but is not often needed. The electrolytes often stabilize without additional medication.

Cortisol replacement should be considered in the same manner that physicians consider replacing thyroid, sex hormones, and even insulin. Imagine that the biological "team players" of the body's system are stressed and functioning poorly. By adding back all these hormones as reserves, the original player (glands) may be considered saved.

Add-back hormonal therapy for cortisol is good medicine.

CONCLUSION: DHEA

There is an observed and irrefutable decline in the levels of anabolic hormones with aging. These anabolic hormones, in order of serum concentration, are DHEA, testosterone, estradiol, and triiodothyronine and human growth hormone. Others have confirmed that these hormones could become the markers of the aging process in the human organism.[58] Moreover, low concentrations of DHEA and DHEA-S are related to the evolution of many diseases typically contracted by older people, above all the diseases of the cardiological, neurological, oncological, and immunological systems, as well as osteoporosis.

It is interesting to note that the cholesterol studies are focusing on the alleged benefits of statins to prevent arterial wall intima thickening. The body prevents intima thickening by use of a natural hormone, DHEA—making DHEA one of the protectors of coronary artery disease.[30]

REFERENCES:

1. Available at: http://www.pdrhealth.com/drug_info/nmdrugprofiles/nutsupdrugs/dhe_0094.shtml.
2. Ishikawa M, Shimizu T. Dehydroepiandrosterone sulfate and induction of labor. *Am J Perinatol.* 1989 Apr;6(2):173-5.
3. Selye, Hans. *The Stress of Life.* McGraw-Hill, Inc. 1956.
4. Jefferies, William McK. *Safe Use of Costisol.* CC Thomas Publisher. 3rd ed. 1956.
5. Available at: http://www.wikipedia.com. [Cushing's syndrome].
6. Straub RH, Schölmerich J, Zietz B. Replacement therapy with plus corticosteroids in patients with chronic inflammatory diseases- substitutes of adrenal and sex hormones. *Z. Rheumatol.* 2000 59 S2:II:108-18.
7. Bredikhin TF. Prolongation of homotransplant viability under the influence of thio-TEPA and thio-TEPA combined with hydrocortisone. *Biull Eksp Biol Med.* 1969 Aug;68(8):90-3.
8. MacLaren WR, Frank DE. Continuous steroid hormone treatment of chronic asthma. I. Cortisone and hydrocortisone. *Ann Allergy.* 1956 Mar-Apr;14(2): 183-93.
9. Available at: http://www.pbs.org/newshour/bb/health/july-dec02/jfk_11-18.html.
10. Available at: http://www.wikipedia.com.
11. Fradella CE, Mosso L, Gómez-Sánchez C, et al. Primary Hyperaldosteronism in Essential Hypertensives: Prevalence, Biochemical Profile, and Molecular Biology. *J Clin Endocrinol Metab.* 2000 May;85(5):1863-7.
12. Young R, Sinclair R. Huristes.II: Treatment. *Australias J Dermatol.* 1998 Aug;39(3):1517.
13. Nakamura S, Yoshimura M, Nakayama M, et al. Possible Association of Heart Failure Status With Synthetic Balance Between Aldosterone and Dehydroepiandrosterone in Human Heart. *Circulation.* 2000 Sept 28;110:1187-93.

14. Available at: http://www.nlm.nih.gov/medlineplus/ency/article/000369.htm.
15. Genazzani AR. Inglese S, Lombardi I, et al. Long-term low-dose dehydroepiandrosterone replacement therapy in aging males with partial androgen deficiency. *Aging Male.* 2004 Jun;7(2):133-43.
16. Available at: http://www.pubmed.org. [DHEA].
17. Galindo-Sevilla N, Soto N, Mancilla J, et al. Low serum levels of dehydroepiandrosterone and cortisol in human diffuse cutaneous leishmaniasis by Leishmania mexicana. *Am J Trop Med Hyg.* 2007 Mar;76(3):566–72.
18. Kurtis JD, Mtalib R, Onyango FK, Duffy PE. Human resistance to Plasmodium falciparum increases during puberty and is predicted by dehydroepiandrosterone sulfate levels. *Infect Immun.* 2001 Jan;69(1):123-8.
19. Kasperska-Zajac A, Brzoza Z, Rogala B. Lower serum concentration of dehydroepiandrosterone sulphate in patients suffering from chronic idiopathic urticaria. *Allergy.* 2006 Dec;61(12):1489-90.
20. Gallagher P, Watson S, Smith MS, Young AH, Ferrier IN. Plasma cortisol-dehydroepiandrosterone () ratios in schizophrenia and bipolar disorder. *Schizophr Res.* 2007 Feb;90(1-3):258-6.
21. Yehuda R, Brand SR, Golier JA, Yang RK. Clinical correlates of associated with posttraumatic stress disorder. *Acta Psychiatr Scan.* 2006 Sept;114(3):187-93.
22. Daniell HW. DHEAS deficiency during consumption of sustained-action prescribed opioids: evidence for opioid-induced inhibition of adrenal androgen production. *J Pain.* 2006 Dec;7(12):9017.
23. Nordmark G, Bengtsson C, Larsson A, Karlsson FA, Sturfelt G, Rönnblom L. Effects of dehydroepiandrosterone supplement on health-related quality of life in glucocorticoid treated female patients with systemic lupus erythematosus. *Autoimmunity.* 2005 Nov;38(7):531–40.
24. Cutolo M. Sex hormone adjuvant therapy in rheumatoid arthritis. *Rheum Dis Clin North Am.* 2006 Nov;26(4):881-95.
25. Jeffries W. McK. Mild adrenocortical deficiency, chronic allergies, autoimmune disorders and the chronic fatigue syndrome: a continuation of the cortisone story. *Medical Hypotheses.* 1994 Mar;42(3):183-189.
26. La Montagna G, Baruffo A, Buono G, Valentini G. Dehydroepiandrosterone sulphate serum levels in systemic sclerosis. *Clin Exp Rheumatol.* 2001 Jan-Feb;19(1):21-6.
27. Tellez N, Comabella M, Julià E, et al. Fatigue in progressive multiple sclerosis is associated with low levels of dehydroepiandrosterone. *Mul Scler.* 2006 Aug;12(6);487-94.
28. Genedani S, Rasio G, Cortelli P, et al. Studies on homocysteine and dehydroepiandrosterone sulphate plasma levels in Alzheimer's disease patients and in Parkinson's disease patients. *Eurotoxic Res.* 2004 6(4):327-32.
29. Nachshoni T, Ebert T, Abramovitch Y, et al. Improvement of extrapyramidal symptoms following dehydroepiandrosterone () administration in antipsychotic treated schizophrenia patients: A randomized, double-blind placebo controlled trial. *Schizophr Res.* 2000 Nov 15;79(2-3):251-256.
30. Fukui M, Kitagawa Y, Nakamura N, et al. Serum dehydroepiandrosterone sulfate concentration and carotid atherosclerosis in men with type 2 diabetes. *Atherosclerosis.* 2005 Aug;181(2):339-44.
31. Howard J.M. Common Factor of Cancer and the Metabolic Syndrome may be Low. *Ann Epidemiol.* 2007 Apr;17(4):270.
32. Glei D.A, Goldman N. Dehydroepiandrosterone sulfate (DHEAS) and risk for mortality among older Taiwanese. *Ann Epidemiol.* 2006 Jul;16(7):510-5.
33. Casson PR, Faquin LC, Stentz FB, et al. Replacement of dehydroepiandrosterone enhances T-lymphocyte insulin binding in postmenopausal women. *Fertil Steril.* 1995 May; 63(5):1027-31.

34. Van Vollenhoven B, Park JL, Genovese MC, West JP, McGuire JL. A double-blind, placebo-controlled, clinical trial of dehydroepiandrosterone in severe systemic lupus erythematosus. *Lupus*. 1999 8(3):169-70.
35. Available at: http://www.hopkins-arthritis.org/arthritis-info/rheumatoid-arthritis/rheum_treat.html.
36. Available at: http://www.medscape.com/viewarticle/482792.
37. Available at: http://www.whale.to/drugs/remicade9.html.
38. Arlt W, Hammer F, Sanning P, et al. Dissociation of serum dehydroepiandrosterone and dehydroepiandrosterone sulfate in septic shock. *J Clin Endocrinol Metab*. 2006 Jul;91(7): 2548–54.
39. Solerte SB, Precerutti S, Gazzaruso C, et al. Defect of a subpopulation of natural immune cells in Graves' disease and Hashimoto's thyroiditis: normalizing effect of dehydroepiandrosterone sulfate. *Eur J Endocrinol*. 2005 May;152(5):703-12.
40. Sahelian R. *A Practical Guide to DHEA*. Avery Publishing Group. 2002.
41. Huang LR, Coughtrie MW, Hsu HC. Down-regulation of dehydroepiandrosterone sulfotransferase gene in human heptocellular carcinoma. *Mol Cell Endocrinol*. 2005 Feb 28;231(1-2):87-94.
42. Labrie F. Adrenal androgens and intracrinology. *Semin Reprod Med*. 2004 Nov;22(4):279-80.
43. Jefferies W. McK. *Safe Uses of Cortisol.* CC Thomas Publisher. 1955.
44. Available at: http://www.amphastar.com/cortrosynwhatis.htm.
45. Gupta S, Aslakson E, Gurbaxani BM, Vernon SD. Inclusion of the glucocorticoid receptor in a hypothalamic pituitary axis model reveals bistability. *Theor Biol Med Model*. 2007 Feb 14;4:8. Available at: http://www.tbiomed.com/content/4/1/8.
46. Schultte KH, Myers JA. *Metabolic Aspects of Health*. 1933.
47. Dickstein G, Shechner C, Nicholson WE, et al. ACTH stimulation test: Effects of basal cortisol, time of day, and suggested new sensitive low dose. *J Clin Endocrinol Metab*. 1991 Apr;72:773-8.
48. Lovallo WR, Al'Absi M, Blick K, Whitsett TL, Wilson MF. Stress-like adrenocorticotropin responses to caffeine in young healthy men. *Pharmacol Biochem Behav*. 1996 Nov;55(3):365-9.
49. Gurnell E.M. A Longer Term Trial of DHEA Replacement in Addison's Disease. *Endocrine Abstracts*. 2002 4:OC24.
50. Kim SS, Brody KH. Dehydroepiandrosterone replacement in addison's disease. *Eur J Obstet Gynecol Reprod Biol*. 2001 Jul;97(1):96-7.
51. Cherniske, Stephen. *Caffeine Blues: Wake Up to the Hidden Dangers of America's #1 Drug.* Warner Books. 1997.
52. Available at: http://www.wilstar.com/caffeine.htm.
53. Hines GA, Smith ER, Azziz R. Influence of insulin and testosterone on adrenocortical steroidogenesis in vitro: preliminary studies. *Fertil Steril*. 2001 Oct;76(4):730-5.
54. Unnikrishnan AG, Kumaravel V, Nair V, et al. TSH receptor antibodies in subjects with type 1 diabetes mellitus. *Ann N Y Acad Sci*. 2006 Oct;1079: 220–5.
55. Turken O, NarIn Y, DemIrbas S, et al. Breast cancer in association with thyroid disorders. Breast Cancer Res. 2003 5:R110-R113.
56. Cutolo M, Sulli A, Pizzorni C, et al. Circadian rhythms: glucocorticoids and arthritis. *Ann N Y Acad Sci*. 2006 Jun;1069;289-99.
57. Kodama M, Kodama T. Four problems with the clinical control of interstitial pneumonia, or chronic fatigue syndrome, using the megadose vitamin C infusion system with dehydroepiandrosterone-cortisol annex. *In Vivo*. 2006 Apr;20(2): 285-91.
58. Haller U, Hepp H, Winter R. Antiaging or better aging: a contribution to the prevention of aging. *Gynakol Geburtshilfliche Rundsch*. 2003 Apr;43(2):69–70.

CHAPTER 5

THE BIOLOGY
OF
REPRODUCTION

"Every living creature has two primary drives: first, to sustain its own life (which includes seeking food, shelter, and safety), and second, to pass on that life to a new generation."[1] If a near perfect being could exist, no matter how long its life span, it would fail in its prime directive if it did not reproduce. Yet doctors, scientists, theologians, and anthropologists have not thoroughly considered how the biology of reproduction affects each human being's ability to stay healthy, weather disease, and continue to reproduce.

In nature there are two distinct types of reproduction: Either the life form relies on proliferative reproduction with hundreds of fertilized eggs or seedlings left to the wild with hope that some survive (plants, fish, amphibians, spiders, and birds) or the parent becomes the nurturer and protector of its few young. The highest life forms, mammals, go so far as to carry their young to viability. As man is a mammal, one would expect a Darwinian selection of the fittest; first mankind has to survive to reproductive age and then traverse a second selection process as adults to compete successfully and be able to impregnate, reproduce, and protect their young within a potentially hostile environment.

In the scheme of life, there are two factors that affect each living life form's ability to reproduce: genetic and environmental. Man, by means of his genetic, mental, and neuro-endocrine-immunological superiority, is the dominant life form on this planet at this time. But the second factor, environment, has a potentially more significant interplay.[2] If greenhouse gases and global warming change the environment drastically, if there is a pandemic of biblical proportion, then there will in all probability be a dramatic decrease in the numbers of human beings occupying the earth.[3]

Health, wellness, survival, and reproduction rely on genetic and environmental factors.[2,4-6]

GENETICS AND ENVIRONMENT

Every disease reviewed in this book recognizes that the bio-identical hormone and nutrient are of primary importance for survival and reproduction from both a genetic and an environmental consideration. Could one's efforts to ignore hormone replacement and nutritional supplementation be considered indifference to the prime directive to stay healthy and reproduce? Examples gleaned from selective chapters are listed in summary below:

1. Vitamin D. The dark skin that proves protective against sunburn and dehydration in the African plains becomes a negative genetic phenotypic factor in an environment of limited sun exposure. Together there is an impeded production of vitamin D. This combination possibly contributes to disease states, somewhat selective to blacks in the Northern and Southern Hemispheres (hypertension,[7] heart disease,[8] stroke[9]). Meanwhile, a deficiency in vitamin D in every genetic population is associated with increases in 17 different human cancers, the most prominent being colon cancer.[10] Historically and "recent case reports" highlight the resurgence of rickets in certain groups of breastfed infants. Infants residing in the North, irrespective of skin color, and dark-skinned African-American infants residing anywhere in the United States are most vulnerable to nutritional rickets if they are exclusively breastfed past age six months without vitamin D supplementation.[11] By example, then, increased hypertension, cancer, and heart disease in the adult and rickets in children would negatively impact the ability of these genetically and environmentally vulnerable individuals to reproduce in the non-equatorial environment.

The answer is overwhelmingly simple: take 2,000 to 5,000 IU of vitamin D daily. Toxicity is rare and serum vitamin D blood samples can be followed until an adequate level is reached. (See chapter 1.)

2. Human Growth Hormone. Individuals with idiopathic and postsurgical growth hormone deficiency have not only short stature and immunologic deficiencies but are also at increased risk of heart disease, cancer regrowth, and premature death.[12] Optimized growth relies on the pubescent growth spurt. Continuously low levels of growth hormone before adulthood contribute to short stature and unhealthy internal organ systems.

While Dr. Lichten does not recommend hGH replacement for healthy adults, his experience and that of the medical literature does propose that the severely afflicted individual who is in a state of catabolism breakdown may benefit from a short course replacement with hGH and then re-evaluation. For many others, optimal nutrition and adequate sleep as suggested in the Appendix may bring markers for hGH, specifically insulin-like growth factor-1 (IGF-1), into a more normal range.

The answer to maintaining optimal environmental nutrition may be as simple as taking a balanced vitamin, mineral, protein, and essential fatty acid supplement and getting plenty of REM sleep. An optimal IGF-1 level can be treated with supplements and, when necessary, by daily injection. (See chapter 2.)

3. Thyroid Hormone. Individuals with both low and high levels of thyroid hormone suffer increased mortality. Recent studies show that hypothyroidism as well as hyperthyroidism are associated with increased incidence of ischemic stroke.[13]

Discussed previously is the association of hypothyroidism and congestive heart failure, called dropsy.[14] Uncontrolled hyperthyroidism, called thyroid storm, can lead to heart failure and death.[15] Thyroid disease is most definitely an environmental factor overlaid on a genetic predisposition, as 50% of children in the Midwestern United States and Canada had evidence of goiters prior to the use of iodized salt[16] at the beginning of the 20th century. There is an associated increased risk of autoimmune disease and cancer in those with thyroid antibodies. Thyroid disease is associated with decreased performance, slowed response, and decreased fertility.[17]

While Broda Barnes, M.D. in 1939 stated that clinically upward of 50% of the Unites States population suffers from hypothyroidism based on low basal body temperature, replacement of thyroid hormone is prescribed for less than 10%[13] based on modern laboratory testing. Therefore, the development of thyroid disease needs to be addressed with the supplementation of appropriate amounts of necessary minerals prior to disease development and thereafter, with appropriate bio-identical thyroid hormone replacement that will bring both clinical laboratory parameters and basal body temperature into the normal range.

The answer to mineral replacement may be quite simple: Take the appropriately balanced mineral/vitamin preparation as suggested in the Appendix. To this, affected individuals may add extra minerals: daily iodine, selenium, zinc, and magnesium. The amount needed is upward of 1,000 mcg of iodine, 200 mcg of selenium, 30–50 mg of zinc, and 1,000 mg of magnesium or even more. To the vitamin package is added appropriate levels of B vitamins, digestive enzymes, and the ubiquitous vitamin D to improve absorption. (See chapter 3.)

4. Adrenal Hormones. Individuals with low levels of cortisol have Addison's disease and suffer from extreme fatigue. Those individuals with excessive production of cortisol develop Cushing's disease, which is associated with increased central body fat, insomnia, immune deficiencies, and extreme muscle weakness. The overproduction of aldosterone, the normal salt-balancing adrenal hormone, results in salt loss and fatigue. Surgical removal of the adrenal glands results in death within one week. In clinical practice, the low levels of DHEA and cortisol contribute to the large numbers of individuals suffering from adrenal exhaustion and fatigue. With adequate DHEA and balanced cortisol, the morning and afternoon caffeine binging becomes unnecessary. (See chapter 4.)

But this answer is more complicated. It seems that the adrenal gland concentrates vitamin C in the production of adrenal hormones. Based on the work of Linus Pauling and others, since the human animal cannot manufacture vitamin C, he or she needs 6,000 mg of vitamin C daily. Unless supplemented with powder in liquid drinks, this amount is virtually unobtainable in a standard diet.

5. Pancreatic Hormones. The pancreas produces two hormones, insulin and glucagon. Insulin is necessary for the body to process sugar, move it into the cell, and store it as glycogen. Glucagon allows the stored glycogen (in muscle and the liver) to be reconverted to glucose. The rate for developing diabetes is higher in certain populations that are genetically more at risk.

Using Mendelian genetics, one could postulate that 25% will not become diabetic no matter what they eat. For the remaining 75%, their diet and environmental factors control whether they become diabetic or not.

Recognizing the risks of being diabetic is a strong impetus for both men and women to change their diet and exercise program. The state of diabetes control is affected by levels of individual hormones, especially testosterone and thyroid replacement. In case reports in this text, the internal environment of balanced bio-identical hormones creates the optimal condition to minimize diabetic potential from a hostile environment. (See book 3.)

6. Ovaries and Testes: Estrogen, Progesterone, and Testosterone. There are seven chapters dedicated to how changes in bio-identical hormones can cause disease and in fact prevent or reverse certain disease states. A healthy, reproductive male and female with an active sex life will have a more optimal health and wellness constitution then the older, retired, and sedentary individuals not having effective sexual contact. It is the need for reproduction of the species that demands the maintenance of optimal reproductive hormonal levels.

Over the past 100 years, great strides in medicine have reduced the death of the mother in childbirth from 1,700 in every 100,000 as seen today in primitive Afghanistan to six in every 100,000 in Canada.[18] Therefore, there will be a greater number of mothers alive to take care of offspring, and that is a positive for the human prime directive.

WHAT CAN EVERYONE DO?

The food sources have such little nutritional value[19] that it is now mandatory to take vitamins and minerals. Even eating twice as many vegetables and fruits will not replace what is absent. And as John A. Myers, M.D.[20] showed in epidemiological studies more than 70 years ago, mineral deficiencies affect the plants and livestock, as well as the humans who eat both.

So, first and foremost, replace minerals and vitamins. The amounts of minerals needed are often 5–10 times greater than the RDA. So, if you did, hypothetically, take too much of the balanced minerals and vitamins, the excess would be lost in urine and stool anyway.

The important aspect to remember here is that every chemical reaction in the body depends on minerals and vitamins. If you have a genetic defect, you need more, not less of these substances. Whether it is vitamin D to prevent childhood rickets, or vitamin C to prevent scurvy, teeth loss, and illness, we as a nation need much more supplementation of vitamins, minerals, proteins, herbs, and essential fats. And the reason is that we do not get sufficient nutrition from our food. *Simple, dangerous, and life-shortening.*

Dr. Lichten screens for mineral deficiencies with serum samples of magnesium in the red blood cells and other trace minerals. If a person is low in magnesium, they are low in all minerals. The appropriate vitamin-mineral preparation covers the basic deficiencies.

In today's world there are societies that live years longer than most Americans. These societies do not have modern medicine, life-support, open-heart surgery, or MRIs. Although many factors have been suggested,[21] Dr. Lichten, and Myers and Pauling before him, believe it is the natural minerals and vitamins in the diet.

By taking in additional minerals, perhaps we can re-create what nature produces naturally. Or at least we can try.

REFERENCES

1.   Available at: http://www.touchstonemag.com/archives/article.php?id=18-05-027-f.
2.   Kokot F. 25-hydroxyvitamin D in patients with essential hypertension. *Clinical Nephrology* 1981; 16(4): 188–92.
3.   LaGuardia S.P. Secondary hyperparathyroidism and hypovitaminosis D in African-Americans with decompensated heart failure. *American Journal of Medical Science*. 2006; 332(3): 112–8.
4.   Poole KES. Reduced Vitamin D in Acute Stroke. American Heart Association. *Stroke*. 2006; 37:243.
5.   Gant WB. An estimate of cancer mortality rate reductions in Europe and the US with 1,000 IU of oral vitamin D per day. *Recent Results in Cancer Research*. 2007; 174:225–34.
6.   Rajakumar K. Reemerging nutritional rickets: a historical perspective. *Archives Pediatric and Adolescent Medicine*. 2005; 159(4): 335–41.
7.   Rostand SG. Ultraviolet light may contribute to geographic and racial blood pressure differences. *Hypertension*. 1997 Aug;30(2 Pt 1):150-6.
8.   Qureshi AI. Free thyroxine index and risk of stroke: results from the National Health and Nutrition Examination Survey Follow-up Study. *Medical Science Monitor*. 2006; 12(12): CR501-CR506 Epub.
9.   Available at: http://www.suite101.com/article.cfm/womens_thyroid_disease/35085.
10. Available at: http://www.suite101.com/lesson.cfm/19330/2898/5.
11. Available at: http://www.saltinstitute.org/37.html.
12. Available at: http://www.thyroid-info.com/articles/fertilitythy.htm.
13. Barnes B. Hypothyroidism. 1939.
14. Available at: http://www.qualitymeasures.ahrq.gov/summary/summary. aspx?ss=1&docid=8020.
15. Available at: http://www.unicef.org/pon96/leag1wom.htm.
16. Available at: http://www.prcdc.org/summaries/aidsinafrica/aidsinafrica.html.
17. Gore A. An Inconvenient Truth. 2006.
18. Available at: http://www.urbanherbalwoman.com/articles/Chemicals_Mimic_2006.html.
19. Available at: http://www.hmc.psu.edu/healthinfo/i/infertility.htm.
20. Schutte K., and J.A. Myers. *Metabolic Aspects of Health*. 1933.
21. Available at: http://www.abcnews.go.com. Finding the Keys to Longevity January 18, 2007.

NOTES

BOOK TWO

Understanding THE ROLE *of* NATURAL ESTROGEN

CHAPTER 6

ESTROGEN
AND
MENOPAUSAL
DISORDERS

WOMEN, MENOPAUSE, AND RELATED DISORDERS

Estrogen was discovered and manufactured in Europe in the 1930s. Its origin for commercial products was from *pregnant mare urine*, hence the name Premarin®.

First marketed in the United States in 1942, Premarin® was soon prescribed to treat the hot flashes of an aging female population. It did not gain popularity until Robert A. Wilson, M.D., wrote the best-selling book *Feminine Forever*.[1] Supported by a national book-signing tour, women soon clamored for estrogen replacement therapy—ERT. The initial complication from elevating estrogen levels in the postmenopausal female was breakthrough uterine bleeding that could become very heavy; known as metromenorrhagia. Physicians figured out that Upjohn's synthetic progestin, Provera®, would control the bleeding problems. Wyeth-Ayerst added this synthetic progestin, medroxyprogesterone acetate (MPA), to its best-selling

Premarin® and marketed the combination as Prempro®, which became one of the most prescribed medications of the 1980s, 1990s, and into the first part of the 21st century. There were 67.2 million[2] prescriptions filled for Premarin®/ Prempro® in peak years in the United States.[2]

Concerns were raised by Barbara Seaman, however, in her book entitled *Women and the Crisis in Sex Hormones*,[3] written just 10 years after Wilson's. She questioned whether the increase in these synthetic estrogens could cause breast cancer, strokes, and blood clots. Conflicting studies pitted the epidemiologists who showed that premature and surgical menopause increased the incidence of heart disease, strokes, and Alzheimer's in women against the naturalists who showed that Prempro® caused an increase in strokes, heart disease, breast cancer, and deep-vein thrombophlebitis.

COULD THEY BOTH BE CORRECT?

Both performed laudable scientific studies. To understand each side's position, the following reviews first the scientific studies of women who went through a premature or surgical menopause and the complications and hormonal difficulties that they had in their lives. Secondly, the material will present the statistics from both arms of the Women's Health Initiative (WHI) and the results this study has had on the practice of medicine in the United States. To this, Dr. Lichten's adds his knowledge and experience of treating 150,000 women patients' visits over 35 years in private gynecologic practice.

Personal Perspective

Kelly D. was 28 years old when she was first seen for hot flashes, irritability, insomnia, and a lack of sex drive. She had seen a number of other physicians who prescribed tranquilizers, sleeping medication, and antianxiolytic-like drugs. Kelly D. refused to take these medications, as they further "zoned" her out, and she was unable to function at her job in a meaningful manner.

After listening to Kelly D., Dr. Lichten drew the Appendix-listed laboratory profiles to measure the six basic endocrine systems. To his surprise, Kelly had evidence of a full-blown nonsurgically induced menopause: high FSH and LH signaling that the pituitary wanted more ovarian hormones and an estradiol level less than 35 pg/ml, showing that there would be no more estrogen released, no more eggs for pregnancy and no more progesterone production, ever. To be sure, Dr. Lichten repeated the laboratory tests again, two weeks later. They were consistent. Kelly D. had premature menopause at the age 28.

Kelly D. understood that she would never have a child of her own, but, being unmarried, her immediate concern was being able to function. Dr. Lichten discussed various hormonal regimens, and she tried oral estradiol, the estradiol patch, oral natural progesterone, and injections of testosterone. Finding fault with each of these delivery systems, she was last offered the estradiol pellets and the FDA-approved testosterone pellets. This worked best: no complaints of ups-and-downs mood swings, no complaints of insomnia, good libido and an absence of depression. As Kelly turned 40 this year, she reports a level of comfort with the pellet program because it offers stability to her life.

And although a woman who experiences premature menopause should be fearful of osteoporosis, Kelly's osteoporosis screen shows that her bone density is that expected of a 25-year-old woman.

Katrin F. came to Dr. Lichten on referral from her mother-in-law. She had been raised in Europe, had borne two children, and was so lethargic and physically ill that the family had opted for a full evaluation in Minnesota. However, five days of testing and tens of thousands of dollars later, no answer was forthcoming. Placed on antidepressants and antianxiolytics for sleep, Karin F. was no better than before.

Katrin F. appeared as a pale, thin Caucasian female. Securing a detailed history was difficult due to her European upbringing. She was trained not to complain, and she did not. She allowed Dr. Lichten to draw the obligatory endocrine battery of laboratory tests, receive an intravenous vitamin and mineral infusion, and planned to return to the office in five days to discuss the laboratory findings.

Katrin F. at 42 had stopped menstruation three months previously. She had a history of irregular menses for the previous two years. The laboratory tests showed that she was experiencing premature menopause at age 42. And, to be sure, Dr. Lichten redrew the FSH, LH, estradiol, progesterone, and prolactin two weeks after the initial blood draw. With the results confirmed, he approached the subject of hormonal replacement.

Dr. Lichten discussed the role hormones had in life, energy, sleep, and happiness (including depression and sex drive). She confided she had none and didn't feel much emotion and was just trying to get through the day and take care of her children and husband. While replacing her minerals and deficient magnesium with weekly IVs, Dr. Lichten started Katrin F. on a small dose of Depo-Estradiol®, 2.5 mg, with 25 mg of testosterone intramuscularly. She felt better, but the injection wore off on the fourth day. So he repeated the injections, increasing the dosage gradually and extending the time between injections to seven days. After one month, the laboratory tests were repeated: The FSH and LH were appropriately low, the estradiol level was over 150 pg/ml, and the testosterone was now over 200 ng/dl. Her libido and take-charge personality had blossomed, so the bio-identical testosterone topical cream was substituted for the injections.

Prescription estradiol patches were substituted for the estradiol injections. Bio-identical progesterone was prescribed to modulate the obligatory menstrual cycle. The progesterone caused uncomfortable nausea and crampy, menstrual periods. After rechecking blood values, the patient elected to try the estradiol and testosterone pellets. The pellets solved the problem and allowed Katrin F. to live a completely normal life, with only a rare, light menstruation.

Now Katrin F. was concerned over the Women's Health Initiative and all the bad press and negativity voiced about estrogens. Dr. Lichten explained to her, as appears in greater detail at the end of this chapter, that certain estrogens are a necessary part of every woman's life. A woman needs estradiol her whole life, and without this life-giving hormone, her body and mind will, metaphorically, wither and crumble. And what good is your body if your mind is gone from Alzheimer's disease, your bones crumble from osteoporosis, and your heart and body are too weak to go on?

Needless to say, Katrin now demands to have her estradiol and testosterone replacement.

UNDERSTANDING THE BIOLOGY OF MENOPAUSE

In the 10 years before the complete cessation of menstruation and reproduction, there are profound hormonal issues affecting the maturing woman. From 35 to 50 years of age she will lose a good portion of her other active hormones: thyroid (triiodothyronine), DHEA, hGH, as well as her sex hormones. After becoming less fertile in her late 30s or early 40s, the amount of progesterone hormone produced may drop by 80%. This drop in native progesterone hormone leaves unopposed estrogen to trigger more bouts of PMS and uterine bleeding. Then the estrogen levels drop from ages 40 to 50 by one-third initially, and then by 80% at menopause. The drop in testosterone levels at this time reaches below 50% of her baseline. This disrupts not only the interrelated sex hormones but also every aspect of the hypothalamic-pituitary-adrenal HPA axis.[4] That is why every hormone is in disarray.

The estrogenic hormone that is key to a reproductive woman is estradiol-E2. Produced by the ovary, its fluctuating harmonics with the pituitary hormones of follicle stimulating hormone (FSH) and luteinizing hormone (LH) is the key to triggering ovulation and the continuation of the human species. The estrogenic hormone of menopause is estrone-E1. This is produced from the breakdown of DHEA from the adrenal. The primary estrogenic hormone of pregnancy is estriol-E3. Each hormone is uniquely different and applicable to different times in a woman's life cycle.

These profound changes of shifting from a predominantly estradiol-E2 estrogenic hormone to estrone-E1 affect every aspect of the woman's being. Although there are more than 150 menopausal symptoms, key symptoms noted are hot flashes, insomnia, cardiovascular disease, strokes, and dementia. Osteoporosis and muscle atrophy are discussed in a separate chapter.

THE BENEFICIAL EFFECTS OF
ESTROGEN SUPPLEMENTATION

The beneficial effects of estrogen are reviewed in the next group of scientific studies. These studies confirm that estrogen replacement therapy (ERT) offers statistically significant improvement for certain medical conditions. As the North American Menopause Society (NAMS) reiterates in its position statement:[5]

"The benefits of hormone therapy outweigh its risks in healthy peri-menopausal and early postmenopausal women with menopause-related symptoms and a low baseline risk of stroke."

HOT FLASHES: Hot flashes are caused by spikes of pituitary LH released in response to the low levels of estrogen, progesterone, and testosterone The hot flush is associated with a change in skin conductivity as well as an increase in surface temperature that may exceed 10 degrees Centigrade.[6] Major disruptions of sleep are confirmed in 80% of menopausal women with severe menopausal/ hot flashes symptoms.[7] The worst symptoms occur with surgical versus natural menopause. It is undoubtedly argued that sleep quality is an important determinant of health status and the quality of life for women during and beyond menopause.[8] These vasomotor flushes and the concurrent insomnia are associated with five to 15 years of forgetfulness, insomnia, depression, and loss of sex drive. Better resolution of these symptoms are seen when both estrogen and testosterone were prescribed together.[9]

CARDIOVASCULAR SYMPTOMS: Although women have their first heart attack at least ten years later than their male companions, heart disease remains the leading cause of death in women.[10] In women who had premature removal of their uterus and ovaries, those who were treated with "add-back" ERT had 50% fewer fatal heart attacks versus the nonintervention group over the ensuing 10 years.[11] In a large study of women with confirmed coronary artery disease, ERT was associated with a lower mortality.[12]

Women whose heart catheterization showed major coronary disease and were taking add-back ERT recorded a 3% mortality against a 40% mortality in the non-ERT group in a 10-year follow-up.[12]

In the large Finnish study of 53,000 person-years, in which more than 7,944 women followed for an average of seven years, the absolute risk for an acute myocardial infarction (MI) was 50% lower is those who were present ERT users.[13]

STROKES: In the same Finnish study, the cardiovascular risk of strokes was similarly less in ERT users. Risk basis for death from other coronary artery disease was 1.0 for non-ERT users and 0 for ERT users. Death from stroke was 1.2 for non-ERT users versus 0.15 for current ERT users. And absolute risk for sudden cardiac death was 1.6 in never users, 1.0 in former users, and 0 in current users ($p<0.001$).[13] Since most initial strokes are nonfatal, the difference in degree of severity would allow seniors to remain self-sufficient at home versus being confined in an assisted-care facility.

ALZHEIMER'S DISEASE: In clinical studies of early Alzheimer's patients, the first memory loss is that of smell and visual stimulation. ERT was able to improve memory function for these testing parameters.[14] Based on numerous studies, long-term ERT may eliminate or prevent development of Alzheimer's in up to 60% of women patients. [15]

OSTEOPOROSIS: Chapter 9 is devoted to reviewing osteoporosis, a preventable disease associated with a high percentage of hip fractures and, thereafter, an expected 20% mortality within one year.[16] In Dr. Lichten's practice, the premenopausal and menopausal hormonal-replacement protocols incorporate the estradiol and testosterone pellets placed subcutaneously. They remain the mainstay of treatment, not only because of their outstanding results seen in studies in England, Europe, and Australia, but also because of the vast positive experiences documented in Dr. Lichten's office practice.

REDUCED CANCER RISK: This applies to uterine, ovarian, and colon cancer. In the WHI it was expected that there would be a reduced risk of uterine cancer, as medroxyprogesterone acetate (MPA) is used to reverse endometrial thickening hyperplasia and early uterine cancer. Similarly, studies have linked use of hormonal suppressants like MPA to a reduction in angiogenesis to a reduction in ovarian cancer in animals.[17] The observation of a reduction in the incidence of colon cancer[18] and diabetes in menopausal women on estrogen was to many a surprise.

REDUCED DIABETES RISK: "Women who are considering the risks and benefits of hormone therapy should be informed of the link between hormones and a decreased risk of diabetes, especially if they are at risk for the disorder"—this according to Dr. Wulf Utian, executive director of the North American Menopause Society in Cleveland.[19]

Personal Perspective: Alzheimer's Disease

One of Dr. Lichten's patients asked him to see her mother who had experienced extensive mental deterioration due to Alzheimer's disease. She had not spoken in one year and was mostly wheelchair-bound. As a favor to the patient who obviously dearly loved her mother, Dr. Lichten saw this elderly and frail woman. Not able to take much of a history, Dr. Lichten drew the laboratory tests and pieced together what information he could from the family.

Dr. Lichten offered the family the treatment program used to boost the natural healing powers of the body: IV mineral-vitamin nutrition; oral supplements; larger doses of estrogen, testosterone, and DHEA; small doses of bio-identical thyroid; and the right form of liquid vitamin D. In this case, the elderly woman had extremely low insulin-like growth factor (IGF-1). When the symptoms are severe and the IGF-1 levels extremely low, there may be an opportunity to prescribe hGH for three to six months. The family persisted and privately funded the purchase of low-dose prescription hGH.

After a series of treatments twice weekly for six weeks, the patient turned to Dr. Lichten on this one spring day, looked him right in the eye, and said, "The flowers are beautiful today." The daughter and Dr. Lichten looked again, amazed. "What did you say, mother?" Dr. Lichten's patient asked. And she answered again, "The flowers are beautiful today, don't you think?" And they all agreed that it was a beautiful day.

After another visit at which the mother turned to Dr. Lichten to say "Thank you," the initial successes were lost forever as she reverted into being noncommunicative. But the daughter, seeing his consternation, told him that she had been given an unbelievable gift: the chance to talk with her mother "one more time."

It is Dr. Lichten's opinion that Alzheimer's disease and osteoporosis are preventable. When we realize that women are giving up so much of their quality life to this unnecessary ERT fear, it makes him so angry. Yes, women do die of breast cancer, but is it estrogen that causes it? The literature has many questions. And if it is estrogen, is it the kind the body produces or the synthetic estrogens in our livestock, our drinking water, and our plastics that has triggered the breast cancer epidemic? Dr. Lichten feels that a normally balanced endocrine system with appropriate upper-normal ranges of bio-identical, thyroid, DHEA, estradiol, progesterone, and testosterone offers women the best chance for a long and healthy life.

POINT AND COUNTERPOINT: THE WHI AND THE PROBLEM WITH THE WHI

The Women's Health Initiative consisted of two parts, called arms. The first arm of the WHI treated women who were 20 years postmenopausal with Prempro®, combination Premarin® and Provera®. Prempro® had shown a strong increase in breast cancer, stroke, and cardiovascular complications.[20] The second arm consisted of Premarin® alone. This part of the WHI study of 10,739 women was stopped prematurely because the Premarin®-only arm experienced an increased risk of ischemic stoke[21] and failed to show the cardiovascular benefits expected. The release of the second part of the WHI offered very confusing results. Where the first part of the WHI using Prempro® had shown very significant increases in breast cancer, especially in thin women, not one but three separate analyses of the WHI part-two data showed that the estrogen-only arm had a 23–33% *decrease* in breast cancer as compared to controls. [22] If estrogen was the cause of the scare over breast cancer, then why was the part two Premarin®-only data showing up to 33% less breast cancer?

COUNTERPOINT:
THE PROBLEM WITH THE WHI

Prior to the Women's Health Initiative, a number of studies had found that ERT intervention with Premarin® or Prempro® had a number of encouraging and discouraging outcomes.

MPA-Provera® is not a natural substance, not a bio-identical progesterone, but a derivative from petroleum. It is called a progestin, which means it looks and acts in the body sort of like progesterone. Since MPA-Provera® suppressed the bleeding from the uterus even better than natural progesterone, most doctors would prescribe this synthetic agent to prevent heavy menstrual bleeding in postmenopausal women. It works wonderfully. It can be used to stop postmenopausal breakthrough bleeding and even reverse early cases of endometrial cancer. Dr. Lichten uses MPA when he needs to, for short-term metromenorrhagia control. MPA is a recognized carcinogen, banned in most countries as a contraceptive since the 1960s. Recently, the European Union banned MPA from food entering their countries.[23] The advisory panel requested in 1985 that Depo-Provera® not be approved as a contraceptive[24] in the United States. The literature reports that Upjohn secured approval of the Dutch government for Depo-Provera® and continues to bring Depo-Provera® back into this country where it is used for that very same purpose.

Other than the misguided and billion-dollar expense of the Women's Health Initiative, there have been a number of studies that looked at the complications and cancer potentials of synthetic estrogens and progestins.[13, 25-30] The major flaw of the WHI was to select women that were on average almost 20 years older than comparable studies of women in menopause and many of whom might already have subclinical coronary artery atherosclerosis before starting hormone therapy. This only amplified the risk factors while negating any beneficial effects that could be realized when ERT is started appropriately at menopause.

NEGATIVE EFFECTS OF PREMPRO®
MENOPAUSAL REPLACEMENT

Gambrell,[31] one of the United States' leading gynecologists, stated recently: "There are no new data in the Women's Health Initiative. The Collaborative Study of Hormone Factors in breast cancer showed a non-significant increased risk after 5 years. H.E.R.S. showed an increased risk of cardiovascular disease in hormone therapy (HT) users with previous heart disease. The Cache County study indicated that estrogen therapy initiated after age 60 increased the incidence of Alzheimer's disease.[32] The daily synthetic progestin in the hormone therapy group decreased the estrogen receptors in the coronary arteries and minimized the beneficial direct effect of estrogen. It also decreased progesterone receptors in the endometrium, thus making it less endometrial-protective.

"The WHI was contrary to previous studies of estrogen therapy because women with specific menopausal symptoms were excluded, were older, had never used estrogen and had long-term estrogen deficiency. It takes healthy tissue to allow an effective response to estrogen and maintenance of health. Maximal benefit of HT may require early onset of treatment, near the time of menopause. However, it is never too late to arrest the progression of osteoporosis and decrease the risk of fracture." [31]

The confirmed risk of menopausal estrogen replacement is the development of uterine bleeding, abnormal thickening, and uterine endometrial (lining) carcinoma. Every gynecologist recognizes the need to perform a diagnostic test (D&C) on any woman with abnormal uterine bleeding after menopause and especially those on ERT.

This endometrial cancer is one of the least risky of all cancers. Although its incidence may be tenfold higher in women on ERT, it should not be a cause of death. MPA for periods of time of three to six months may completely reverse the cancer. Hysterectomy will remove the cancer. For those women who are subject to heavy menstrual bleeding before entering the menopause, endometrial ablation by resectoscope has eliminated the development of cancer in almost every single case. With no viable endometrial lining tissue, endometrial cancer is a remote possibility.

Having now explained that the major cancer scare from ERT is uterine cancer and that the risk is minimal, the focus of continuing concern of the WHI was the development of breast cancer and cardiovascular risks.

The second part of the WHI, limited to Premarin® only, showed a slight decrease in breast cancer. Without MPA, the risks dropped in paired groups from as much as a 26-fold increase to a 33% decrease below controls. As comparable large studies form Europe showed,[30] there is a negligible risk of breast cancer and a small increase in thromboembolic events like blood clots, but the numbers are relatively small. Despite these contradictory findings from this huge European study done under the auspices of the German government, it was the Women's Health Initiative that got everyone inappropriately scared.

It is recognized that since the WHI scare, up to two-thirds of women have discontinued estrogen replacement therapy, even stopping the minimal use of topical estrogen vaginal creams. Concurrently with this, prescriptions for insomnia, stress, depression, weight gain, and irritability have skyrocketed.

But giving credence to the increased risk of synthetic hormones and morbidity, Dr. Lichten recognizes that hidden in the medical literature exists a form of treatment that offers a better and safer way. But it is not a focus of the major pharmaceutical companies or the medical research centers. Perhaps it is because the treatment is generic and there are no patents on natural or bio-identical hormones. The answer to ERT may very well be subcutaneous natural estradiol and testosterone pellets.

THE BRITISH STUDY: HOGWASH TO THE WHI

Dr. Kurt Barnhart and his associates at the University of Pennsylvania presented to the Society for Gynecologic Investigation in 2007 the records of the women in the United Kingdom General Practice Research Database (GPRD), including 13,658 women aged 55–79 taking estrogen/progestin hormone therapy against 20,654 younger women on ERT and 30,102 controls aged 50–55. In Europe, the patients took 0.625 mg daily of conjugated estrogen and 150 mcg of norgestrel (not MPA-Provera®, as in the WHI study). A similar drug in the United States is available, called norethindrone, sold under the brand name Aygestin®. Not only was the hazard ratio for myocardial infarction insignificantly different from the younger women's but also death from all causes was significantly lower in the older subjects taking ERT than controls. The statistical significance was a hazard ratio of 0.75 versus 1.0. (meaning 25% lower mortality). As clearly stated by Barnhart: "You could have a stroke or have breast cancer or you could be protected from colorectal cancer, but really it matters what happened to you, and it looked like there was a lower death rate. I don't know why." [32]

To Dr. Lichten, the answer is obvious: The WHI used Wyeth-Ayerst's brand of synthetic progestin, medroxyprogesterone acetate (MPA), Provera®, a known carcinogen. The British used Aygestin® (norethindrone), which is used in oral contraceptives and taken by millions of women every day. Aygestin® is available in the United States from Duramed pharmaceuticals. It is almost twice as expensive as Provera®. Based on the Barnhart study, changing the ERT from Prempro® to conjugated estrogen and norethindrone would reduce risks significantly, albeit at a justifiable increased cost.

THE MEDICAL BENEFITS UNREALIZED

As stated by Wolf Utian, M.D.,[33] president of the North American Menopausal Association in 1994, the fact is that less than 15% of women who qualify for estrogen replacement therapy (ERT) take estrogen/ Premarin®. This was before the WHI scare. In Dr. Lichten's practice, he too found 30 years ago that only a third or less of women would tolerate Premarin® for extended periods of time. Most would take another form that consisted of bio-identical estradiol in a patch, cream, gel, or pellet.

Even though thousands of women receive prescriptions for estrogens, many thousands also fail to realize the benefits. Statistically, up to half of all women discontinue the medication within six months or fail to fill the prescription at all. These same women took oral contraceptives in their 30s and 40s without complaint, however. While they understood the benefit of oral contraceptives, for some reason they do not understand the benefits of estrogen replacement. Unless they had experienced the rare side effects of oral contraceptives, they should have no qualms about adding ERT into their menopausal lives. Remember again that oral contraceptives use norethindrone and its derivates, not medroxyprogesterone acetate (Provera®).

BREAST CANCER: IS THE SCARE REAL?

Consensus: When analyzing the WHI study in the Premarin®-only protocol, the risk of breast cancer is less in the Prempro®-only group.[34] Again, the synthetic progestin MPA-Provera® may be the only logical answer for the increased risk of breast cancer.

It is not that women forgot the benefits of oral contraceptives and estrogen; rather, they become obsessed with the fear of breast cancer. Breast cancer strikes one in eight women in their lifetime — almost all over 50. And the fear of cancer is the primary inhibition women have to taking supplementary estrogen.

In the last 35 years, more than 40 epidemiological studies have been performed to gather information about the risks of taking estrogen and developing breast cancer. Most studies show either no increased risk or slight increase with prolonged estrogen use. And to the physician, this information is both comforting and reassuring that prescribing estrogen is in the best interest of our female patients. But relating our security with estrogen replacement to our patients is not enough.

Dr. Lichten explains to his patients that even if estrogen would ever so slightly increase the risk of cancer, very few women would have their lives shortened by that disease. The net gain, however, from using estrogen to prevent cardiovascular disease, stroke, osteoporosis, and senility add so much more quality life years. Why not take advantage of living longer and living better — with estrogen?

SUMMARY OF RISKS AND SIDE EFFECTS OF ESTROGEN USE

1. Breast Cancer: Yearly mammograms, self-examination. Early diagnosis limits the risks. ERT may be prescribed for women free from breast cancer for five years.
2. Adenocarcinoma of the Uterus: Rarely aggressive lesions. Discovered by breakthrough bleeding or uterine thickening on ultrasound. Reversible often, with short-term progestin therapy.
3. Resumption of menses can be adjusted by changing ratio of bio-identical ERT and bio-identical progesterone (not Provera®).

THE ALTERNATIVE FORMS OF ESTROGEN

In the United States, most women associate estrogen with the Premarin® oral pill. But there are five forms of bio-identical estradiol that offer alternatives that are often better tolerated than Premarin®.

1. **VAGINAL ESTRADIOL CREAM:** It can deliver the lowest levels of systemic estradiol. By using 1/2 to 2 grams daily, the vaginal and bladder symptoms are relieved, with small amounts being absorbed. The estrogen level is usually measurable well below half the level of an average 40-year-old woman.

2. **PATCH:** Women who want to take a bio-identical estrogen preparation may start with natural estradiol (E2) in the transdermal patch. Clinical studies show a relief of vasomotor symptoms and a continuation rate of 88% with the matrix patch.[35]

3. **GEL:** Other patients may elect to use a *natural* estrogen body cream. Once only available through compounding pharmacies, Estrasorb® is now available by prescription. As the predominant estrogen is estradiol, it is absorbed with once-a-day applications to the skin. It may be reasonably effective at blocking hot flashes, especially when used with natural, bio-identical progesterone capsules of Prometrium® or bio-identical, compounded progesterone cream (4%) applied nightly. Continuation rate is much below that of the estradiol patch.

4. **PELLETS:** An old technique from the 1950s and 1960s is returning into use. This technique places compressed pellets of natural estrogen under the skin of the hip via a minor office procedure. In exchange for the two minutes it takes the physician to place these pellets, most women can remain hormonally stable for one to three months. This therapy is ideal for women who suffer with migraine headaches, mood swings, or breast tenderness that occurs when hormonal levels spike and drop. Estradiol pellets are not FDA-approved and are available only to physicians from compounding pharmacies. The pellets often are the ideal treatment modality for women when patch and capsule are not tolerated.

5. **ORAL CAPSULES:** Lastly, oral ingestion of any estrogen causes a rapid peak that lasts for about four hours and then a long period with relatively little or no estrogen. This is not natural and contributes to the symptoms associated with both too much and too little estrogen. Therefore, oral estradiol can be used but not in individuals for whom the estrogen fluctuation increases mood swings, headaches, or physical symptoms.

PARENTERAL ESTROGEN: WHY IT IS BETTER

Parenteral means that the delivery system is not oral. Parenteral includes transdermal patches, skin creams, vaginal creams, injections and pellet delivery systems. In every case, the first pass of the hormone is through the tissues of the body, not the liver. Oral hormones have detrimental effects on the liver, including increased risk of liver tumors.[36] Of all the different parenteral delivery systems, the pellets keep the hormone levels the most stable for months; the injections peak in 3–4 days and dissipate over 14 days, the patches keep hormones low for 3–7 days, and the topical gels or creams have an initial high level followed by a low level for 8–12 hours. The creams really need to be reapplied every 12 hours.

Fifty years ago, wealthy European women came to see Dr. Robert Greenblatt at the Medical College of Georgia to have long-acting estradiol and testosterone pellets placed every six months. Based on information gleaned from his publications and his colleagues, Dr. Lichten had three-month compounded estradiol and testosterone pellets manufactured to his specifications. These are the same pellets Dr. Lichten has used for more than 20 years.

In Conclusion

The failure of women to take estrogen is a combination of a fear of estrogen and negative experiences with oral estrogen. By trying either the transdermal estrogen patch or the natural estrogen gels or pellets, many more women will discover the beneficial effects of this hormone. With estrogen and the supplementation of all the bio-identical, anabolic hormones, which may be the keys of "antiaging" medicine, hopefully women will live a longer and better life!

THE MISSING BREAST CANCER LINK: IS IT ESTROGEN OR A MINERAL DEFICIENCY?

Linus Pauling, one of the greatest medical minds of the 20th century, alleged stated more than 50 years ago that "you can trace every sickness, every disease, and every ailment to a mineral deficiency." [37]

Though the Linus Pauling Institute denies this was Pauling's position statement, new evidence raises the question whether the statement might be true for breast cancer. More than 30 years ago, Stabel[38] in *The Lancet* restated the observation of John Myers[38] (1933) that geographic differences in iodine intake dramatically influence the risk of breast and other cancers. In countries that take in seaweed as a major staple of their diet, there is less than one-quarter the incidence of breast,[40] thyroid, and prostate cancer. [39] Guy Abraham,[41] through loading tests, determined that the minimum intake of iodine and iodide should be greater than 10,000 mcg per day. Current recommendation on daily iodine requirement of 150 mcg is so low that virtually 100% of Americans are low in iodine and, therefore, at increased risk for breast, thyroid, and prostate cancer.

SERMS: SELECTIVE ESTROGEN RECEPTOR MODULATORS

Once the information from the WHI Premarin®-only study demonstrated that Premarin®—conjugated equine estrogen— decreased the risk of breast cancer, decreased the risk of colon cancer, and decreased the risk of diabetes, why would women accept having their estrogen[21] taken away, only to give hot flashes, Alzheimer's disease, osteoporosis, and heart disease a head start?

Since it is established that the progestin is the major contributing factor to the deep-vein thrombophlebitis, the breast cancer increase, and the cardiovascular disease, why is the product still the most-prescribed ERT today?

Into this artificial confusion over the dangers of ERT comes a host of expensive new products called SERMS—Selective Estrogen Receptor Modulators. Tamoxifen®, the first SERM is used to block estrogen receptors for individuals with breast cancer. As SERMS act differently, the benefits must be considered separately:

Tamoxifen® (generic for Novadex®)—blocks receptors in breast; stimulates receptors in the liver, lowering cholesterol; stimulates receptors in bone in treatment of osteoporosis; stimulates lining of uterus; and may lead to bleeding or thickening. Because it is such a weak estrogen, it is acting more as an antiestrogen.

Raloxifene® (generic for Evista®)—is prescribed for osteoporosis. In the RUTH Trial, Raloxifene®, like Tamoxifen®, has the ability to improve blood cholesterol levels by lowering low-density lipoprotein (LDL) cholesterol (bad cholesterol) and increasing high-density lipoprotein (HDL) cholesterol (good cholesterol). For this reason, researchers wanted to test whether it could reduce women's heart problems. The results of the RUTH Trial were released in July 2006[42] and showed that after more than five years of follow-up, no real improvement in heart problems was noted. The subsequent study of Raloxifene® by Barrett-Connor showed a 49% increase in fatal stroke.[43]

Emphatically understand that SERMs may offer much less benefit to the menopausal woman than a bio-identical estradiol or even Premarin®, yet at a high financial cost and potential risk.

Unless dealing with a breast cancer or cancer *in situ* and recommended by the oncologist, Dr. Lichten does not routinely use SERMs in medical practice.

The problem with all standard estradiol products is that they may not realize an adequate serum estradiol level to relieve the hot flashes, stabilize bone loss, or prevent migraine. Consistent data in the literature shows that the threshold for the hot flush is below 60 pg/mL; osteoporosis 70 pg/mL; and to prevent migraine might be as high as 100 pg/mL. The estradiol 0.1 mg patch may bring serum estradiol levels from 70 to approximately 100 pg/mL. But absorption varies from individual to individual, which affects serum hormone level.

If the standard product does not deliver adequate blood levels, the physician may have to increase the strength of the product or have the patient use twice the dosage. Because of the scare from the WHI and the general fear of estrogen and steroids, women are being denied adequate estrogen to protect their bodies from the ravages of disease: heart disease, osteoporosis, Alzheimer's, and insomnia, let alone hot flashes. As demonstrated in the future chapter on testosterone, adequate dosages are not the absolute number that appears on the laboratory report but the bio-available number that is calculated based on the ratio of total hormone to binding globulin.

The second benefit of compounding creams is that the pharmacist can mix two or three products into one cream: estradiol, progesterone, and testosterone—and this may be cost-saving. But just as Dr. Lichten often uses the estradiol patch together with estradiol vaginal cream, he may prefer that progesterone be applied to the breast and the testosterone cream applied to the hair area of the *mons veneris* below the bikini line. Compounded creams and gels, especially those for men with testosterone, are one-fourth the price of commercial Androgel® and Testim® and equal or stronger in potency.

In conclusion, in reference to progesterone and testosterone for women, there may be fewer complications, fewer side effects, and lower costs when these products are compounded. As discussed previously, the compounding pharmacists should not hesitate to contact the national compounding pharmacy organization, the PCCA, about formulations, different bases, and new formulations. These pharmacists are specialists whom Dr. Lichten consults with regularly: whether to make up a skin lotion for a specific medical condition, to increase the strength of topical agents for nail fungus, or to find a better delivery system for topical ketoprofen for muscle pain or various testosterone compositions to avoid mild hirsutism and unwanted hair growth.

Estrogen, specifically estradiol, is the life-sustaining hormone of women. To modulate this hormone is the key to treating a litany of medical problems: menstrual bleeding, PMS, migraine, and menopause. To restrict, remove, and fail to replace this hormone is the equivalent of castration in the male; it is inflicting on her a potentially miserable and downhill slide until she dies.

Say yes to bio-identical estrogen—estradiol. For it is with estrogen that nature created woman in all her splendor!

Estrogen Preparations
Product generic dosage/ frequency quantity
Estrogen
Prempro® 1.25/10mg
Premarin® CEE 1.25 mg
Cenesta® 1.25 mg estradiol
Estrace® oral estradiol 1 mg
Vivelle patch 0.1 mg
Climara® 0.1 mg
injectable Depo-Estradiol® 5 mg/ cc/wk 5 cc
Estrace® vag 0.1 mg
Estrasorb® 4.35 mg

SERMs
Product generic dosage/ frequency quantity
Nolvadex® tamoxifen 20 mg
Evista® raloxifen 60 mg

Progestins and Progesterone
Product generic dosage/ frequency quantity
Progestin
Provera® medroxyprogesterone
medroxyprogesterone 10 mg
Aygestin® norethindrone 5 mg

Progesterone
Prometrium® 100 mg
Progest® 3% 20 mg/ pump
Pro Fem 2.5% two ounce jar

Testosterone preparations
Product generic dosage /frequency quantity
Estratest® E2+methyl testosterone 1.25 mg/2.5 mg
Oxandrin® oxandrolone 2.5mg
Depo-Testosterone® testosterone
Cypionate® 200 mg/mL per week

REFERENCES:

1. Wilson, Robert. Feminine Forever. New York: M. Evans, 1966. 19.
2. Available at: http://www.bloomberg.com/apps/ news?pid=20601087&sid=axHrXNeT_Pso&refer=home
3. Seaman B, Seaman G. *Women and the Crisis in Sex Hormones.* New York: Bantam, 1977.
4. DeLeo V, et al. Hypothalamo-pituitary-adrenal axis and adrenal function before and after ovariectomy in premenopausal women. *European Journal of Endocrinology.* 1998; 138(4): 430–5.
5. Utian W. NAMS Releases Updated Position Statement on HT. *OB-GYN News.* 2007; 42(4):1.
6. Ravnikar V, et al. Vasomotor flushes and the release of peripheral immunoreactive luteinizing hormone-releasing hormone in postmenopausal women. *Fertility & Sterility.* 1984; 41(6): 881–7.
7. Ohayon MM. Severe hot flashes are associated with chronic insomnia. *Archives Internal Med.* 2006; '66(12): 1262–8.
8. Landis CA, et al. Sleep and menopause. *Nursing Clinics of North America.* 2005; 39(1); 97–115.
9. Bachmann GA. Vasomotor or flushes in menopausal women. *American Journal of Obstetrics and Gynecology.* 1999; 180 (3 Pt 2): S312–6.
10. Available at: http://www.cdc.gov/women/lcod.htm
11. Samsioe G. Cardioprotection by estrogens: implications of observational studies. *Intl J Fert Menopausal Stud.* 1994 39 S1:20-7.
12. Sullivan JM, Vander Zwaag R, Hughes JP, et al. Estrogen replacement and coronary artery disease. Effect on survival in postmenopausal women. *Arch Intern Med.* 1990 Dec;150(12):2557-62.
13. Sourander L, Rajala T, Räihä I, et al. Cardiovascular and cancer morbidity and mortality and sudden cardiac death in postmenopausal women on oestrogen replacement therapy (ERT). *Lancet.* 1998 Dec 19-26;352(9145):1965-9.
14. Guthrie JR, Dennerstein L, Taffe JR, et al. The menopausal transition: a 9-year prospective population-based study. The Melbourne Women's Midlife Health Project. *Climacteric.* 2004 Dec;7(4):375–89.
15. Waters R. Estrogen to prevent Alzheimer's. *Health.* 1997 11:(1):1940–2.
16. Barclay L. Four-Item Score May Predict Hip Fracture, Mortality Risk in Elderly. *Women Annuals of Family Medicine.* 2007; 5:48–56. Available at: http://www.medscape.com/viewarticle/551685
17. Xie SZ, Wang J, Li DZ, Wang Y. Medroxyprogesterone acetate therapy against antiangiogenesis of transplanted ovarian cancer in nude mice. *Di Yi Jun Yi Da Xue Xue B.o.* 2004 Jul; 24(7):8213.
18. Hulley SB, Grady D. The WHI Estrogen-Alone Trial- Do Things Look Any Better? *JAMA.* 2004 Apr 14;291:1769-71.
19. Utian W. Women Should Know HT Is Tied to Lower Risk of Diabetes. *OB-GYN News.* 2007; 42(4):1
20. Chlebowski RT, Hendrix SL, Langer RD, et al. Influence of estrogen plus progestin on breast cancer and mammography in healthy postmenopausal women: the Women's Health Initiative Randomized Trial. *JAMA.* 2003 Jun 25;289(24):3243-53.
21. Hendrix S, Wassertheil-Smoller S, Johnson KC, et al. Effects of Conjugated Equine Estrogen on Stroke in the Women's Health Initiative. *Circulation.* 2006 May 23;113:2425-2434.
22. Stefanik ML, Anderson GL, Margolis KL, et al. Effects of Conjugated Equine Estrogens on Breast Cancer and Mammography Screening in Postmenopausal Women With Hysterectomy. *JAMA.* 2006 Apr 12; 295:1647-1657.

23. Available at; http://europa.eu/rapid/pressReleasesAction.do?reference=IP/02/1065& format=HTML&aged=0&language=EN&guiLanguage=en.
24. Public Board of Inquiry Advises That Depo-Provera Not be Approved for Use as Contraceptive in U.S. *Family Planning Perspectives*. 1985 Jan-Feb;17(1):38-39.
25. Persson I, Thurfjell E, Bergstrom R, et al. Hormone replacement therapy and the risk of breast cancer. Nested case-control study in a cohort of Swedish women attending mammography screening. *Int J Cancer*. 1997 Sep 4;72(5):758-61.
26. Persson I, Yuen J, Bergkvist L, et al. Cancer incidence and mortality in women receiving estrogen and estrogen-progestin replacement therapy--long-term follow-up of a Swedish cohort. *Int J Cancer*. 1996 Jul 29;67(3):327-32.
27. Palmer JR, Rosenberg L, Clarke EA, et al. Breast cancer risk after estrogen replacement therapy: results from the Toronto Breast Cancer Study. *Am J Epidemiol*. 1991 Dec 15;134(12):1386-95; discussion 1396-401.
28. Bergkvist L, Adami HO, Persson I, et al. The risk of breast cancer after estrogen and estrogen-progestin replacement. *N Engl J Med*. 1989 Aug 3;321(5):293-7.
29. Persson I, Adami HO, Bergkvist L, et al. Risk of endometrial cancer after treatment with oestrogens alone or in conjunction with progestogens: results of a prospective study. *BMJ*. 1989 Jan 21;298(6667):147-51.
30. Dinger JC, Heinemann LA, Möhner S, Thai do M, Assmann A, et al. Breast cancer risk associated with different HRT formulations: a register-based case-control study. *BMC Womens Health*. 2006 Sep 12;6:13.
31. Gambrell RD, Jr. The women's health initiative reports in perspective: facts or fallacies? *Climacteric*. 2004 Sep;7(3):225-8.
32. Zandi PP, Carlson MC, Plassman BL, et al; Cache County Memory Study Investigators. Hormone replacement therapy and incidence of Alzheimer disease in older women: the Cache County Study. *JAMA*. 2002 Nov 6;288(17):2123-9.
33. Utian W. NAMS. 1994.
34. Clark JH. A critique of Women's Health Initiative Studies (2002-2006).Nucl Recept Signal. 2006 Oct 30;4:e023.
35. Akhila V, Pratapkumar. A comparison of transdermal and oral HRT for menopausal symptom control. *Int J Fertil Womens Med*. 2006 Mar-Apr;51(2):64-9.
36. Giannitrapani L, Soresi M, La Spada E, et al. Sex hormones and risk of liver tumor. *Ann N Y Acad Sci*. 2006 Nov;1089:228-36. Review.
37. Available at: http://lpi.oregonstate.edu/
38. Stadel BV. Dietary iodine and risk of breast, endometrial, and ovarian cancer. *Lancet*. 1976 Apr 24;1;(7965):890-1.
39. Schultte KH, Myers JA. *Metabolic Aspects of Health*. 1933.
40. Aceves C, Anguiano B, Delgado G, et al. Is Iodine a gatekeeper of the integrity of the mammary gland? *J Mammary Gland Biol Neoplasia*. 2005 Apr;10(2):189–96.
41. Abraham G, Abraham GE. The safe and effective implementation of orthoiodo supplementation in medical practice. *The Original Internist*. 11:17-36, 2004. Available at: http://www.helpmythyroid.com/IOD50.htm.
42. Mosca L, Barrett-Connor E, Wenger NK, et al. Design and Methods of the Raloxifene Use for the Heart (RUTH) Study. *Am J Cardiol*. 2001 Aug 15;88(4):392-5.
43. Barrett-Connor E, Mosca L, Collins P, et al. Effects of Raloxifene on Cardiovascular Events and Breast Cancer in Postmenopausal Women. *N Eng J Med*. 2006 Jul 13;355:125-1376.

CHAPTER 7

MENSTRUAL PAIN, PMS, AND MOOD DISTURBANCES

As Dr. Lichten explains menstrual pain, PMS, and migraine, he speaks as a man writing this chapter for women. Dr. Lichten starts the discussion to an audience of both men and women. "Please understand that I am doing you a favor. As a male, it is difficult enough understanding how your body works. But as a gynecologist for now 35 years, I recognize that a woman's life is a million times more difficult. We know that if the human race left childbearing and childbirth up to men, humankind would have ended 5 million years ago. So, for the sake of our species, men, try to understand your partner in reproduction and that the changes she endures is a necessary part of every man's existence."

UNDERSTANDING THE MENSTRUAL CYCLE

A woman's menstrual cycle begins with her first day of menstrual (blood) flow.

This menstrual "period" is a result of a drop of two primary female hormones, estrogen and progesterone. Estrogen thickens the lining and gives a woman her womanly shape: breasts, hips, smooth skin. Progesterone's function is to mature the lining of the uterus, called the endometrium, after an egg has implanted. If pregnancy has not occurred, the withdrawal or drop in progesterone level results in menstruation. Therefore, this estrogen–progesterone cycle prepares the uterus (womb) for pregnancy every month.

The estrogen levels are low from day 1 to day 10 of a normal 28-day cycle. Due to stimulation from the pituitary (master gland), there is release of FSH (follicle stimulating hormone) and LH (luteinizing hormone). This causes a surge of estrogen from the ovary, occurring on days 10–13. This surge of estrogen triggers release of the developing egg (ovum) from the ovary. This occurs two weeks prior to the onset of menstruation; therefore, day 14 of a 28-day cycle. To laypeople, this is called "egg" day, as the 2–3 days before and this day are the best days to become pregnant.

Once the egg/ovum has been released, the ovarian cyst collapses and begins to manufacture progesterone. Progesterone has multiple effects:

1. Progesterone changes the mucus of the cervix preventing additional sperm from traveling into the uterine cavity.
2. Progesterone matures the lining of the uterus to prepare the lining for the fertilized ova (egg) to implant in the next four days.
3. Progesterone tones down the emotional irritability that may occur from the effect of unopposed estrogen on the female brain.

This roller-coaster hormonal cycle is visualized thus: Estrogen peaks day 11–13, drops at 14–16, then slowly increases to maximum on day 23 and slowly falls to day 28. In reference to progesterone, the levels are low until day 18, when it increases to its maximum on day 23 and slowly falls to day 28. So this is why a gynecologist will measure the progesterone level on days 23–25. If it is high, it is proof of ovulation.

"If only we men could understand our female partners' internal wiring," many a man has confided in me. Hormones' ups and downs, to a great degree, parallel women's *changes*. Understanding this roller-coaster pattern may make some changes in personality more predictable and more understandable to the spouse. And, for the doctor, understanding hormones make these changes more treatable.

MENSTRUAL PAIN AND ENDOMETRIOSIS

The medical term for menstrual pain is *dysmenorrhea*. This comes from the Greek: *dys* meaning painful, *men* referring to monthly, and *rrhea* meaning flow.

Dysmenorrhea refers to the cyclic pain that occurs in reproductive women in the days before and during the onset of menstruation. The pain can be so severe that many a young woman has had her appendix removed inadvertently. And, for young girls, still shocked by the monthly bleeding that has forced them into womanhood, the pain is often physically and emotionally unbearable.

Since Freud in the 1920s, women have born the stigma of being "hysterical," emotional, and of having somehow psychologically induced into women symptoms of menstrual pain, premenstrual distress, and migraine. Leading gynecologists like Meigs[1] in the 1940s showed that the menstrual pain would disappear when either the hormones of menstruation were modulated or surgical removal of the ovaries completed. Yet the extensive scientific works of past professors are completely ignored even today, and women are considered to have some genetic defect (the extra X chromosome) as the cause of an alleged psychological weakness.

Fortunately, pioneering work by Penny Budoff, M.D.,[2] documented in her book *No More Menstrual Pain and other Good News* in the 1980s, brought attention to this misunderstood and undiscussed malady. The treatment is now available at every corner drugstore in the form of ibuprofen. Taking up to 2,400 mg of ibuprofen for 4–5 days per month will relieve the pain for more than half of affected women—safe, simple, and readily available.

No girl should go through her teen years without it.

For some women, this treatment is not enough. The nausea, vomiting, and rocking on the toilet takes a tremendous toll. And, from one woman to another, there is a sense of disbelief and that the other is "faking it." Each woman has only her own self as a point of reference, yet to the gynecologist, the cause of all three maladies is the same: the hormonal fluctuation. And, in truth, all three symptom complexes are grouped under one medical term, *molimina*. Molimina means literally all the symptoms that occur at the end of the menstrual cycle. Laypeople call this pain with menstrual flow "menstrual cramps;" mood changes before menstruation "premenstrual syndrome;" and the migraine pain either before or during menses "menstrual migraine."

Since the 1960s, the birth control pill, properly called an oral contraceptive (OC), has been readily available. Since the OC introduces an artificial level of hormones, the OC pill, in fact, may be used to treat this menstrual pain disorder. And, as the dosage of estrogen has decreased by 80% from the first OC pills, the amount of bleeding and side effects has decreased accordingly.

So a young woman with menstrual pain and heavy menstrual flow can now have a very light or nonexistent menstruation. And even better are the newest OC pills, which allow for withdrawal menstrual bleeding only once every three months.[3]

There are still some women who cannot tolerate either ibuprofen or oral contraceptives—or they find that other over-the-counter products like Midol® and prescription medication for pain such as Toradol®, Stadol®, or Vicodin ES® are ineffective even for short-term use. Many of these women will be diagnosed as having a medical and or surgically treatable disease: endometriosis.

ENDOMETRIOSIS

Endometriosis is a medical condition in which the cells of the endometrial lining (normally inside the uterus/womb) grow outside the uterus, on the ovaries, the wall of the uterus, and/or the pelvic cavity. It has been shown that for some women, the uterus does not empty properly into the vagina and can back-flush the menstrual debris through the tubes to the abdominal cavity, where these cells may implant and grow. This endometriosis can be almost microscopic dustings of black, red, white, or yellow blebs, or thick, brown concrete encasements, destroying the woman's entire reproductive system. In a gynecologic practice, whether the patient is a 14-year-old African-American teen or a 55-year-old Caucasian grandmother, endometriosis is part of the differential diagnosis for unremitting, cyclic lower abdominal pain.

The diagnosis of endometriosis is made as part of an outpatient surgical procedure that introduces a laparoscope through the lower part of the umbilicus (navel) under anesthesia. With a diameter similar to that of a ballpoint pen, the instrument allows visualization, photographic documentation, and treatment of most cases of endometriosis. Since Dr. Lichten first connected a laser to the laparoscope in Michigan in 1982, thousands of gynecologists have been trained to use the laser to vaporize endometriosis, cut adhesions, and even remove and destroy affected tissue.

Personal Perspective

Dr. Lichten met Jody in his third year of private practice. She was at that time 23 years of age, intelligent, and articulate. His initial interaction was interrupted by her startling outburst of "I want a hysterectomy, now!" She explained that she had been treated by more than 25 physicians since the age of 14 for severe, unremitting menstrual cramps. Two laparoscopies failed to find anything, so they referred her to not one but three psychiatrists, four internists, neurologists, gastroenterologists, and she tried a variety of chiropractors, naturopaths, faith healers, and a shaman. To no avail: Every month she spent a full seven days on the cold floor in severe, white-knuckle pain. Nausea and vomiting would occur and she would miss work. Even Percodan® would only drug her. She had made this rational decision because "living like this is not living, period!"

Intrigued and empathetic, Dr. Lichten began a three-year journey to find her cure. First, Jody allowed Dr. Lichten to take a complete history, again, and to review all doctor's notes and procedures. Everything was negative, including the laparoscopy reports. So, being a young doctor with three years of private-practice experience, Dr. Lichten, 27 years ago, asked to repeat the laparoscopy. And when looking closely at the walls of the abdominal cavity, ovaries, and uterus, he also did not find any endometriosis.

So, still believing this was endometriosis, Dr. Lichten started the only drugs available in 1982, Danazol®[4] and then megesterol acetate.[5] Danazol® is an antiestrogen to suppress estrogen and endometriosis, while megesterol acetate is a synthetic progestin that also suppresses the estrogen and endometriosis by inhibiting release of FSH and LH. Both caused severe side effects for Jody: nausea, depression, and weight gain. They were quickly discontinued.

Jody's employer called again, as she was lying and crying on the floor, and so Dr. Lichten asked him to have her brought into the office. He had nothing left to offer, except . . . the concept that her pain was coming from cervical contractions and he could block that pain with lidocaine (Novacaine®) just like doctors do during labor. This is called a paracervical block, and in the 1970s and 1980s, every obstetrician-gynecologist was fully trained to perform this on laboring women.

Dr. Lichten explained to Jody what he was going to do. She understood that this same technique of anesthesia was used for pain relief during pregnancy, terminations, D&Cs, and labor. She agreed. Dr. Lichten warned her that the effects would wear off in 45–60 minutes, as happens when these anesthetic blocks are used for labor pain. She said 45 minutes would be "better than nothing."

The paracervical block caused Jody to almost pass-out. Cold and dehydrated, he had his office staff treat her with orange juice and cookies for 45 minutes. She did report that there was no pain. NO PAIN! And Jody went home to call Dr. Lichten one hour later.

In one hour, Dr. Lichten heard from an elated Jody. Still no more pain! And she felt like the weight of the world had been lifted from her shoulders. "Can you make this permanent?" she asked. And then a thought went through Dr. Lichten's mind, and he said, "Yes!"

Dr. Lichten had read that a doctor had taken biopsies of the uterosacral nerves through a laparoscope while looking for infection in the nerves to the cervix. If a biopsy could be performed, then a surgical destruction (cautery heat to charring) would be so easy. And bleeding would be minimal and easily controlled. So Dr. Lichten scheduled Jody for another outpatient laparoscopic surgery.

Again, he found no endometriosis. But in his planned surgery, Dr. Lichten took the cautery graspers and cauterized right against the cervix. This is the place surgeons put instruments when performing a hysterectomy. The procedure took very little time and Jody went back to the recovery room. Dr. Lichten did not know whether this would cause more pain, so he performed that same paracervical block before starting the surgical procedure.

Jody was elated. No pain day one. No pain after her next menstrual period. No pain reported when asked about the next and the next. The surgery had been a tremendous success, but for how long?

When last they spoke, Jody had been pain-free for 23 years.

THE PEER REVIEWED AND PUBLISHED LUNA STUDY

If surgery is performed for dysmenorrhea or for sexually active women with complaints of pain with deep penetration during intercourse, Dr. Lichten will perform a procedure he discovered/invented in 1982 for Jody. The procedure uses the laser or cautery to cut through two-thirds of the uterosacral ligaments. The uterosacral ligaments are the V-shaped support that connects the back of the uterus-cervix to the sacrum and contains most of the nerve supply to the lower uterus and cervix. Called LUNA, for laparoscopic uterine nerve ablation,[6] Dr. Lichten was honored by his colleagues and called a "LUNA-tic" because he insisted, rightly so, that menstrual pain was real. LUNA made pelvic pain treatable, and this was directly opposite to the common genre of rationalizing women's pain as some part of hysteria.

Historically, Dr. Lichten's chairman did not believe that any surgical operation other than hysterectomy would block the pain of menstruation, even though the work of Balweg[7] was nationally recognized for treating endometriosis. So he and the head of anesthesiology created an institutional review board (IRB) protocol. The double-blind controlled study would compare LUNA versus no LUNA in those patients with a pelvis free of disease and who were also free of psychological impairment. Although Dr. Lichten would perform the surgery, a psychiatrist would evaluate the women for pain before and after, and an associate gynecologist would see the patient postoperatively. Of 39 women volunteers, only 21 met the criteria; 15 would be excluded for having pelvic pathology and/or endometriosis, and three could not complete the psychological testing.

Eleven women had LUNA surgery, and nine had dramatic relief of pain initially, while six remained pain free-for six months. In the NO LUNA group, no one was pain-free at six months, proving that women with menstrual pain are not imagining their pain. As the chairman did not believe the results, he had his secretary call the patients to see if the data was correct. It was true, and Dr. Lichten published the study in the *Journal of Reproductive Medicine* in 1987. Subsequently, the effectiveness of LUNA was confirmed in 35 studies reproduced across the world. Except for one or two naysayers, gynecologic surgeons accept LUNA as a simple, safe, and cost-effective option to treat women with menstrual pain and endometriosis at the time of laparoscopy. It became the fifth-most-often-performed procedure in the 1990s for gynecologist laparoscopists.

In subsequent research, Dr. Lichten discovered that women with menstrual pain have a block or pseudo-obstruction to the egress of menstrual blood through the cervix. Their bodies act as if someone had put a cork "bottle stop" in the cervix, forcing the contractions to become up to four times stronger than necessary to deliver a baby! These intense contractions are the reason for the intense pain, retrograde menstruation, and the development of endometriosis. "Pelvic pain is real" is the undeniable scientific conclusion. And when medication fails, there is a simple doctor's-office paracervical block and thereafter outpatient surgical treatment for most of the afflicted.

"No More Pain and Other Good News" is today's news headline for menstrual-pain-suffering women. And, if one or two outpatient surgeries are not effective, then there exist three medications that can lower estrogen levels to control the disease. The prescription medications are Danazol®, Lupron®[9], and Synarel®. Danazol® costs approximately $300 a month for capsules, while the once-a-month Lupron® injection is almost $600.

In clinical studies, there is a definite cost benefit to Danazol®, which can be taken for many years, while Lupron®/Goserelin® is limited to six months and has a much higher discontinuation rate.[8] As the following examples will illustrate, Dr. Lichten will often try Danazol® for all problems related to molimina (that-time-of-month malady).

METROMENORRHAGIA:
HEAVY MENSTRUAL BLEEDING

Whereas endometriosis affects younger, childless women, there is a condition that affects predominantly older women with children. The medical term is *adenomyosis*, and it results in very heavy, cramping-type menstrual flow. Just as endometriosis may be medically or surgically treated, so can adenomyosis. The surgery is simply different.

The problem from aging and childbirth is that the uterus develops large varicose-like veins. These veins are not just outside the uterus but also in the uterine walls. The anatomic aspects find a soft, squishy uterus with a bluish tint on the surface. This is secondary to the veins and stasis of venous blood.

When the condition is found early, it will respond to low-dose Danazol®. When the condition is advanced, a drug of choice may be luprolide acetate if a higher dosage of Danazol® will not control the bleeding and pain.

But with the invention of an outpatient surgery by Goldrath[9] in 1980, 80% of hysterectomies for adenomyosis and metromenorrhagia can be avoided.

Goldrath was one of the first gynecologists to utilize a laser attached to an operating instrument. Goldrath had a special hysteroscope designed for him to look inside the uterus (*hyster* = uterus; *scope* = scope). When there were polyps in the uterine cavity, he attempted to burn their base and remove them. He developed a technique of using the YAG laser to pinpoint burn spots across the endometrial cavity. It took almost two hours, but most had minimal bleeding for years after.

Goldrath taught Dr. Lichten his technique in 1983. But Dr. Lichten's former chief resident at Ohio State had modified a urologic instrument used in resection of the excess prostate tissue through the urethra. This resectoscope worked very well and destroyed the entire lining in the uterus in an average of 20 minutes. This procedure enabled the removal of polyps and also large leiomyomata (fibroids).

Combining the knowledge of Goldrath and others, a retrospective study of Dr. Lichten's resectoscope patients brought the best results: a five-year follow-up showed less than 15% needed hysterectomy.

With newer techniques, a five-year follow-up in another surgeon's hands may be compatible.[10] In any case, a successful endometrial ablation precludes a hysterectomy. And the downside is the loss of one day in the best of surgical hands to give up, potentially, menstrual flow for life. And the key to performing the surgery was to suppress the endometrial lining completely. And Goldrath had used Danazol® first to suppress the endometrial lining of the uterine cavity.

PMS

Although one-third of American women have dysmenorrhea, there are millions of others whom suffer with other symptoms at that "time of month". Many have changes in their psychological and physical makeup: the medical term is *molimina*, the bad things that occur with menstrual flow. Laypeople call this complaint PMS. Women call this "Putting Up with Men's Stuff," rather than considering PMS as an imbalance of her endocrine system.

Historical Perspective

"Premenstrual distress" was first described by Franks[11] in 1931. He identified the four characteristics of this disorder as follows:

1. Anxiety and irritability
2. Depression
3. Food cravings
4. Fluid retention, bloating, and headache

However, in writings dating from the Golden Age of Greece more than 2,300 years ago, writers referred to the personality changes in their wives as the changing swells of the sea; calm some days and violent the next! Unrecognized until 1959[12] when a woman decided to solve her issues with her problem boyfriend by pinning him between her car and a lamppost, PMS is definitely a medical condition that demands our attention.

As Dr. Lichten started his third year in practice, he was accepted as the youngest member of a four-man group. As such, the low man on the totem pole is privileged to take care of all cases that are troublesome and time-consuming. That is why he was assigned to see the woman in the University Hospital lockdown. It seems she had attacked her husband and sent him to the hospital with a broken arm.

Trepidatious at the very least, Dr. Lichten was led to a secluded part of the hospital psychiatric wing. There he imagined, based on television shows, that there would be a guard or some Plexiglas separator between him and this dangerous felon. No, they said as they led the doctor through the door and locked it behind him. The chill of the guard's voice saying, "Call out if you need us" was not reassuring. So here stood Dr. Lichten surprised to see facing him a petite, youthful, blond-and-blue-eyed woman of 30, about five-foot-two and no more than 110 pounds.

She saw the fear in the doctor's face and smiled and said that he need not worry (as she started menstruating in the lockdown) and would he please sit down? Surprised, Dr. Lichten did so and asked her to tell her story.

It seems that in the few days before her menses, she has a dramatic Dr. Jekyl/Mr. Hyde transformation. Usually meek, happy, and pleasant, she turns seemingly overnight to a screaming, hateful shrew that was more prone to throwing objects than not. It just happened that her husband was not quick enough and she broke his arm. And he was six-foot-plus and 230 pounds. And she did it with only her bare hands!

Armed with the necessary information, and so grateful for her menstrual period, Dr. Lichten returned to the hospital to perform a literature search of this disorder. It soon came to his attention that Katrina Dalton[12] in England had written about treating the woman who killed her boyfriend during the PMS frenzy and had become docile as soon as her menses started. Dr. Lichten's case exactly, or so he thought. So the suggested treatment was bio-identical, natural suppositories of progesterone for three weeks out of every hormonal cycle.

Dr. Lichten explained to the woman in lockdown the next day that progesterone is naturally produced to counter the effects of estrogen in the second half of the menstrual cycle. Further searching showed that estrogen, when unopposed in rat studies, could actually cause seizures. So, before discharge, the young lady and Dr. Lichten discussed the use of progesterone suppositories, which were produced by the first compounding pharmacy in Michigan. And she did well.

The story would have been forgotten if Dr. Lichten had not gotten extensive local and national attention for his treatment for menstrual pain. Suddenly, he was not inundated with the 15- to 30-year-old no-children-yet women with dysmenorrhea, but 30- to 50-year-old women with pelvic discomfort and the extremes of moods of PMS. These patients were not surgical candidates, and if laparoscopy was performed, LUNA really didn't help.

The discovery of the treatment for PMS came by accident. One of the women who had come to Dr. Lichten with severe PMS, anxiety, depression, and food cravings also had severe menstrual cramping and extremely heavy menstrual flow. She refused a hysterectomy, which Dr. Lichten proposed, as most gynecologists are still trained to do. Instead of surgery, she requested and he agreed to prescribe for her Danazol® for the heavy menstrual bleeding and waited. And she came back one month later to state that not only had the heavy flow dwindled to almost nothing and that her PMS mood swings, the anxiety and depression, not to mention the salt cravings, had all magically disappeared!

Dr. Lichten proceeded to treat a large number of women with PMS successfully with low-dose Danazol® and other nutritional supports, feeling it was relatively easy. So, for the first and last time, there was a joint meeting of the hospital psychiatrists and gynecologists. Dr. Lichten presented the information on Danazol® as an alternative to standard psychiatric medication for PMS. It would have been a lonely fight if the literature and patient videotapes had not been available.

To educate the doctor even more was a pleasant, mid-thirties mother of two who became the key participant in a TV news story they ran on PMS. This quiet woman had chased her husband around the house brandishing a cleaver before starting therapy!

In the subsequent years, as Dr. Lichten was readying his

patients' data for publication, he would learn that separately two gynecologists, one Canadian and one Scottish[13-14] had found that Danazol® treated **PMS** effectively. Well done! So when Dr. Lichten's colleagues asked why he didn't use Prozac®, Paxil®, Elavil®, Desyrel®, Xanax®, Ativan®, and Klonopin® for these psychiatric disorders, he showed them the studies. When the pharmaceutical representatives showed him the numbers of monthly prescriptions from his colleagues, he could only shrug his shoulders. It seemed that both male and female gynecologists refused, unfortunately, to consider **PMS** as a hormonal disorder.

But, as word spread of a doctor who believed that menstrual pain and **PMS** were real, and that the doctor didn't believe in tranquilizers, antidepressants, and antianxiety medication for his women patients, the symptomatology associated with **PMS** became even more diverse. There are supposedly 150 symptoms associated with **PMS**, and the only common factor is that the symptoms occur in the week before and during the menstrual flow. Dr. Lichten believes he may have seen the worse when one woman presented with menstrual-related epilepsy and the next presented with a menstrual-related collapsed lung.

Ms. TD. was a tall, big-boned woman in her 40s who came to see Dr. Lichten to treat her **PMS**. Her complaint was quite extreme. She explained that "my right lung collapses with my menstrual period." And she had menstrual periods almost every month. When the collapsed lung occurred, she had to be taken to the emergency room and have a chest tube placed. This is not the thing anyone wants to do, and definitely not every month.

Dr. Lichten started the Danazol® therapy and waited. No menses, no lung problems. After six months, she asked him to explain. Dr. Lichten explained that there were fewer than 100 cases in the literature of endometriosis[15] invading through the diaphragm and being present in the lung parenchyma (lining). She told her that the surgeons at one time had operated and tried to send off tissue, but nothing had come of it. Dr. Lichten told her that was not his plan.

She approved a laparoscopy, and Dr. Lichten found endometriosis in the pelvic cavity and on the uterus. Nothing was seen near the liver edge or diaphragm, but close-up visualization often failed to show any "holes" to the lung. But Dr. Lichten had an answer, and that was endometriosis, which had caused severe cramping and bleeding. She hadn't mentioned these symptoms, as they were minimal compared to the collapsed lung. But it was devastating anyway. Before choosing hysterectomy, she stopped all medication against medical advice and experienced another collapsed-lung episode. Fortunately, hysterectomy and appropriate bio-identical hormone therapy were balanced to keep her estrogen levels low. This program worked well, and she had no more episodes of collapsed lung or related complaints over these last 15 years. The literature years later would point out that fully one-third of women with spontaneous pneumothorax or collapsed lung would have it on the right side, with endometriosis implants and the treatment, post-operatively would be hormonal suppression.[15]

When Denise initially consulted Dr. Lichten, she failed to tell him she had severe PMS and menstrual pain. The treatment he started was bio-identical progesterone, spironolactone, and nonsteroidal anti-inflammatory agents (NSAIDs). But after the first consultation, Dr. Lichten got a call from the emergency room that Denise had had a grand mal epileptic seizure.

When Dr. Lichten visited Denise, she was still postictal (post-seizure), i.e., dazed and confused from the seizure. From her husband Dr. Lichten learned that the seizures would occur suddenly, she would fall down, bite her tongue, and lose control of her urine. She would have no memory of what happened and would awaken with a severe headache. It would take 10 hours for her to be functional and 24 hours to recover enough to take care of the house and return to work. And Dr. Lichten learned that Denise's occurrences of seizures had occurred every month with every menstrual cycle for the previous three years.

Now, seizures are serious stuff, so Dr. Lichten insisted that she see a well-trained neurologist, who tried everything medically over the next three months—all to no avail. She continued to seize with the onset of every menstrual period.

So Denise and Dr. Lichten decided to treat her seizure as a PMS event. With most patients, Dr. Lichten's protocol is to start with 200, 300 or even 400 mg of Danazol® daily, but with Denise he started with 800 mg and then increased the dosage until the daily amount was 1,200 mg daily. Dr. Lichten acknowledged that this is 50% over the recommended dosage, but since the seizure posed so great a risk, it seemed prudent to try that dose, with the patient's permission, and then closely monitor liver enzymes. Liver enzymes can become elevated with high doses of many pharmaceutical drugs. And high-dose Danazol® proved safe and effective, as Denise would have no seizures or PMS or menstrual flow for the next 24 years. Note that after the seizures were controlled, Dr. Lichten continued to reduce the medication slowly. At this time, she is taking only 100 mg of Danazol® daily, and that may be unnecessary. But neither Denise nor Dr. Lichten will risk a recurrence of those horrific seizures. On Danazol® she simply remains seizure-free.

Scientific Perspective

Into Dr. Lichten's office in 1985 came a psychology student working on her Ph.D. Diane B. was in her 40s and told Dr. Lichten how she wanted him to help her with her dissertation. The problem was she was looking for a pediatrician not a gynecologist. But being that both were interested in scientific studies, Dr. Lichten discussed other Ph.D. topics with Diane B., including PMS. Now, at that time, and not all that different today, women were considered the "weaker sex" and unable to handle the stress of everyday life. As a male, Dr. Lichten readily admits being unable to do the housework, care for the children, and cook the meals without expecting a complete physical and mental breakdown. So, with neither Dr. Lichten nor Diane B. believing that PMS was a psychological disease, the clinical study of PMS as a hormonal or a cognitive disorder was born.

Half the PMS patients were to come from Dr. Lichten's patient base. All patients would have a history and psychological examination performed by Ms. B. Dr. Lichten required them to complete a questionnaire similar to that of Robert Reid, M.D., because it generated a value score for the various elements of PMS. He also requested that all patients have hormonal blood work on day 3 and day 23 to delineate the expected low-hormonal week (day 3) and high-hormonal week (day 23). All information would be tabulated at the end of the study.

The two learned, later, as they tabulated the data, that the standard psychiatric tests had been standardized on men. So the Eysenck psychological tests is formulated to see every woman as abnormal. The standard Hamilton-Beck depression tests were not superior to the simple Reid questionnaire, and so the cognitive intervention was really not very effective.

Nevertheless, they found that a large number of the women with PMS by Reid's questionnaire criteria also had abnormal hormonal parameters. What are expected as normal are low levels of estradiol, FSH, and LH at day 3 of the menstrual cycle. What are expected as normal are elevated levels of estradiol and progesterone and low levels of FSH and LH at day 23.

But most of PMS women had high levels of estradiol and low levels of progesterone on day 23. This is what Katrina Dalton implied 20 years earlier. It explains why if bio-identical progesterone capsules, suppositories, or rectal liquid proved ineffective that Danazol® could potentially be helpful, because it would suppress excess estrogen, thus alleviating the "estrogen dominance" phenomenon (i.e., too much estrogen in relation to progesterone). But PMS would still remain classified as a psychiatric disorder, no matter what Dr. Lichten said, what Diane B. noted in her dissertation, and Robert Reid would publish later.[16]

The most interesting findings were women who had high levels of estradiol with or without progesterone on day 3. The data was rechecked and the dates were correct. Neither Dr. Lichten nor Diane B. can explain why these women would have menstrual flow at the wrong hormonal time phase. These women responded positively to Danazol® therapy and not to Prozac®, Paxil®, and other selective serotonin uptake drugs (SSRIs).

So, for the layperson and the doctor, any distressing symptom that is found at the time of menstruation is considered molimina. By changing the estrogen and progesterone levels, using Danazol®, for example, to balance and lower the hormonal levels, the symptoms may be completely controlled. Therefore, menstrual bleeding and cyclic pain, PMS and mood disorders, seizures, collapsed lungs, and a host of other maladies may disappear with the disappearance of the menstrual flow. It is worth a try.

DEPRESSION AND TESTOSTERONE HORMONE REPLACEMENT

Although not often considered by physicians, the focus on the cause of depression may be low levels of the hormones; specifically testosterone[17] and triiodothyronine-(T3).[18] Barbara Sherwin, Ph.D., wrote almost 20 years ago that testosterone was as important if not more important in treating depression in the menopausal and surgical menopausal women. Testosterone, she wrote, had positive effects on depression, libido, and self-imagery. Of the testosterone preparations available in Canada, she chose testosterone and estradiol pellets[19] as the ideal prescription replacement form because of their constant release and similarity to bio-identical hormone patterns.[20]

CHRONIC PELVIC PAIN

These symptoms of menstrual pain, heavy menstrual bleeding, strange premenstrual symptoms, and migraine are devastating to a woman, no matter what her age. With each of these disorders, Dr. Lichten has outlined how he diagnoses and treats these conditions associated with the menstrual period: (1) establish that the medical complaint is related in time to the menstrual flow and that the disease process will respond to hormonal suppression with Danazol®, megesterol, or luprolide acetate (Lupron®); and (2) block mitigating mechanical muscle trigger points in the lower back and/or abdomen that may have developed from auto accidents, falls, or childbirth.

Into the practice came Carol, who sought relief from chronic pelvic pain that prevented her and her husband from taking long bicycle rides across Michigan. The increased pelvic pain from riding the bicycle had left her in a hotel room one day during the previous year because she could not continue. She wanted relief and she wanted it yesterday.

Step one in Dr. Lichten's pain protocol is to determine if the pain can be relieved by an active intervention. As most patients have seen numerous doctors, adding one more pill rarely works. These patients do not respond to a placebo. If the pain can be relieved by some intervention from a medical hormonal or anesthetic pain basis, then this is overwhelming evidence that the pain is not psychosomatic and can be treated and cured. Just as if the disease were caused by hidden endometriosis, higher-dose Danazol® or luprolide acetate will stop the pain by the second cycle. If the pain is relieved, laparoscopy with transection of the uterine sacral nerves is performed. The laparoscopy will document any abnormalities of the pelvis, any disease, and whether the laser surgery can bring any long-term relief. Step two is to determine if the trigger points were missed.

TRIGGER-POINT INJECTIONS

It is beyond the scope of this book to cover an entire field of medicine. Let it be said that for thousands of years, the Chinese had used acupuncture to treat pain disorders. Now, acupuncture is much more complicated than trigger points, but acupuncture shares the idea of sticking a needle into a tight muscle to get it to relax. The difference is that American physicians add lidocaine (Novocain®) to spread out over a one-inch-square area so as not to miss the exact spot.

In the chapter on migraines, the greater occipital nerve block is one of the trigger points that can be injected to stop and prevent migraine. But for chronic pain, the pain triggers may be in the lower abdomen, the groin, and/or the back and may include sciatica (pain down the leg). For treatment, Dr. Lichten will palpate the muscles lateral to the spine, the sacrum, and the sciatic notch. All tender spots are injected and pain results documented.

If pain persists, and trigger injections prove to not be effective, the next step becomes an epidural segmental block. The anesthesiologist can place an epidural (continuous) anesthetic in the space around the spine. This is commonly done for painless childbirth. Once in place, the anesthesiologist can slowly increase the level of anesthetic until the level reaches above the navel. If no relief is forthcoming, the pain is probably psychological. But since most women's pain is relieved below that level, the pain is real and treatable first by the anesthesiologist with a long-acting steroid. And for those women in whom the segmental block was temporarily effective, and the long-lasting blocks not so, hysterectomy may well prove to be safe and effective almost 100% of the time.

Medications discussed in this chapter

Dysmenorrhea

Ibuprofen (OTC) 200 mg–2,400 mg/day
Ketoprofen 5 mg/1–4 daily
Toradol® ketorolac 30 mg/ml injections
Ketorolac® injections

Endometriosis Severe dysmenorrhea

Danazol® 200 mg (1–4/daily)
Megace® megesterol acetate 20 mg/1–2 daily
Luprolide® Acetate 3.75 mg/injection monthly

Premenstrual Syndrome

Danazol® 200 mg/2–3 per day
Spirolactone® 100 mg/1–2 per day
Luprolide® Acetate 3.75 mg/injection monthly

REFERENCES:

1. Ingersoll FM, Meigs JV. Presacral neurectomy for dysmenorrhea. *New England Journal of Medicine.* 1948; 238:357–12.
2. Budoff P. *No More Menstrual Cramps and Other Good News.* Penguin Press. 1981.
3. Archer DF. Menstrual-cycle-related symptoms: a review of the rationale for continuous use of oral contraceptives. *Contraception.* 2006; 74(5):359–66.
4. Freidlander RL. The treatment of endometriosis with Danazol®. *Journal of Reproductive Medicine.* 1973; 10(4):197–9.
5. Kistner RW. Newer synthetic progestins for the treatment of endometriosis. *Progress in Gynecology.* 1970; 5:283–302.
6. Lichten EM, Bombard J. Surgical treatment of primary dysmenorrhea with laparoscopic uterine nerve ablation. *Journal of Reproductive Medicine.* 1987; 32(1): 37–41 Updated.
7. Balweg ML. *Overcoming Endometriosis.* 1987. New York City.
8. Sculpher M, et al. A cost effective analysis of goserelin compared with danazol as endometrial thinning agents. *British Journal of Obstetrics and Gynecology.* 2000; 107(3):340–6.
9. Goldrath MH. Hysteroscopic endometrial ablation. *Obstetrics and Gynecology Clinics of North America.* 1995; 22(3):559–72.
10. Lethaby A, et al. Endometrial destruction techniques for heavy menstrual bleeding. *Cochrane Database Systemic Review.* 2002; (2):CD001501.
11. Franks J. *Neurology.* 1931.
12. Dalton K, et al. JR *College General Practitioners.* What is PMS? 1982; 32(245):717–23.
13. Deeny M, et al. Low Dose Danazol® in the Treatment of Premenstrual Syndrome. *Postgraduate Medicine.* 1991; 67:450–54.
14. Derzko CM. Role of danazol in relieving the premenstrual syndrome. *Journal of Reproductive Medicine.* 1990; 35(1 S):97–101.
15. Marshall MB, et al. Catamenial pneumothorax: optimal hormonal and surgical management. *European Journal of Cardiothoracic Surgery.* 2005: 27(4):662–6.
16. Hahn PM, Reid RL. A randomized, placebo-controlled, crossover trial of danazol for the treatment of premenstrual syndrome. *Psychoneuroendocrinology.* 1995; 20(2):193–209.
17. Hohlagschwandtner M, et al. Correlation between serum testosterone levels and peripartal mood states. *Acta Obstetrics Gynecology Scandinavia.* 2001; 80(4):326–30.
18. Posternak M, et al. A pilot effectiveness study: placebo-controlled trial of adjunctive triiodothyronine (T3) used to accelerate and potentiate the antidepressant response. *Internal Journal of Neuropsychopharmacology* 2007; 1–11.
19. Sherwin BB. Affective changes with estrogen and androgen replacement therapy in surgically menopausal women. *Journal of Affect Disorders.* 1988 Mar–April; 14(2):177–87.
20. Sherwin BB. Effects of hormone implants on psychological disorders in the climacteric. *Lancet.* 1987; 1(8540):1038–9.

CHAPTER 8

HEADACHE AND MIGRAINE DISORDERS

MIGRAINE

On a busy patient day in 1983, Dr. Lichten was stressed and surprised when a patient grabbed his arm to talk. "Yes," she said. "I am fine. But I want you to hear my story before running out of the room." Shocked by her directness, he sat down and listened. Little did he know that this would change his medical direction and offer new insight to a disease that dates back to the dawn of mankind.

"I have very severe headaches," said this 45-year-old, heavy-set woman. "Before then, I was happy, energetic, and full of life. After my last childbirth, the most severe headaches started. I had this young baby and I was in the bathroom, throwing up, lying down in the dark room with the pillow over my head, and suffering day after day. I was incapacitated for two to three days, and sometimes five days, every month. And no medication and no handful of Excedrin® would change my pain. Until you."

"I am a gynecologist," Dr. Lichten said. "And I don't treat headaches. I am so pleased that I could be of assistance," he said as he scurried for the door.

She grabbed his arm again and held on until he sat back down in his chair. "You don't seem to understand: I didn't stay here looking for an answer. I went to Chicago, New York, Connecticut, and even Los Angeles. No one helped in any way. Just you."

Again, Dr. Lichten said "Thank you" and gave her a six-month prescription instead of the normal three months and wished her adieu.

And life would have been hectic but uneventful if the same story line had not been repeated that very same afternoon.

When the second patient said, "You relieved my headaches," Dr. Lichten sat down and listened. This woman's headaches had started in her teen years even before the onset of her first menstrual flow. She recognized them as premenstrual and tried everything to avoid having headaches. First there were the ibuprofen NSAIDs, then oral contraceptives, ergotamine, Percodan®, propranolol, seizure medications, and then lots and lots of caffeine, but nothing really worked.

She had made the rounds of five of the most well-known facilities that specialize in headaches and migraines. And here she sat in front of Dr. Lichten and thanked him. So he listened and he listened and he listened some more until he gleaned this simple lesson: No, Dr. Lichten was not a neurologist, or a pain specialist. He was, however, a real doctor who wanted to be a healer not a prescription writer. Not because he was smarter, not because he was better. No, simply because he listened and he wanted to understand simply why.

Historical Perspective

So that night he went to the hospital library and found the guru's book on headache, first written in 1950 by Wolff.[1] In *Headache and other Head Pain,* Harold Wolff, M.D., had single-handedly developed the field of headache and migraine research. Over 30-odd years, he explored every angle to explain migraine and was the first to champion the idea of a vascular event based on blood flow through the carotid vessels into the head. That is, he explored every angle but one: hormonal. Yet, when you look back at literature that is more than 30 years ago, you can find the truth in his book, unwashed by the need to prove that "this" pharmacological drug is the newest and best. Here in the first 70 pages of Wolff's textbook was the answer: *Women have six times as many severe headaches as men,* and this ratio is present in the reproductive years, from 11 to 50 years of age. Before and after a woman's 'reproductive career,' the epidemiologists find that the incidences of migraine by gender are approximately the same. It is the hormones of reproduction that cause these migraines: menstrual migraines, ovulation migraines, hormonal migraines, and postpartum migraines.

The second discovery in Wolff's later editions edited by Dalessio was that there was much confusion between the neurologists on what constituted a "migraine" and a "headache." Based on the Greek origin of the words, migraine refers to a headache on one-side of the head—*hemikrania*. The French modified the Greek-Latin word to *migraine,* and the English changed it to *megrim* and then accepted *migraine* in the 15th century. Since burr holes, called trepanations, have been found in skeletons dating back 12,000 years, perfected by the Incas 3,000 years ago, and written about by Hippocrates 2,300 years ago, it's clear that migraine headaches have been a medical disease that dates back well before man gained the skills to write.

Wolff's third discovery: With no clear understanding of the physiological cause of migraine, the neurologists were apt to try anything and record the results as percentage improvement. So the treatments in Ann Arbor first focused on blood pressure medications (beta blockers), the treatments in Chicago on antiseizure medication, while the treatment in Los Angeles could be lidocaine and Phenobarbital®. And they all had good results in some patients because there is an additional 25% who respond to any or no treatment (called the placebo effect). And that is why Dr. Lichten's index patients had gone to four or five centers to try to find the one treatment that would work for them.

And then a menopausal patient appeared in Dr. Lichten's office. While taking oral estrogens, the severe migraine attacks recurred, only worse and on a daily basis. Here she was caught between severe night sweats and mood swings and severe migraines. No one had the answer, so she came to Dr. Lichten. And he listened.

Dr. Lichten reasoned that if the estrogen was triggering migraines, and the antiestrogen Danazol® was effective, then every estrogen-stabilizing agent should work. Well, it did. Sort of. The patient had no more migraines, but the menopausal symptoms were still there on Danazol®. So he offered her another option. "What if we use a natural estradiol pellet?" he asked. "This will give you stable estrogen levels, which should relieve your flashes but will not be prone to the highs and lows of taking an estrogen by mouth. Oral estrogen is in and out of your bloodstream in four to eight hours. The downside is, if I am wrong, you could have migraine headaches for a whole month." Dr. Lichten waited for her answer.

Helen G. tried the pellets and never had another migraine attack from hormones in the next 20 years. Now she still gets tension headaches, but they are few and far between.

TWO DIFFERENT MEDICAL TREATMENTS: ONE HYPOTHESIS

Two seemingly diabolically opposite treatments work:

1. Lower the estrogen level in reproductive-age women.
2. Raise the estrogen level in postmenopausal women.

The answer came from reviewing the literature with the terms *hormones* and *migraine*. And there was B.W. Somerville, M.D., an Australian neurologist who already had the answer.

In 1972, Somerville[2] had asked the same question, "What is the hormonal change that triggers migraines at menstruation?" There were only two choices, estrogen and progesterone. Somerville injected one hormone and then the other into women with migraines before the first day of flow. Then he observed what happened, scientifically.

The women who received progesterone had their onset of menstruation delayed. This showed that the primary function of progesterone withdrawal was the onset of menstrual flow. The migraine occurred on the expected day, not the menstrual flow day.

Women who received estrogen injections recorded their menses on the expected day. And they had no migraine initially. Then, a week later, they had a much worse migraine. So bad, in fact, that they probably screamed something quite unladylike to Somerville.[3]

But Somerville was brilliant in being able to deduce the cause of this scientific evaluation. He did more experiments and published more scientific papers until he had covered every conceivable hormonal event. This is the key to finding the truth. It is called the scientific method, and it is the basis of all good medical research, because a hypothesis is not proved until it is observed to be 100% correct. These are Somerville's three postulates[3]

1. A drop in estrogen levels precipitates migraine attacks.
2. A period of estrogen priming is a necessary precursor to the hormonal migraine.
3. Migraine attacks may be prevented by a stable estrogen milieu.

Somerville explained that changes in hormones during the reproductive years for women contribute to migraine. Furthermore, more migraines occur in the week before menstruation, because the last two weeks are the time of estrogen priming. The rapid peak of estrogen at midcycle preceding ovulation will rarely trigger a migraine. And third, migraine attacks may be prevented by a stable estrogen milieu.

Eureka! Stable estrogen milieu existed in the reproductive woman on Danazol®. Stable estrogen milieu existed in the postmenopausal woman on estradiol pellets. Dr. Lichten's patients were proving Somerville's postulates.

But why hadn't Somerville provided a cure for hormonal migraine, well before Lichten's trials and errors? The answer was simple, and it was the gynecology literature that held the answer. Greenblatt[4] had kept women migraine-free for up to 20 years on estradiol pellets. It seemed the only difference was that Somerville's[5] pellets were manufactured in Europe and Greenblatt's were manufactured in the United States.

So, after hunting down the manufacturer of the Organon® pellets from Europe, as well as the drug manufacturer in the United States, Dr. Lichten traveled to New York to talk to Frank, who was the manufacturer for the estradiol pellets.

Before speaking to Frank, Dr. Lichten called his professor, Frederick P. Zuspan, M.D. Dr. Zuspan is considered to be one of the most influential gynecologists of this century. Not only was he involved in the original use of magnesium sulfate to control toxemia of pregnancy, he also performed one of the first sex-change operations, was the founder of the high-risk pregnancy fellowships, chairman of OB-GYN at three major university programs, and also editor of three of the four gynecology journals. Loved by patients, feared by colleagues, he will always remain one of Dr. Lichten's closest friends.

When Dr. Zuspan was chairman of the OB-GYN department at the Medical College of Georgia, he and Dr. Greenblatt traveled to rural areas to lecture the state gynecologists. They heard each other's lectures so often, that, for fun, they would give the other doctor's lectures. So Dr. Lichten asked Dr. Zuspan to tell him what Greenblatt had taught the medical doctors twenty years earlier.

Once armed with this knowledge, Dr. Lichten then went to meet Frank, a 78-year-old Italian who created the once-a-day sustained-release pain-relief tablet for the army in the Korean War, only to have the patent stolen by a pharmaceutical company. Brilliant and self-trained, there are not many like Frank. He and Dr. Lichten got along fine.

What Frank explained to Dr. Lichten was that the European pellets were compressed but not to the pounds-per-square-inch that Frank incorporated in his American pellet design. And the equipment Frank used was 30 years more modern than the European.

So the absorption rate of Frank's pellets would be uniform, while the European pellets fractured and crumbled, Dr. Lichten reasoned. That explained why Greenblatt's pellets worked and Somerville's pellets failed to prove effective (in step 4) despite the scientific method. Simple. Safe. Effective.

Returning to Michigan, Dr. Lichten organized the IRB protocol for the study of Danazol® in the treatment of migraine. The best studies are double-blind, meaning that one group gets the active ingredient and the other gets blanks, called placebos. With a hospital-supervised IRB in hand, Dr. Lichten contacted the manufacturer of Danazol®, Sterling-Winthrop Laboratories. Intrigued by the documented observations, they asked Dr. Lichten to file with the overseeing federal commission for a new drug investigational permit, called an NDA. Lichten did so and it was granted.

And then something unusual happened. The permit was pulled and no explanation was offered. Dr. Lichten was studying a drug that was FDA-approved 20 years earlier and for four capsules per day for nine months of continuous use; Lichten wanted to use only two capsules a day for two months. Six months went by without an answer except that Sterling withdrew their offer for placebo and never contacted Lichten again.

Now Dr. Lichten is a persistent person, so he called again. This time he contacted his friend who was surgeon to Carl Levin, a senator from Michigan. It took five months for Senator Levin to get an answer back. The answer was not from the government director. He informed Lichten in writing that there were presently (1980s) enough medications for headache (Valium®, Elavil®, and Inderal® were prescribed at that time) and not to pursue the double-blind study. Dr. Lichten got the message.

Dr. Lichten changed the protocol to be an elimination study. Try drug A. If you don't get better, you get drug B. Then C, D, and finally Danazol®, drug E. Of the 145 women who entered the study, only a few got better or dropped out in steps A through D. The study had 131 women left to take Danazol® for two months.[5] And of these, 67 felt so good taking Danazol® that they continued it for a full year —headache-free. Many had had migraines for 10 years or longer!

Armed with this new knowledge, Dr. Lichten joined the American Headache Society. He was originally greeted with skepticism, because this was neurology nirvana. They warmed to him when he showed a true interest in what they had to say. At least they were kind at the first meeting.

At the second meeting, Dr. Lichten had submitted the published article on Danazol® and how he was able to control menstrual migraine. One neurologist in particular was adamant that Dr. Lichten not be allowed to speak. It seems that a large number of his patients had left to become Dr. Lichten's patients because of a TV news story. But Dr. Lichten did speak, and a whole gaggle of neurologists circled around to thank him and tell how they had tried to treat migraine hormonally but had not found the success that Dr. Lichten had reported.

But internists and neurologists did not follow Dr. Lichten's lead. It seems that there is a fear among some doctors of treating women with hormones and how they might have to treat them should their patients experience abnormal bleeding. The Women's Health Initiative report in 1999 and 2002 did much to worsen this position.

So the neurologists never treated with Danazol®. They instead kept to their regimens of using abortives like sumatriptan (Imitrex®), beta-blockers, antihypertensives such as propranolol (Inderal®), and nonsteroidal anti-inflammatory agents such as Toradol® injections. And, of course, they used antidepressants and neuronal stabilizers like amytriptyline (Elavil®), Prozac®, and Topamax®. Patients suffering from the most severe headaches never seemed to get the cause of their migraine treated.

After the first lecture to the neurologists, Dr. Lichten tried again, with a second publication showing that luprolide acetate,[6] a once-a-month injection that suppressed estrogen like Danazol® did, would work as well. It did, but the luprolide acetate (Lupron®) had worse side effects. Point proved: Migraines are hormonal events.

Then Dr. Lichten presented that hysterectomy was effective at treating menstrual migraine but only with ovarian removal. Point proved: Migraines are hormonal events.

And then Dr. Lichten performed a simple, scientific study that many neurologists still reference in their peer-review studies. This was a study similar to Somerville's in which the IRB protocol was to give the same estrogen injection that Dr. Somerville used but to give it to menopausal women. The study plan would observe and then document what happens when estradiol injections are given to women with and without a history of migraine during their reproductive years. This significant bit of history, whether they had hormonal migraine, was hidden in the charts and away from any investigator's eyes.

All women were given the same dose of estradiol injection initially. Somewhere between the third and fourth week, one group of women reported severe migraines, while the others did not. And when the code was broken, every one of the women who had a migraine had a previously documented history of menstrual migraine.[7]

What Dr. Lichten's study proved is that for migraine, women needed to be both:

1. genetically prone, and
2. experience an estrogen withdrawal from a significantly higher level.

In all discussions of disease today, it is commonplace to speak of the equal roles of genetics and environment just as others had stated previously. When Dr. Lichten was asked by a young doctor one day if he knew at what blood level each of the test subjects had noted headaches, he said, "Yes, it was 50 pg/ml." "How did you know?" the student asked. "Because you should always know what results are expected before you begin, and Somerville said the estradiol threshold for his four patients was 40 pg/ml. + 10 pg/ml." The basis of the scientific method is that results are reproducible no matter who does the study.

So, if Somerville reported his threshold level for estradiol and migraine was 40–50 pg/ml, then everyone's results should be the same.

With this new knowledge, Dr. Lichten measured blood levels of estradiol before and after migraines and soon could determine what dosage of estradiol pellets and estradiol patches would be sufficient to keep the estrogen levels stable and above the 50 pg/ml. threshold. And this methodology has worked well for hundreds of his patients treated over the past 20 years.

A fifth paper was presented by Dr. Lichten to the International Headache Society in Madrid in 1999 and abstracted in Cephalgia.[8] All the volunteers were migraineurs severely affected by menstrual and hormonal events. The study confirmed that the use of monthly estradiol pellets eliminated more than 80% of the sumatriptan (Imitrex®) drug usage for 27 of the 30 women. With oral sumatriptan drugs costing $14 per capsule and with many patients taking 20 to 30 per month, the cost savings pale in comparison to the improvement in lifestyle. The estradiol pellets have changed the medical intervention of migraines to *proactive* rather than reactive. That is the role that Dr. Lichten sees for the use of bio-identical and natural hormones: "Bring these six sets of life-giving hormones into the normal range and watch a number of diseases disappear."

As a gynecologist, Dr. Lichten was pleased to participate in the Menopause Symposium held by Reid-Rowell (now Solvay Pharmaceuticals) in 1990.[9] This symposium booklet was distributed to almost all gynecologists in the United States.

Recently, Dr. Lichten was proud to read that the director of the large Headache Centre, Institute of Neurology, University of Parma, Italy, wrote in *Cephalgia*[10] of their established plan to treat menstrual migraine. Their policy is as follows:

"Because of its patho-physiological and clinical peculiarities, true menstrual migraine (MM) requires an ad hoc management different from that of other migraines. The paucity of well-conducted, controlled clinical trials and the lack of a universally accepted definition of MM have meant that the treatment of MM is still largely empirical. In our clinical practice, we adopt a sequential therapeutic approach, including the following steps: (i) acute attack drugs (sumatriptan, ergot derivatives, NSAIDs); (ii) intermittent prophylaxis with ergot derivatives or NSAIDs; (iii) estrogen supplementation with percutaneous or transdermal estradiol (100 mg patches); (iv) antiestrogen agents (Danazol®, tamoxifen)."[10]

And the other large women's headache center at Turin[11] has a similar policy stating:

"Moreover, menstrual migraine-MM can be prevented by a variety of hormonal manipulations, including oral contraceptives, which may be administered with an extended-dosing strategy; estrogen replacement therapy; antiestrogen agents (Danocine®, tamoxifen); gonadotropin-releasing hormone agonists followed by oestrogen add-back therapy."[11]

If you are a woman with menstrual migraine, consult with your gynecologist and neurologist about prescription estradiol hormonal patches, pellets, or antiestrogens such as Danazol®. A gynecologist should treat the drop in estrogen at menstruation with the estradiol patch. If this is not successful, he should discuss treating with Danazol® as if he were treating endometriosis. If the above is not ideal, and the gynecologist is not comfortable in inserting estradiol pellets, Dr. Lichten maintains his office in Birmingham, Michigan, as a resource for patients who need hormonal stabilization. Or take a nice vacation to Italy. They seem to understand very well there.

But with new knowledge comes new problems. It seems that only 15% of women with severe headaches have pure migraine. J.R. Couch, M.D.,[12] a key American neurologist, states that tension components have an active role in 85% of migraine, and the subdivisions of chronic daily headache (CDH) may include a tension-type headache (TTH). Although Dr. Lichten's initial success with Danazol® was gratifying, the second wave of patients did not do as well on hormonal intervention alone.

In the corner of the American Headache Society meetings and the International Headache Society was a quiet man who was willing to teach. His name was Dr. Sjaastad.[13]

Dr. Sjaastad had a different opinion on severe headaches. While migraines occur for a short 24- to 48-hour period of time in the vicinity of the menstrual flow, chronic tension headaches (CTH) occur throughout the month. These headaches can be one- or both-sided and range from mild to severe. The severe CTH was indistinguishable from migraine.

Dr. Sjaastad explained how Wolff had determined that migraines start from dysfunction in the carotid artery. Sjaastad explained that the carotid node was innervated from spinal root nerves C2-3. But being in the front half of the body, the nerves that connect back to the brain were from one branch—the anterior (front) root or division of the spinal nerves.

CTH and CDH, he reasoned, started from the back of the neck at the junction of the neck muscles and the skull. This region is called the occiput, and the nerve that comes out to innervate the skull's occipital muscles is called the occipital nerve. It originates from the dorsal (posterior) root of spinal nerves C2-3. This is what Sjaastad calls cervicogenic headaches (CGH).

This is what Sjaastad told Dr. Lichten he did next: Sjaastad injected that region with lidocaine, not to block the sensory nerve but to relax the muscles that were in spasm around the sensory nerve. This is an application of the legendary work of Janet Travell, M.D.,[14] who used these local anesthesia injections and trigger-point injections to propel John F. Kennedy out of his wheelchair and into the White House 40 years ago. Let it be remembered that Chinese acupuncturists used needles for pain management 2,500 years before Travell and Sjaastad.

So Sjaastad showed Dr. Lichten the anatomical muscles that support the head, that each muscle groups refers pain differently, and how and where to block it. And with this extra knowledge, Dr. Lichten went back to the United States to treat those patients who had not been helped by hormonal therapy.

The key points about muscle contraction and tension headaches is that they are everywhere in our society. They occur with the whiplash, the slip and fall, the secretary poured over her computer, the woman with bad posture, and the woman with skinny bra straps and large breasts. Any activity that causes undo strain on the five layers of muscles that support the skull on the narrow vertebral column will cause strain. Persistent strain leads to muscle spasm, which traps the muscle and irritates the nerves.

Think of the trigger point as the knot in a piece of wood. Muscles knot up around the nerve. And with the tightening of that knot of muscle, the nerve is irritated. Chronic muscle irritation begets chronic pain. And taking any medication that causes muscle spasms—including caffeine (Excedrin®), nicotine, sumatriptan (Imitrex®), and Fiorinal® with Codeine—will create a rebound muscle tightening and continuation of headaches.

Sometimes, when one reads the medical literature, it is clear that many doctors themselves are confused about what a headache is. Hilton[18] described the concept of headaches originating from the cervical spine in 1860. In 1983 Sjaastad introduced the term "cervicogenic headache" (CGH).[13] Diagnostic criteria have been established by several expert groups, with agreement that these headaches start in the neck or occipital region and are associated with tenderness of cervical paraspinal tissues.[17] Prevalence estimates range from 0.4–2.5% of the general population to 15–20% of patients with chronic headaches. CGH affects patients with a mean age of 42.9 years, has a 4:1 female disposition, and tends to be chronic. The main differential diagnoses are tension-type headache and migraine headache, with considerable overlap in symptoms and findings between these conditions.[14]

Sjaastad[15] simplified the process of diagnosing whether the headache was of cervicogenic origin. He listed four criteria that separated CEH from migraine:

1. Unilateral side worse, but opposite side also affected.
2. Neck involvement.
3. Nonclustered occurrence (vs. clustered hormonal migraine with hormonal event).
4. Relief with injection of the occipital branch of the cervical C2-3 root.

He injected either local anesthetic or a saline solution into the muscle knots that surrounded the occipital nerve. This nerve comes out laterally from the cervical vertebrae at C2-3, wraps around the base of the skull, and innervates the muscles of the back of the skull, called the occipitalis muscles. Aspiration establishes that the needle is not in a vessel, and then slow injection is performed in at least two directions. Most physicians report that pain relief is almost instantaneous.

Few neurologists are trained in performing occipital nerve or trigger blocks. The International Headache Society makes the diagnosis based on questionnaires and history. The problem with this concept is that these questionnaires are not specific at diagnosing CDH[21], which makes up half of the chronic-headache population.

The more specific symptoms for migraine were severity, photophobia, phonophobia, and vomiting. IHS criteria for chronic-tension-type headache have a very low sensibility; only 45% of these headaches meet criteria and 62% of the CDH has analgesic overuse. CONCLUSIONS: IHS criteria distinguish accurately between migraine and tension-type headache. Symptoms do not differentiate the different kinds of CDH. So, in simplicity, there were just three kinds of headaches in a migraine-headache practice:

1. **Migraine:** 6:1 ratio of women to men; reproductive years, severe nausea, vomiting, sensitivity to light and sound; lasts 24 to 48 hours. Pain above eyes and one side of forehead. Caffeine may be helpful.

2. **Tension:** 4:1 ratio of women to men; up to 10 to 14 days or more per month; less severe, more chronic. Pain present in neck region where it can spread to temples and forehead. May originate with an automobile accident, sudden fall, or bad posture. Head forward position associated with inability to move shoulder backward past neutral (unable to bring scapulas together). Responds to deep heat and muscle relaxers. Caffeine contraindicated. CTH. CDH. CGH. All these are variations of the same theme: tension neck pain.

3. **Cluster headaches:** Severe attacks; rare in women. Cycles of severe headaches for days or weeks. Seasonal. Some patients will bang head against wall until unconscious. May cause suicide. Extremely rare.

In 23 years of treating headaches, only a handful of headache/migraine patients have failed to respond when treated as having both migraine and headache. Treat patient initially with hormonal stabilization for migraine and treat concomitantly the muscle contraction with anesthetic blocks. The ones who failed to respond included 10 women who needed to have breast reductions, one fractured vertebra headache from a headstand yoga pose, one acoustic neuroma, on octogenarian with an osteoporosis-related fracture, and one brain tumor diagnosed by CT/MRI imaging.

Those who failed to respond to hormonal and anesthetic injections were referred to a neurologist to rule out more serious causes of their malady.

Dr. Lichten's migraine headache protocol starts with an initial history and physical examination with questions as follows. There should be almost a 90% separation based on history alone:

1. **Migraine:** first occurred with a hormonal event
   a. Women: 6:1 ratio
   b. Age: 11 to 50 (the reproductive years)
   c. Migraine: at menses, oral contraceptives, postpartum, menopause
   d. Location: forehead and temples, above eyes
   e. Days per month: In the beginning, lasted 1–2 days
   f. Timing: days before and during the menstrual period
   g. Characteristics: one-sided, severe, sharp, stabbing, cutting
   h. Other symptoms: nausea, vomiting, sensitivity to light and noise
   i. Medication: caffeine initially may be helpful; oral contraceptives may worsen head pain at time of menstrual flow

2. **Tension or Cervicogenic Component:**
   a. Women 4:1
   b. Age: reproductive and menopausal years
   c. Headache: may occur after a traumatic event:
      (i) automobile accident or whiplash or fall;
      (ii) rebound from caffeine or other prescription medications
   d. Location: back of neck, radiating to temples and forehead

e. Days per month: often 10–14 days or more
f. Timing: no relationship to menstrual cycle
g. Characteristics: bilateral, moderate, achy characteristics
h. Other symptoms: fewer complaints of nausea, vomiting, light
i. Medication: muscle relaxers most helpful

When Marge B., a 39-year-old Caucasian female, came into the office, she answered the questionnaire and the physician's additional questions to delineate how much of her complaints are migraine and how much are those of a cervicogenic or tension component. Most women with chronic-headache disease benefit from a thorough evaluation that both diagnoses and treats.

In Dr. Lichten's experience, it seems that the first type of headache in women is usually hormonal. This begins in the teens, 20s, and 30s. As delineated above, the hormonal events are just part of everyday life: starting to menstruate, starting oral contraceptives, getting pregnant, delivery, postpartum, and menopause. In each case, there is a normal fluctuation of estrogens up and down. Now, from the work of Somerville, the drop of estrogen precipitates the migraine. And from the work of Lichten, there has to be a predisposing genetic makeup. Therefore, the first and easiest headache to treat is always hormonal, whether with an estradiol patch before and during menstruation or with the estrogen stabilization that Danazol® offers.

It seems that the misdiagnosis and mistreatment of hormonal migraine is a primary cause of adult chronic daily headaches. The simplest treatment for a headache most people believe is to take a cup of coffee or other caffeinated product. The caffeine causes a vasoconstriction, which treats the vasodilatation of migraine temporarily. Then the effects of caffeine wear off and the headache rebounds and pain recurs. But in the meantime, the muscles in the body and especially the neck tighten and this may progress to chronic daily headaches. A full 62% of patients with chronic daily headaches are addicted to pain medication. So headache patients need to know that taking caffeine for 1–2 days a month is acceptable, but 4–10 cups of coffee a day may lead to an addiction as the tolerance builds, especially if one is genetically inclined.

All headache and migraine disorders are treated from the first visit when the patient is in pain, per Sjaastad, with a series of three occipital nerve blocks; C6 trigger points; and, if pain is not relieved, other anesthetic blocks to the appropriate area: mandible, sphenopalatine, sternocleidomastoid, trapezoid-supraspinatus, and subscapular as defined by the corresponding trigger points.

Marge B., for example, had experienced headaches since her teen years. She could not take oral contraceptives because they worsened the headaches. The really severe migraine attacks began after the second childbirth. Her migraines were full blown, with nausea, vomiting, severe photophobia/ phonophobia (sensitivity to light and noise), and she was scheduled to leave town that night for an ice skating competition. Her vision was blurry, with moving lights, called scotomas, in the left eye. Even if she had a history of responding to sumatriptan injectable, it might have left her "hung over" and unable to function. Instead, following the protocol, Dr. Lichten identified the irritated nerve root and injected appropriate anesthetic into the muscle/ nerve complex and reevaluated for pain relief as follows:

1. Identified tender occipital notch (back of neck at base of skull) — injected greater occipital nerve (GON) on affected side (left). Pain relief good, tenderness remains lateral to GON. Injected the accessory occipital nerve of affected side.

2. Identified tender occipital notch on contralateral side (opposite side) —injected greater and lesser occipital nerves on secondary side. Pain relief better, but tenderness noted at C6 vertebrae on both sides.

3. Identified tender C6 lateral root on both sides —injected both trigger points. Pain relief better, but tenderness remains in suprascapular region, with deep tender trigger over scapular notch (shoulder).

4. Local anesthetic injections of trapezoid-suprascapular muscles prevent spasm as deep palpation identifies the location of the scapular notch. Sterile anesthetic technique allows 2-inch needle to penetrate behind the scapular, and with injection of 4 cc of 2% lidocaine mixture, patient has full and complete relief of pain.

Explanation: Sjaastad and Travell were pioneers in the identification of trigger points and referred pain. In the 25 years spent in pain management, Dr. Lichten learned that all muscle groups are interrelated. In the case of headaches and migraines, most early migraine headaches can be treated by a single injection of the occipital nerve or its accessory component.[19,22,23] This is repeated three times in practice over two weeks to break the cycle and start muscle retraining through physical therapy.[23] However, as migraine headaches continue to become more and more severe, the head is stilted just like a broken arm, and this spasm causes more muscles to be recruited into stabilizing the head. That is why the second location for migraine headache is at C6. When C6 is affected, it can cause a frozen scapular complex to develop. This can lead to a frozen shoulder, tears and even surgery.[21] That is why a comprehensive physical examination needs to be performed by the physician who is prepared to treat migraines and headaches and offer pain relief by performing the aforementioned nerve blocks.

After identifying the muscle component, Marge B. was placed on the estradiol patch to stabilize fluctuations of estrogen 10 days before until 10 days after menses begins. And if she did not do well, she would be treated with prescription Danazol® twice daily for 25 days on and off for three. She did well and went on to win the national competition in her sport.

Her brother-in-law was not as fortunate. Paul B. had injured his neck in an automobile accident 15 years earlier. They called it whiplash and sent him to physical therapy for a period of 12 weeks. Better, he returned to work only to have occasional sharp jabbing pain in his neck. He tried hot showers, warm heat, exercises, topical Ben-Gay® ointment, and when the pain became more severe, Vicodin® pain pills. One Sunday, Dr. Lichten got a frantic call from Paul B.'s brother stating that his doctor had scheduled him today for an emergency MRI of the neck and shoulder and that the neurosurgeon was on call. What was the emergency, Dr. Lichten asked? "The smallest movement of my right arm gives me tearing pain from my shoulder to my head. And I mean terrible!"

So Paul B. came to the office, driven by his brother. Here was a 50-year-old somewhat overweight male holding his right forearm with his left arm to stabilize it. The slightest jar sent him writhing in pain. The presumptive diagnosis was a frozen shoulder.[21] So after getting the history, Dr. Lichten sat him down in the chair to palpate for trigger points in tender muscles and the respective dermatome innervated by the specific cervical nerves. This was performed after determining that the routine neurological and ophthalmologic examinations were normal.

He also had a head-forward position. Dr. Lichten asked what he did all day and he told he worked at a computer. He was tender over the greater occipital nerve (GON) on the right side of the back of the head, so this was injected first. He reported at least a 30% relief of the pain in his arm and the ability to move his fingers a little bit without pain. Dr. Lichten then palpated C6. It was exquisitely tender. So this was injected and an additional 30% of pain relief was noted. He was able to move his arm up and down without wincing. And then before proceeding, he injected the left GON and the C6. This did not make any difference in his pain.

Dr. Lichten next infiltrated the trapezoid and supraspinatus muscles that connect the neck and the shoulder girdle. This was helpful, in that the muscles were no longer in spasm but severe pain remained. Then Dr. Lichten positioned the patient so that he might pass the 2-inch-long needle behind his right scapula.[21] The injection went well, as the placement of the needle was performed without difficulty. And 100% of his shoulder pain was now gone.

Dr. Lichten was amazed, and when Paul B. shook his hand with that right hand, Dr. Lichten saw stars! It seems that the emergency MRI that was a prerequisite to surgery was no longer needed.

Dr. Lichten wondered if the results would be temporary or permanent. Paul B decided to avoid surgery and return for another series of blocks within the week. He had some tingling in his thumb that lingered and some pain with movement of his hand, but he was back to work and no longer needed pain medication. After the second block gave him complete relief, he came back for the third block two weeks later.

Paul B. has now gone back to golfing. Dr. Lichten can't say his game has improved but he was without a spinal fusion and the problems that cervical root surgery can bring. Paul B. became a good patient and follows the vitamin, mineral, and hormonal regimens that best serve his age. And he appreciated the fact that these blocks are AMA CPT-coded and reimbursable under normal conditions and normal health insurance plans.

GON blocks may relieve migraines, opthalmic migraines (with/ or without blindness), muscle contraction headaches, and some report even relief from cluster headaches.[20,23] They are very effective in the emergency room in differentiating migraine headaches from major neurological disorders. When Karen D. came in for a severe headache, she didn't get any relief from the GON, the accessory occipital nerve block, or the C6 block. Dr. Lichten asked her to get a second opinion with a neurologist that day and an MRI the next. The young neurologist said it was migraine, but the MRI showed a fracture at C5. The senior neurologist said he had seen this neck-fracture headache just twice before, and in both cases these women were doing headstands in yoga class. Karen D. scheduled cervical fusion with an orthopedic specialist in Philadelphia. She had an uneventful and pain-free recovery.

Then Karen D. was attacked by a student and thrown against a blackboard. Karen D. suffered a subdural hematoma and reinjured her neck. This time she was operated on locally, and there was not enough bone, so they transplanted some from her hip to support the fractured bone in her neck.

When Dr. Lichten next saw Karen D., she had a V-shaped defect in the back of her neck and intense daily headaches. Percodan® was not strong enough to relieve the pain, but she had refused the morphine prescriptions. Instead she saw Dr. Lichten and insisted that she receive the nerve blocks.

Physically, Karen D. was severely restricted. She could not rotate her neck to look toward her shoulder, and her head position was that of a woman in a collar. She could not or would not drop her chin down. So Dr. Lichten started with her in a sitting position.

The first blocks were in the GON and accessory nerves to relieve the tight band-like pain. Then Dr. Lichten proceeded down the V-shaped defect in her neck, always staying outside the V, where the muscle and scarring were still present. C4, C5, C6, and C7 were injected with standard Travell technique. Karen began to relax.

After completing the GON, accessory, and trigger-point injections, Karen D. had some mobility in her neck, both lateral and up and down. She was advised of the special blocks for the shoulder girdle and scapula and was willing to be injected.

The block on the left scapula worked magic, and Karen D. began to cry. "I have been in pain for eight months," she said, "and you made it completely go away."

After the three block series was completed, Karen D. is ready to return to teaching school. She had some recurrent pain, as is expected in her scarred neck. So she comes in every three months for blocks and injections of dilute BOTOX[24] in the occipital and neck regions. If needed, dilute BOTOX could be placed behind her scapula.[26] She had been told she would have to retire, but little miracles happen every day.

BOTOX®

The use of BOTOX® for headaches is a direct offshoot of these anesthetic blocks. BOTOX® is a muscle poison that is bio-identical to that produced by the bacterium *Clostridrium botulinum*. As such, it is not expected to find its way into the human body, as large doses could be fatal. But it is used in ophthalmology to rebalance weak eye muscles, which led Carruthers[25] to use it to paralyze frown lines. It has been FDA-approved for cosmetic uses since 1989. New applications and off-label drug use allow it to be used for additional medical as well as cosmetic indications.

Although there were reports of success with BOTOX® in both migraine and tension-type headaches, controlled studies show minimal improvement at best.[26] Lichten uses BOTOX® only in select patients who establish success with the anesthetic blocks yet whose results are not permanent or long-lasting. BOTOX® is commonly used in the occipital muscles and diluted for use in the neck, scapula, and other select muscle groups. Without a thorough knowledge of the anatomy, the anesthetic blocks, and the experience of clinical practice, BOTOX® remains an expensive and often less-than-ideal treatment modality for headache patients.

In Summary

The medical management of migraine and headache depends on incorporating two additional modalities: (1) hormonal modulation and (2) trigger-point injections. Although hormonal modulation is a keystone to the practices of gynecology, and trigger-point injections are a keystone to the practice of physical medicine, neither of these disciplines typically are involved in the treatment of the *whole* headache patient. Those who do treat the majority of headaches, neurologists and internists, are inherently fearful of hormonal modulation because of the extended responsibility for treating a woman's breakthrough bleeding should an estrogen imbalance occur. Since it is only the rare neurologist who routinely performs occipital nerve blocks or trigger-point injections, this leaves most headache doctors with a cacophony of prescriptions as their only option, garnering dubious benefits at best.

CLUSTER HEADACHES

The cluster headache is different, in that it is six times more prevalent in men, usually aged 20–40. There is no typical appearance, as some describe the sufferer as the large, red-faced, bulbous-nosed truck driver, and others as the compulsive executive. In either case, the most severe forms of these vascular, pounding headaches occur in clusters that occur up to eight times a day for weeks and then suddenly disappear. The attacks are often seasonal and will abruptly wake an individual out of a deep sleep.

Although much has been written about the contributing factors of alcohol intake, heavy smoking, air travel, bright lights, foods, and nitroglycerin, the true origin of cluster headaches has eluded physicians to date.

Personal Perspective

As his wife painfully described Paul T.'s episodes, "I have seen him trying to get to the bathroom with a pillow over his head and his whole body appearing to be tied in a ball; hitting his head against the wall, pulling on his hair and crying out to get anything to stop the pain. His face contorted and flushed red and his eye watering, so pitiful and so helpless. Why can't the doctors do more than give him shots of Demerol® and tell him the attacks will pass? Can he tolerate even one more attack or will he do himself permanent harm?"

Into Dr. Lichten's office came Paul T. one day. When asked what brought him to the office, he stated that he had severe headaches that were described by the neurologists as clusters. Having not seen such an individual before, Dr. Lichten asked him to describe the episodes. "I jump out of bed somewhere after 1:00 a.m. in such pain that I have hit my head against the wall to stop the pounding. It feels worse than a jackhammer going off; and it does not stop! The attack stops suddenly and then restarts, sometimes going in cycles for days or weeks. The medications do not work, and even Demerol® cannot stop the pain. If I didn't know they would stop, I would have jumped out of the window long ago."

Dr. Lichten's laboratory profile applies to all patients seen in the office. The profile for Paul T., this big truck-driving mountain man, showed a very low *testosterone* level at 197 ng/dl, coupled with an elevated *sex hormone-binding globulin* (SHBG). Needless to say, his free androgen index was even lower than most men at 80 years of age.

Dr. Lichten explained to Paul and his wife that the use of testosterone patches and even injections would bring an unwanted fluctuation to his already low testosterone. Dr. Lichten suggested use of the testosterone pellets monthly to keep the testosterone levels elevated above a threshold that might exist to precipitate the cluster. Since the drop in estradiol triggers the migraine in women, Dr. Lichten reasoned, the drop in testosterone below a specific threshold may trigger clusters in men. Paul and his wife agreed to the use of the FDA-approved bio-identical testosterone pellets.

Every month for three years, Paul returned regularly for his testosterone pellets. Then suddenly he disappeared for one year. When he returned he educated the doctor: In that three-year period, he was free from clusters, unheard of in his family. But he got lazy and within three months off the pellets was skewered by the renewed cluster attack. He vowed never to be without his testosterone pellets again.

Into Dr. Lichten's practice have come a few men and a woman with cluster headaches. Although the treatment with hormonal stabilization has been inconsistently beneficial to female patients with estradiol pellets, the few men have reported good success in preventing cluster attacks on testosterone pellets.

Again, a literature search confirmed the repeated observations that low testosterone levels are found in men and cluster headache.[27-29] Only Klimek[30] tried using oral and injectable testosterone to abort the migraine attack in 1985. He reports great success in reducing the number of attacks from 308 to 94 the second week and then to approximately 14. Yet no one else had established a protocol for using a stable testosterone milieu in men with cluster attacks. And when Dr. Lichten approached this topic with the ranking hierarchy of the Headache Society and others, the hormonal connection via the continuous release of testosterone from pellets was not considered seriously.

In researching this topic, there appears an article by Stillman in 2006 reported in *Headache*[31] that five of seven cluster-headache men achieved full remission within 24 hours on "pure" testosterone replacement. Stillman treated two women with testosterone and estradiol. It seems that the hormonal stability offered by testosterone replacement in men and testosterone and estradiol in women worked to abort these potentially life-threatening events.

With migraine attacks by definition now a hormonal event in women, and with cluster attacks being a suspected hormonal event in men, it behooves each physician who treats these individuals to understand the role of hormones.

Hormones are not just for reproduction. Hormones affect insomnia, muscle aching, Raynaud's, weight gain, fatigue, diabetes, heart disease, osteoporosis, and Alzheimer's disease to name but a few. It is time to add migraine and cluster to hormonal diseases and treat them as such.

PREFERRED PRIMARY MEDICATION THERAPIES FOR MIGRAINE AND TENSION HEADACHE

Medication **Generic Dosage/Frequency Quantity**
Ibuprofen OTC 200 mg/ 1–12 per day
Orudis® Ketoprofen 75 mg
Toradol® 10 mg 100
ketorolac injection 30 mg/ ml
Excedrin® limited use

Hormonal Modulation **Dosage/ frequency Quantity**
Danazol® 100–200 mg
Estradiol patch .1 mg
Aldactone® Spirolactone 100 mg/2x day
Neurotoxins
BOTOX® 100 IU

Anesthetic Pain Blocks for Chronic Tension and Cervicogenic Headaches

1. Greater occipital nerve block
2. Accessory occipital nerve block
3. Trigger-point injections
4. Supraspinatus and trapezoid triggers
5. Subscapular nerve block
6. Masseter nerve block
7. Sternocleidomastoid block
8. Sphenopalatine block

Simple, Relatively Safe Primary or Secondary Migraine-Headache Treatments Medication Over-the-Counter Dosage/Frequency Quantity

Aspirin 325 mg/ 1–6xday

Antinausea
Benadryl®
Periactin® cyproheptadine 4 mg
Atarax® hydroxyzine 25 mg
Vistaril® hydroxyzine 50 mg
Compazine® prochlorperazine 10 mg
Phenergan® promethazine 25 mg

Secondary Migraine-Headache Treatments
.

NSAID Medication Generic Dosage/Frequency Quantity
Ansaid® flurbiprofen 100 mg/1–3 daily
Toradol® keterolac 30 mg injection
Indocin® indomethacin 75 mg

Caffeine
Excedrin® 65 mg
Fiorinal® 50 butabarb
Plus codeine 30 codeine
Esgic® 50-500-40

Abortives
Cafergot® suppositories 1–100 mg
Midrin® 325-100-65
Bellergal-S® bellergal .6-40-.2
DHE-45® injection

5-HT1 Block
Imitex® sumatriptan 100 g/ 4x week
nasal 20 mg/act
Relpax® 40 mg
Zomig® oral/ nasal 5 mg
Zomig® Nasal 6.5 mg
Frova® 2.5 mg

Addicting & Pain Meds
Demerol® meperidine 50 mg
Stadol® butorphanol nasal10 mg /2.5ml
Percodan® 40-38-325
Nubain® 20 mg/ml 10ml $ 40.00
Methadone® 5 mg
Lidocaine® patch

Corticosteroids
Prednisone 10 mg

Blood Pressure Beta-Blockers
Inderal® propranolol 40 mg/ day
Tenormin® atenolol 50 mg
Lopressor metoprolol 50 mg
Toprol XL® 50 mg

ACE Inhibitor
Zestril® Lisinopril 10 mg

Calcium Channel Block
Calan® verapimil 80 mg
Catapres® clonidine .1 mg
Corgard® nadolol 40 mg

Seizure Meds
Depakote® 250 mg
Donnatal® phenobarbital 64.8 mg
Tegretal® carbamazepine 100 mg
Trileptal® 300mg
Topomax® 50 mg

Tricyclic Antidepressants
Tofranil® imipramine 25 mg
Elavil® amitriptyline

MAO Inhibitor
Marplan® 10 mg

S. Serotonin Reuptake Inhibitor
Prozac® Floroxitine 20 mg
Pazil® paroxetine 20 mg
Effexor® venlafaxine 37.5 mg
Wellbutren® bupropion 100 mg

Mineral Salt
Eskalith® lithium 450 mg

Excerpted from the National Headache Foundation medication index.

REFERENCES:

1. Wolff HG. *Headache and Other Head Pain*. 1950. Oxford University Press (3d ed), 1972.
2. Somerville BW. The role of estradiol withdrawal in the etiology of menstrual migraine. *Neurology*. 1972; 22:355–365.
3. Somerville BW. Estrogen-withdrawal migraine. II. Attempted prophylaxis by continuous estradiol administration. *Neurology*. 1975; Mar: 25 (3): 245–250.
4. Greenblatt RW, ed. *Menopausal Syndrome*. New York: Medcom Press, 1974:102–110.
5. Lichten EM. Efficacy of Danazol® in the Treatment of Hormonal Migraine. *Journal Reproductive Medicine*. 1991; 36(6):419–425.
6. Lichten EM, et al. The Use of Leuprolide Acetate in the Diagnosis and Treatment of Menstrual Migraine. The Role of Artificially Induced Menopause. *Headache Quarterly*. 1995; 6(4):313–317.
7. Lichten EM, Lichten JB. The confirmation of a biochemical marker for women's hormonal migraine: The depo-estradiol challenge test. *Headache*. 1996; 36(6):367–70.
8. Lichten EM. Estradiol Subcutaneous pellet for the definite diagnosis and treatment of hormonal migraine. *Cephalgia*. 1999; 19(4):332.
9. Lichten EM. *Menstrual Migraine in The Menopause*. Reid-Rowell Symposium, 1990.
10. Granella F. Treatment of Menstrual Migraine. *Cephalgia*. 1997; 17S(20):35–8.
11. Allais G. Advanced strategies of short-term prophylaxis in menstrual migraine: state of the art and prospects. *Neurologic Sciences*. 2005: 26 S(2):125–9.
12. Couch JR. The tension headache component of chronic daily headache. *Current Pain Headache Report*. 2004; 8(6):479–83.
13. Sjastaad O. "Cervicogenic" headache. An hypothesis. *Cephalgia*. 1983: 3(4):249–56.
14. Travell J, Simon D. *Trigger Points and Myofascial Pain and Dysfunction*. Lippincott Williams and Wilkins, 1998.
15. Sjaastad O. et al. Cervicogenic headache: diagnostic criteria. *Headache*. 1990; 20(11):725–6.
16. Pajaron E. The validity of the classification criteria of the International Headache Society for migraine, episodic tension headache and chronic tension headache. *Neurologia*. 1999; 14(6):283–8.
17. Antonaci F, Sjaastad O, et al. Cervicogenic headache: clinical presentation, diagnostic criteria and differential diagnosis. *Current Pain Headache Report*. 2001; 5(4):387–92.
18. Haldeman S, et al. Cervicogenic headaches: a critical review. *Spine Journal*. 2002; 2(2):162.
19. Afridi SK, et al. Greater occipital nerve injection in primary headache syndromes prolonged effects from a single injection. *Pain*. 2006; 122(1–2):126–9.
20. Naja ZM, et al. Repetitive occipital nerve blockade for cervicogenic headache: expanded case report of 47 adults. *Pain Practitioner*. 2006 ;6(4):278–84.
21. Jankovic D, et al. The frozen shoulder syndrome. Description of a new technique and five case reports using the subscapular nerve block and subscapularis trigger point infiltration. *Acta Anaesthesiology Belgium*. 2006; 57(2):137–43.
22. Chiodo A, et al. Cadaveric study of methods for subscapularis muscle needle insertion. *American Journal of Physical Medicine and Rehabilitation*. 2005; 84(9):662–5.
23. Scattoni L, et al. Great occipital nerve blockade for cluster headache in the emergency department: case report. *Headache Pain*. 2006; 7(2):98–100. Epub 2006.
24. Farinelli I, et al. Long-term benefits of botulinum toxin type A (BOTOX) in chronic daily headche: a five-year long experience. *Journal of Headache Pain*. 2006; 7(6):407–12.

25. Carruthers A, et al. Cosmetic uses of botulinum A exotoxin. *Advanced Dermatology.* 1989; 12:325–47.
26. Schulte-Mattler WJ, et al. Botulinum toxin therapy of migraine and tension-type headache: comparing different botulinum toxin preparations. *European Journal ofNeurology.* 2006; 13 S 1:51–4.
27. Kudrow L. Plasma testosterone levels in cluster headache preliminary results. *Headache.* 1976; 16(1):28–31.
28. Nelson RF. Testosterone levels in cluster and non-cluster migrainous headache patients. *Headache.* 1978; 18(5):265–7.
29. Klimek A. Plasma testosterone levels in patients with cluster headache. *Headache.* 1982; 22(4):162–4.
30. Klimek A. Use of testosterone in the treatment of cluster headaches. *European Neurology.*1985; 24(1):53–6.
31. Stillman M.J. Testosterone replacement therapy for treatment refractory cluster headache. *Headache.* 2006; 46(6): 925–33.

CHAPTER 9

HORMONE REPLACEMENT AND OSTEOPOROSIS

OSTEOPOROSIS

Prior to the 20th century, men and women had a life expectancy below 50 years of age.[1] With our economy being primarily based in agriculture until the end of Second World War, the high level of physical activity and work outdoors made osteoporosis a rare disease. If it weren't for the rare parathyroid tumor or untreated hyperthyroidism, the disease would not be predominantly placed in the textbooks of medicine. Today it is expected that 50% of all women will have an osteoporotic fracture during their lifetime.[2] Recent studies from Scandinavia imply that the rate of osteoporosis is increasing faster than expected, leading to an unprecedented increased risk of hip fracture and complications. Falch[3] and others are implying that environmental factors and increasing longevity are contributing to the prominence of this disease. Although it is primarily a disease of women, more and more older men are affected. In fact, one in four men will suffer a fracture from osteoporosis after 60 years of age. The direct and indirect cost of osteoporosis is $60 billion dollars per year in the United States.[4] Pulmonary embolism (thromboembolism) is the most common fatal complication due to hip and pelvic fracture. Of patients with a hip fracture who die, 38% die of pulmonary embolism.[5]

PHYSICAL FINDINGS

While there are forms of osteoporosis from disuse, such as when immobilized or wheelchair bound, the form that medical science is concerned about is called diffuse osteoporosis. This form affects all the bones of the body, though the skeletal and long bones are most affected. At first, X-rays show decreased density but in time there are diffuse small fractures, later followed by X-rays showing evidence of compression vertebral fractures. These are the individuals who are bent over as the fractured vertebrae in the back have collapsed and reshaped the back from straight up to hunched over. Both the long bones and the surface bone formation are affected. The pathophysiology is unknown but the body is absorbing bone faster than laying down new growth.

As the majority of osteoporosis patients are menopausal women, medical specialists divide up osteoporosis into type I and type II. Type I occurs earlier, and the osteoporosis is limited to the long bones and the spine. Type II applies to women who are usually older than 70, and the osteoporosis involves both the long bones (trabecular) and the cortical (surface). Type II is called senile osteoporosis.

The key to treating osteoporosis, and any disease in fact, is finding the cause. The risk factors are:[6]

1. Being female
2. Small, thin body with low BMI
   (body mass index lower than 19)
3. Postmenopausal
4. Family history of osteoporosis
5. Caucasian and Asia races
6. Abnormal absence of menstruation
7. Eating disorders: anorexia, bulimia
8. Long-distant runners
9. Low testosterone levels in men

10. Nutritional deficiencies: vitamin D, calcium
11. Inactive lifestyle
12. Smoking
13. Medications that lower natural hormones
    a. Glucocorticoids: prednisone, steroids for arthritis
    b. Luprolide acetate for endometriosis or heavy menstrual flow
    c. Seizure medications
    d. Aluminum-containing antacids
    e. Chemotherapy for cancer: multiple myeloma
    f. Excessive thyroid medication; thyroid or parathyroid disease
14. Surgical procedures and diseases that affect the gastrointestinal tract:
    a. Gastric bypass
    b. Colitis and Crohn's disease
    c. Cholecystectomy (gall bladder removal surgery)

Everyone needs to be concerned about osteoporosis. There is a simple, out-patient two-minute procedure that can directly measure the bone mineral density (BMD). It is called a dual-energy X-ray absorptiometry (DEXA) machine. With its computer attachments, an exact measurement of bone density is made and compared to thousands of normals. Although it is recommended to have the test at 65 years of age, it should be done at 50 years of age for any woman who has not been on estrogen replacement, weighs less than 127 pounds, is a smoker, eats poorly, and for those who have loose or flabby underarm skin.

The diagnosis of osteoporosis is based on how thin the hip and vertebral bones have become compared to normal values for your respective age. Osteopenia is when the bone density is less than 85% of normal; osteoporosis is when the bone density is less than 75% of normal.

The problem with medical treatment is that doctors wait until there is evidence of osteoporosis before prescribing medication. The pharmaceutical companies that make osteoporosis medications publish studies showing that their drugs decrease the risk of fractures. These drugs, however, have not consistently shown that they can thicken the bones or lay down new bones. The drugs are available at great costs. And the side effects of these drugs include not only severe indigestion but also rare, serious side effects.

Karen M. was Dr. Lichten's physical and massage therapist. An active woman who skied and sailed, she could work daily on six individuals for one hour daily. At 50 she was definitely in excellent physical shape. She walked with just the hint of a limp on her right. Little did Dr. Lichten know, until she sought out his medical expertise, that she had a problem with osteoporosis.

Karen M. had a congenital hip dysplasia from birth and already had five hip-replacement surgeries. At this time, her osteoporosis had been localized to her right hip. Osteoporosis was limited to a large defect of bone that was once surrounding the metal shaft placed in her upper leg (femur). The surgeons had stated that if it weren't for the muscles, the leg would literally "fall off." The surgeons wanted to perform surgery and replace the metal shaft with a much larger one. Karen M. was looking for another answer, as Dr. Lichten had shared with her some of his program's successes with individuals experiencing rapid healing, rapid postoperative recoveries, and maintenance of health well into their 90s. His recovery program consisted of balanced nutrition; comprehensive vitamins, minerals, and essential fatty acids; and prescription anabolic therapies. She was initially looking for a way to recover faster so she could return to work in a few weeks rather than a few months.

When Karen M. brought the X-ray pictures to Dr. Lichten, they were quite impressive. Imagine looking at a bull's eye target. The little black area in the center was the metal shaft, whereas the 5–10 times larger surrounding area was empty of bone! No wonder the surgeons wanted to perform surgery.

Karen M. had another idea after speaking about the risks of the procedure versus the risk of prescribing medication that could improve healing. She clearly understood that the body is a wondrous system that uses the hormone systems to grow, heal, and repair. As described previously the systems are:

Gland Hormone Function.
Vitamin D deposit of calcium in bone.
Pituitary human-growth-hormone-accelerated growth of bone in teen years.
Increased repair and regrowth of muscle/tissue.
Thyroid T3 accelerates Kreb's energy cycle.
Increases serum levels of testosterone and estrogen.
Ovary estrogen increases peripheral and central circulation, reproduction, and repair.
Ovary testosterone increases muscle mass, anabolic function.

Recognizing that the damage to the long bone of the right leg was probably not medically repairable, she started the anabolic program in hopes that it would build muscles prior to surgical intervention. This would be a conservative attempt to improve her leg muscles to hold her leg in place in anticipation of the planned surgery in four months. And the stronger leg muscles would reduce her pain as she tried to remain working in anticipation of a long period of recovery.

The problem with expectations is sometimes you can be wonderfully wrong. Not only did the anabolic-program mixture of high-dose vitamin D, DHEA, small doses of human growth hormone, and moderate doses of bio-identical testosterone make her muscles in her leg stronger, they eliminated her need for surgery: She was destined not to undergo orthopaedic surgery.

What happened was that the increase in circular muscle placed stress on the long bones. This is called cortical bone. But Dr. Lichten believes the longer muscles of the leg were actually placing a strong torque on the long bone, and this torque was the reason her long bones got thicker and stronger. By adding low-dose triiodothyronine (T3) and estrogen as a catalyst to the anabolic mix, Karen M. was able to reduce that white ring of empty space around her artificial hip shaft by two-thirds in six months. The doctors did not know what to say, but she and Dr. Lichten said, "Thank you." Miracles happen.

What is still surprising to Dr. Lichten and the older, more experienced doctors is that no one today seems to remember that testosterone and its more anabolic derivative, nandrolone, were the only therapy available for the elderly in the 1950s to the 1980s. Studies at major universities showed that estrogen and testosterone replacement were able to increase bone density.[7-10] Whether there is fear of the Women's Health Initiative and the implication that estrogens can cause cancer (see chapter 6) or a fear of testosterone causing facial hair growth, these simple hormonal treatments are, for some unknown reason, not offered to affected osteoporotic women.

MISSING BIOCHEMISTRY

Nearly thirty years ago, when Dr. Lichten was just out of residency, it was common knowledge that "treatment of osteoporosis with sex steroids or orally administered calcium with . . . vitamin D . . . arrested or slowed bone loss."[7]

The problems with the medical management of osteoporosis then and now is:

1. Peak bone mass is established in the first three decades of life through adequate nutrition and exercise.[13] Anorexia, extreme exercise, and smoking have negative impact on peak bone mass.
2. Surgical menopause leads to earlier evidence of osteoporosis. Similar concerns are avoidance of indicated estrogen replacement therapy.
3. Sex hormone replacement in the estrogen or testosterone-deficient patient can maintain, and in certain cases augment, skeletal mass and reduce fracture incidence.[14]
4. The route of administration may affect the risk-to-benefit ratio of estrogen on cardiovascular disease morbidity and mortality.[15]

Personal Perspective

The role of estrogen and osteoporosis in women is well established. There is a linear decline in bone mass at all key measurements with every decade after 50. The slope of this decline is less when estrogen replacement therapy (ERT) is part of the medical management.

There is also overwhelming medical science that testosterone has a role in the prevention and treatment of osteoporosis in both men and women.[12,14,20] Two of Dr. Lichten's long-term patients serve to delineate his personal perspective.

Darlene S. is well over 60 but feels and looks 20 years younger. She has been on a program of nutrition, exercise and appropriate hormone replacement for the past 15 years. Her medical regimen includes all the hormones described as anabolic, muscle-building, and necessary for life: vitamin D, thyroid, DHEA, estrogen, and testosterone. She is thin, sinewy, muscularly toned, and able to climb mountains while leaving 18- and 19-year-old teens way behind.

Darlene's BMI shows a bone density of a 20-year-old. It is right off the top of the chart. Considering that she went through menopause more than 25 years ago, her studies are proof that osteoporosis is in her case a preventable disease. The philosophy that runs throughout is that balanced nutrition, comprehensive vitamins, minerals, essential fatty acids, and bio-identical hormonal replacement with a program of exercise are key to wellness. And many of Dr. Lichten's patients live to realize that the best years of life may actually start at 50, 60, 70, or even later.

Mary W. is 74 years old and an Olympic swimmer. When Mary came to Dr. Lichten more than 25 years ago, she was inactive, unhappy, and suffering with a gynecologic problem that necessitated she enter surgical menopause. But after surgery, Mary began a program of nutrition, with extra vitamin D, thyroid replacement, DHEA, estrogen, and testosterone. Mary began to swim for fun. She entered competitions and won. She swam more. At 71 she swam across San Francisco Bay in a half wetsuit, winning with the best time for her division. Today, at 74, she routinely wins 10 swim-meet medals in national competition in 10 different swimming events. She has not had plastic surgery and has to fend off male lifeguards that are her grandchildren's ages. Personally, Dr. Lichten cannot imagine a five-hour, 10-kilometer swim, but it was a test that Mary completed with flying colors. And yes, her bone density is indistinguishable from a 20-year-old woman. Osteoporosis is a preventable disease.

THE ROUTE OF ADMINISTRATION

The difference between Darlene and Mary and the rest of the elderly women in the United States may be the means by which they get their estrogen replacement. In Dr. Lichten's office, he has not used Prempro® since the early 1970s because of complications and risk of associated cancer. Almost 20 years ago, Dr. Lichten began to use natural, bio-identical estradiol in crystalline pellets. These pellets are implanted every 1–2 months in the upper-outer quadrant of the buttocks. The procedure takes approximately 1–2 minutes, and there is no need to take oral estrogen, estrogen patches, or topical or vaginal creams for ERT. Not only does this method of treatment remove one more thing from a busy woman's daily schedule, but it is medically proven to be superior to any other ERT for the treatment of osteoporosis, as demonstrated in multiple studies.[17–19] A three-month pellet will soon be available.

The leading researchers of menopause in the world in the second half of the 20th century were the Studd-Whitehead group in England. Doctors referenced their textbook in residency training. Studd[20] stated in the prestigious *British Medical Journal* in 1988 the results of a nine-year follow-up study comparing ERT to an implant group given estrogen and testosterone implants:

"Subcutaneous oestrogen is more effective than oral eostrogen in preventing osteoporosis, probably owing to the more physiological (premenopausal) serum oestradiol concentrations achieved. It also avoids problems of compliance that occur with oral treatment."[21]

Studd was not concerned with the high levels of serum estradiol achieved with pellets as he measured the level of pituitary releasing hormones (FSH, LH) and had documented that all hormones had reached a balance comparable to premenopausal range. In a second study of another 110 women on estradiol and testosterone pellets for almost nine years, Studd measured total bone density at the spine and proximal femur (hip) and showed that the difference from controls were significant. Statistically significant correlation is a P value less than .05. These studies showed P less than .0001. And the increase in bone density was at every location that BMD could measure. Studd stated this in 1991 in *Obstetrics and Gynecology*, the premier U.S. peer-review journal.[22]

"Subcutaneous estradiol and testosterone prevent postmenopausal osteoporosis and maintain normal bone density for as long as treatment is continued."

And that is why Darlene and Mary have been treated by Dr. Lichten with bio-identical hormones of estradiol and testosterone and with pellets for the better part of their postmenopausal years.

A study was performed in Japan to compare oral treatments

in women with senile osteoporosis. Four treatment groups were identified: (1) control (no treatment); (2) vitamin D; (3) Premarin® .325 for three weeks on, one week off; and (4) pregnenolone, androstenedione, androstenediol, testosterone, estrone, and thyroid. Considering the BMD measurements at the start of the study to be individually 100%, after 24 months group 1 had a BMD that was 96% of baseline; groups 2 and 3 showed transient improvement and return to baseline, while group 4 (with testosterone) showed a 12% increase in BMD when compared to group 1.[23]

When a study of micronized estradiol-E2 and micronized testosterone was performed in the United States, the conclusion was that "Sublingual micronized HRT favorably decreases serum and urine markers of bone metabolism, prevents bone loss, and results in a slight increase in spine and hip bone mineral density. Although the addition of testosterone to HRT for 1 year did not result in added benefit to the spine bone mineral density, it did result in a significant increase in hip bone mineral density. Longer duration of therapy may have further improved these outcomes."[24]

Again, a treatment program that includes all the anabolic hormones showed improvement in bone mineral density in women. Not only can loss of bone mineral density be avoided, but increases in bone mineral density in critical areas can be demonstrated.

THE PROBLEM

As outlined in Chapter 6, on women and menopause, the Women's Health Initiative (WHI) has scared women away from taking hormone replacement during menopause. Remembering that 98% of women's deaths occur from some other disease than breast cancer, the omission of estrogen replacement therapy throws women directly through death's door. Estrogen deficiencies have been closely tied to the development of heart disease, osteoporosis, Alzheimer's disease, and other forms of chronic diseases. The mistaken perspective of the pharmaceutical companies that backed WHI physicians is that they believe that any estrogen, even conjugated horse urine, should be able to reverse these diseases-related deficiencies.

Obviously, estrone is not estradiol and Premarin® (conjugated equine estrogen) is not a purely bio-identical estrogen. Obviously

MPA-Provera® is not Aygestin®, and neither is bio-identical progesterone—period.

From the Women's Health Initiative, it is obvious that the addition of MPA Provera® is linked to the high number of breast cancer cases. This does not occur in either the second part of the WHI[25] study, in which treatment of postmenopausal women occurred without Provera®, or the GPRD study, where Aygestin® was substituted for MAP-Provera® in Britain. In fact, medroxy-progesterone acetate (MPA) is overwhelmingly the statistical carcinogen.

The government, or those interpreting the data, made broad assumptions that "estrogen is estrogen" and mandated that all estrogen manufacturers acknowledge the risks of the WHI study and apply a "black box warning" to their products. As outlined previously, Premarin® is conjugated equine estrogens (CEE) from pregnant mare urine and predominantly estrone (E1).

Estradiol (E2) is the bio-identical hormone of reproductive women and it is present in Estrace® oral tablets and Estrace® vaginal cream. E2 is the only hormonal ingredient in the Climara® and Vivelle® estradiol patch. Premarin®/CEE products as predominantly estrone (E1) are not identical to estradiol (E2) products; they contain completely different chemical compositions. Proof of breast cancer and heart disease risks have not been clearly defined for estradiol-only products. In another analysis of the GPRD study, evaluation of estrogen-only CEE women showed a 50% drop in risk of cardiovascular disease on estrogen alone.[26] They showed some slight increase in both breast cancer and colon cancer.

The key to prevention of osteoporosis and other medically associated diseases of aging women starts with the replacement of bio-identical estradiol (E2) and testosterone.

Furthermore, Davis[27] from Australia writes that women need to be aware that their drop in testosterone occurs well before menopause. When supplementary estrogen is administered, whether it be oral contraceptives or ERT for menopause, there is a concurrent decrease in bio-available testosterone. Testosterone administration can lead to increases in a number of scientifically measureable parameters of sexuality and anabolic effects on bone. They do not adversely affect lipids, especially when given parenterally (implants).[27] Testosterone administration can lead to increases in a number of parameters of sexuality, probably by direct neural effects. Androgens also have anabolic effects on bone, and do not adversely affect lipids, especially when given parenterally.[27]

Yet, even among women using ERT for a mean of 60 months, there was osteoporosis. In fact, half of those with osteoporosis and half of those with risk factors for cardiovascular disease in a large Australian population have used ERT.2[18] ERT alone is not enough to prevent or slow the development of osteoporosis.

And based on the long-term studies of Studd, using pellets that avoid the enzymatic conversion of hormonal applications to the skin may be the best proven methodology for the replacement of estradiol and testosterone. It is just that these studies by Studd[31-32] with pellets and others with micronized hormones[33-34] were predominately performed outside the United States[19-27] and unbiased by pharmaceutically supported studies.

It is true that some women will develop small amounts of facial hair and rarely a deepening voice on androgen therapy.[28] The diuretic spirolactone blocks the enzymatic conversion of testosterone to dihydrotestosterone, which is hormonally responsible for hirsutism and deepening voice. It can be used concurrently with hormonal therapy. It is limited to those individuals who do not have a sulfa allergy.

There are other forms of testosterone that are available in the United States that are FDA-approved and available to treat only men. Treatment of women, however, is an off-label use, as the FDA does not readily recognize testosterone as an appropriate treatment for women for any medical disease. Although the testosterone patch Intrinsa® has found great acceptance in Europe, it was vetoed by the FDA from distribution this year.[29] The complete list of testosterone and estradiol products appears in chapter on menopause (6), and the chapter on andropause (11).

OSTEOPOROSIS IN MEN

Osteoporosis is no longer a disease only of women. As Ybarra[30] has pointed out, "a significant percentage of men are at risk of developing osteoporosis. As testosterone begins to decrease with age, risk of osteoporosis dramatically increases as it does in postmenopausal women."

Statistically, 15–20% of all men will, by the time they are 80, have sustained a forearm, a (back) vertebral body, or femoral neck fracture (hip). Bone-mass loss starts at about the age of 35 and may be regulated by race, hereditary, physical activity, hormonal factors, and mineral intake during the formative childhood and adolescent years.[32]

Secondary risk factors include:

1. Glucocorticoid use (prednisone and corticosteroids)
2. Hypogonadism
3. Smoking and alcoholism[31]
4. Skeletal metastases and multiple myeloma
5. Gastric surgery, antacids, anticonvulsant therapy, sedatives, and sleeping pills
6. Warfarin (Coumadin®) blood thinners and vitamin K deficiency

The problem with osteoporosis in men is that 1.5 million men have osteoporosis at age 65 and another 3.5 million are at risk. It has become apparent that men have a higher mortality secondary to pulmonary emboli from hip fractures, and yet the risk factors for men have not been clearly defined.[33]

In a German study that followed up on the treatment of both primary and secondary hypogonadism in men with add-back testosterone for up to 16 years, it was observed that as serum levels of testosterone increased in the first year to the normal range, the maximum increase in BMD was observed. They stated, however, that "in hypogonadal men BMD can be normalized and maintained in the normal range by continuous, long term testosterone substitution."[34]

When testosterone levels are determined in men with vertebral crush fractures, 20% or more are found to be clearly hypogonadal in one study[35] using the FAI model measurement. The biochemistry of hypogonadal osteoporosis is the same as that for women: lack of the gender-specific hormone is associated with increased bone resorption and decrease in mineralization —both are reversed in men with the addition of testosterone.[34]

The measurements of hypogonadism have changed, and it is more likely that 100% of these men with fractures will have a low free androgen index (FAI) as described by D.C. Anderson[36] and explained in detail in chapter 11, on andropause (male menopause). In all men with chronic disease, and chronic disease represents a strong risk factor for osteoporosis, researchers find evidence of a low FAI.

Let it be said that a testosterone level in a male under 450 ng/dl, the presence of a total estradiol greater than 30 pg/ml, and a sex hormone binding globulin greater than 20 nmol/liter are evidence of a predisposed hypogonadal state. But it is ludicrous to wait until there is a bone fracture to treat. The UK commission suggests treating when the BMD is 1 SD, one standard derivation below the mean for the age. This finds the individual's measurements are in the bottom 16% of individuals matched for age and sex.[45] To Dr. Lichten's way of thinking, this is waiting too long, and he believes treatment must begin when the individual falls below the 75% profile for optimal testosterone levels. Testosterone replacement should begins whenever there is clinical manifestations of hypogonadism, as it is just a matter of time until heart disease, diabetes, and osteoporosis will be manifested. Based on the FAI, Dr. Lichten ascribes to the theory that any free testosterone index less than 0.6 needs to be treated.

GROWTH HORMONE

In the context of reversing signs and symptoms of aging, many people are now aware of the breakthrough work of Rudman in 1991 with human growth hormone.[37] Rudman showed that hGH substitution increased muscle strength, reduced skin wrinkles, and improved the ability to get up and out of a chair and be self-sufficient. Jocenhovel[38] showed that acromegalic men and women had greater density of cortical bone and increased osteocalcin levels (bone turnover). He suggested that "observable increase of bone mineral density in acromegaly suggests a potential use for GH in treating osteoporosis."[38]

Another interesting example of the unrecognized correlation of hGH and bone density was discovered by Barrett-Connor, one of the leading epidemiologists of our time. She found[39] there was a very strong statistical correlation between IGF-1 (measurement correlates to growth hormone) and BMD in postmenopausal women. The statistic was overwhelming as growth hormone was uniquely effective for women and testosterone had a direct effect on men's osteoporosis. "The striking gender difference has not been described previously. Its etiology is unknown. The answer could lead to improved understanding of gender differences in osteoporosis and in response to treatment with IGF-I or growth hormone."[39]

Dr. Lichten's experience with Karen, Darlene, and Mary serve to make the point: Osteoporosis is a treatable and reversible disease. But most of all, it is a preventable disease.

MEASURE THE HORMONAL BLOOD VALUES

REGULARLY take high-potency vitamin-mineral supplements.
REPLACE the missing bio-identical hormones.
TELL your doctor what improvements you have been able to document.
REPEAT the laboratory tests to make sure you are within the normal range.

We need to apply this same logic to men. "The beneficial effects of hormone replacement in nonelderly hormone-deficient individuals and in postmenopausal women raised hope that hormone substitution might prevent or even reverse some of the symptoms of male aging."[40]

PRESCRIPTION MEDICATION

In the field of osteoporosis, there are two natural hormone preparations available commercially. The first is calcitonin, which is extracted from salmon. It is indicated for postmenopausal women who are more than five years into menopause and refuse or cannot take estrogen. Clinical studies show that calcitonin increased bone-mineral density in the forearm, femoral (leg) bone, and lumbar spine. Being that this medication is a natural hormone, and without any significant complications, this is a prescription medication that Dr. Lichten will recommend in addition to the above natural hormonal replacement.

The commercial production of parathyroid hormone is another natural hormone for the treatment of osteoporosis. Both medications improve matrix bone formation and have less effect on cortical bone formation. Because of the potential for electrolyte fluctuation on PTH, prescription and management are left to those doctors who often prescribe these pharmaceutical agents.

OSTEOPOROSIS PRESCRIPTION MEDICATIONS DELINEATED TO SECONDARY STATUS

Product Generic Dosage/Frequency Quantity
Miacalcin® calcitonin 200 u/act daily nasal spray
Forsteo® parathyroid hormone 20 mg/80 ml
injection 1 injection

Osteoporosis Prescription Medications Delineated to Tertiary Status

Product Generic Dosage/Frequency Quantity
Fosomax® alendronate 10 mg
Boniva® 150 mg
Actonel® 30 mg

REFERENCES:

1. http://www.cdc.gov/nchs/data/hus/tables/2003/03hus027.pdf.
2. Melton LJ 3rd, Kan SH. Frye MA., et al. Epidemiology of vertebral fractures in women. *American Journal of Epidemiology.* 1989; 129:1000–11.
3. Falch JA, et al. Epidemiology of hip fractures in Norway. *Acta Orthopaedic Scandanavia.* 1985;56:12–6.
4. Holbrook TL. et al. The frequency of occurrence, impact and cost of selected musculoskeletal conditions in the United States. Chicago: *American Academy of Orthopaedic Surgeons,* 1984.
5. Merck Manual of Geriatrics: Section 2. Falls, Fractures, and Injury; Chapter 22. Fractures http://www.merck.com/mkgr/mmg/sec2/ch22/ch22a.jsp
6. ibid.
7. Riggs BL. Postmenopausal and senile osteoporosis: current concepts of etiology and treatment. *Endocrinology Japan.* 1979; S:31–41.
8. Weinerman SA, et al. Medical Therapy of Osteoporosis. *Orthopedic Clinics of North America.* 1990;21(1):109–24.
9. Lufkin EG, Ory S. Estrogen Replacement Therapy for the Prevention of Osteoporosis. *American Family Physician.* Sept. 1989.
10. Savvas N, Studd JW, et al. Skeletal effects of oral estrogen compared with subcutaneous oestrogen and testosterone in postmenopausal women. *British Medical Journal.* 1988;297(6644):331–3.
11. Garnett J, Studd J, et al. A cross-sectional study of the effects of long-term percutaneous hormone replacement therapy on bone density. *Obstetrics and Gynecology.* 1991;78(6):1002–7.

12. Shiraki M, et al. The effect of estrogen and, sex-steroids and thyroid hormone preparation on bone mineral density in senile osteoporosis—a comparison study of the effect of 1 alpha-hydroxy-cholecalciferol (I1 alpha-OHD3) on senile osteoporosis. *Nippon Naibunpi Gakkai Zasshi*. 1991; 67(2):84–95.

13. Weinerman SA, Bockman RS. Medical therapy of osteoporosis. Orthop Clin North Am. 1990 Jan;21(1):109-24.

14. Miller BE, et al. Sublingual administration of micronized estradiol and progesterone with and without micronized testosterone: effect on biochemical markers of bone metabolism and bone mineral density. *Menopause*. 2000;7(5): 318–26.

15. Hulley SB, et al. The WHI Estrogen-Alone Trial- Do Things Look Any Better? *Journal of the American Medical Association*. 2004; 291:1769–71.

16. Tannen RL. Estrogen affects postmenopausal women differently than estrogen plus progestin replacement therapy. *Human Reproduction* 2007. March 8: Epub.

17. Davis SR. Use of androgens in postmenopausal women. *Current Opinion in Obstetrics and Gynecology*. 1997;9(3):177– 80.

18. MacLennan AH, et al. Hormone replacement therapies in women at risk of cardiovascular disease and osteoporosis in South Australia in 1997. *Medical Journal of South Australia*. 1999;170(11):524–7.

19. Studd JW, Holland EF, Leather AT, et al. The dose-response of percutaneous oestradiol implants on the skeletons of postmenopausal women. *Br J Obstet Gynaecol*. 1994 Sep;101(9):787-91.

20. Studd J, Savvas M, Waston N, et al. The relationship between plasma estradiol and the increase in bone density in postmenopausal women after treatment with subcutaneous hormone implants. *Am J Obstet Gynecol*. 1990 Nov;163 (5 Pt 1):1474-9.

21. Holland EF, Leather AT, Studd JW. The effect of 25-mg percutaneous estradiol implants on the bone mass of postmenopausal women. *Obstet Gynecol*. 1994 Jan;83(1):43-6.

22. Holland EF, Chow JW, Studd JW, et al. Histomorphometric changes in the skeleton of postmenopausal women with low bone mineral density treated with percutaneous estradiol implants. *Obstet Gynecol*. 1994 Mar;83(3):387-91.

23. Holland EF, Leather AT, Studd JW. Increase in bone mass of older postmenopausal women with low mineral bone density after one year of percutaneous oestradiol implants. *Br J Obstet Gynaecol*. 1995 Mar;102(3):238-42.

24. Khastgir G, Studd J, Holland N, et al. Anabolic effect of estrogen replacement on bone in postmenopausal women with osteoporosis: histomorphometric evidence in a longitudinal study. *J Clin Endocrinol Metab*. 2001 Jan;86(1):289-95.

25. Savvas M, Studd JW, Norman S, et al. Increase in bone mass after one year of percutaneous oestradiol and testosterone implants in post-menopausal women who have previously received long-term oral oestrogens. *Br J Obstet Gynaecol*. 1992 Sep;99(9):757-60.

26. Garnett T, Studd J, Watson N, et al. A cross-sectional study of the effects of long-term percutaneous hormone replacement therapy on bone density. *Obstet Gynecol*. 1991 Dec;78(6):1002-7.

27. Vashisht A, Studd JW. Five-year changes in bone density, and their relationship to plasma estradiol and pretreatment bone density, in an older population of postmenopausal women using long-term estradiol implants. *Gynecol Endocrinol*. 2003 Dec;17(6):463-70.

28. Kirschner MA. Hirsutism and virilism in women. *Specific Topics in Endocrinology and Metabolism*. 1984;6:55–93.

29. Tsao A. Can Intrinsa Be a Viagra for Women? *Business Week*. October 28, 2004.

30. Ybarra J, et al. Osteoporosis in men: a review. *Nursing Clinics of North America*. 1996; 31(4):805–14.

31. Fujiwara S. Etiology and epidemiology of osteoporosis in men] *Clin Calcium.* 2006 Mar;16(3):444-8. Review.
32. Eastell R, et al. Management of male osteoporosis: report of the UK Consensus Group. *Q. Journal of Medicine.* 1998;81(2):71–92.
33. Siddiqui NA, et al. Osteoporosis in older men: discovering when and how to treat it. *Geriatrics.* 1999; 54(9):20–2, 27–8, 30 passim.
34. Behre HM, et al. Long-term effect of testosterone therapy on bone mineral density in hypogonadal men. *Clinical Endocrinology and Metabolism.* 1997;82(8):2386–90.
35. Scane ASC, et al. Osteoporosis in men. *Baillieres Clinical Rheumatology.* 1993; 7(3):589–901.
36. Anderson DC. Sex Hormone Binding Globulin Is an Oestrogen Amplifier. *Nature.* 1972;240:38–40.
37. Rudman D, Feller AG, Nagraj HS, et al. Effects of human growth hormone in men over 60 years old. *N Engl J Med.* 1990 Jul 5;323(1):1-6.
38. Jokenhovel F. Differential presentation of cortical and trabecular peripheral bone mineral density in acromegaly. *European Journal of Medical Research.* 1996; 1(8):377–82.
39. Barrett-Connor E, Goodman-Gruen D. Gender differences in insulin-like growth factor and bone mineral density association in old age: the Rancho Bernardo Study. *J Bone Miner Res.* 1998 Aug;13(8):1343-9.
40. Hermann M. Berger P. Hormonal changes in aging men: a therapeutic indication. *Experimental Gerontology.* 2001;36(7):1075–82.

NOTES

CHAPTER 10

PUTTING IT ALL TOGETHER

There have been many stories about patients and their recoveries in this book: There was Jodi with intractable menstrual pain, Denise with PMS monthly seizures, Karen with atypical migraine and a broken neck, Paul with nearly suicidal clusters, Dennis with rapid healing from hip surgery, and of course Anthony, who changed the course of medical treatment for diabetes. Each patient visit, and Dr. Lichten is now well over his 150,000th physician-patient interaction, brings a new level of knowledge and understanding to both the doctor and his patient. The science of medicine begins with an observation, and the greatest part of that is what the patient tells the doctor about his perceived illness. This is called "taking a history," and this takes more than three minutes allocated in the clinic. It takes not only time but also trust. And trust takes a delicate interplay between two equal human beings who have a common goal: improved health.

Dr. Lichten has always rejected the concept that a physician cannot invade a patient's space. But when the patient is reaching out for life and health, to barricade oneself behind a desk appears to the patient as an insurmountable wall. Dr. Lichten will sit on a stool and meet the patient face-to-face. He will shake his or her hand. He will draw the blood and take the blood pressure, listen to the heart and lungs, and check the thyroid for enlargement. He will touch the patient to determine exactly where the pain is reported. He will answer the telephone calls and the e-mails. And more than once, he will gratefully receive a holiday card and appreciate a spontaneous hug from a most satisfied patient.

If only, Dr. Lichten says, we all could do more.

And then, in the summer of 1999, on a Monday morning at 8:30, to be exact, a 16-year-old pixie young girl, 4'6" in height, came to Dr. Lichten's office. She had the brightest shine in her eyes and no hair. After she put her hand braces to the side, she positioned herself on the examination table and looked intently into his eyes and smiled! Surprised by her self-assuredness and her ability to get around unaffected, Dr. Lichten was more surprised by her first statement, "Are you the doctor that is going to make me well?" "I will do my best and try" was his response.

For C.G. had been a normal sprite of a girl, blonde, blue eyed, and weighing barely 22 pounds at two years of age. But then at age four, she had a double whammy: first she contracted a central nervous system complication and coma for a week from a routine vaccination, and then, after recovering from that, she fell against a piece of furniture and sent a splinter of her shattered nasal cartilage into her pituitary stalk. For whatever reason, she started to lose her hair and get weak and sickly. And all these maladies happened within months of the vaccination and the fall. Her mother had taken her to 17 university professors from east to west coast.

Some looked at the hair loss, for which they had no answer. Some looked to the muscle weakness and wanted to treat her for lupus, connective tissue disease, or even muscular dystrophy. No one addressed the fatigue that was forcing C.G. to sleep for more than 14 hours per day. There were no answers to a weakened immune system that was leaving her open to infections. And with the recommendations of methotrexate, 5-FU for skin lesions, and high-dose steroids, her mother did the right thing —she moved the family to Southern California, where the consistently warm weather minimized the havoc forced upon C.G. by a changing environment. And mother never gave up. She made CG self-sufficient and never once commented about her loss of hair, although every other concerned individual had C.G. wondering if she was dying of cancer or some other deadly disease.

On the Friday before the fateful visit to Dr. Lichten, while readying for a move back to Michigan, C.G.'s mother wondered if hGH was a possible answer to C.G.'s small stature and weakened immune system. She had made an appointment to see Dr. Lichten just four days before her move back to Michigan.

So, surprised by C.G.'s directness, Dr. Lichten returned to the problems at hand. "All diseases that are not genetic, I believe are affecting the endocrine system. The endocrine system has six major glands, and any major disruption of these glands results in an imbalance and illness. It is a physician's responsibility to first correct these imbalances and then address whatever disorders persist. And hGH is one of them."

The endocrine glands and their associated medical symptoms and normal range of blood tests have appeared previously:

INITIAL LABORATORY ASSESSMENT

GLAND- LOCATION	SYMPTOMS	HORMONE MEASUREMENT
Pineal- hypothalamus	Insomnia, mineral deficiency	Vitamin D 0,25 OH
Pituitary- cortex	Growth Hormone deficiency	IGF-1 (insulin like growth factor –1)
Thyroid- neck	Cold hands, feet, lethargy	T3 and T4 free, TSH, T3r
Adrenal- abdomen	Severe Fatigue, skin changes	DHEA and cortisol
Ovaries- abdomen	No menstrual period, no secondary sex changes, a.k.a. pubic hair, breast buds, etc.	Estrogen Progesterone Testosterone
Pancreas- abdomen	Diabetes, obesity	Insulin

1. C.G. did not get adequate sunlight, as seen with her lily-white, almost albino, thin skin.
2. C.G. did not have adequate human growth hormone, as demonstrated by many fine wrinkles over her face, neck, and forehead. Her small stature and poor immunity were a major cause of her disease state, affecting thyroid, adrenal, and her childlike body development.
3. C.G. had cold hands and cold feet and a low body temperature, as she preferred the weather in California.

4. C.G. had extreme fatigue and needed to nap for hours every afternoon. Her fatigue prevented her from even studying at home.
5. C.G. had no evidence of puberty, as she was well into her teen years without development of any secondary sexual traits typical of her gender and age.

The laboratory tests were drawn and the following interpretations were noted:

GLAND- HORMONES	NORMAL RANGE	LABORATORY	LABORATORY PATIENT'S VALUE
Pineal- hypothalamus	Vitamin D 0,25 OH	20-200 ng/mL	35
Pituitary- cortex	Insulin like growth factor –1	182-780 ng/mL	114
Thyroid- neck	TSH T3Free T4 Free: reverse T3: Thyroid antibodies Thyroid Peroxidase antibody	0.4- 5.50 miu/L 230-420 pg/dL 0.8-1.8 ng/dL 0.19-0.46 ng/mL <20 iu/mL <35 iu/mL	5.6 245 1.1 0.25 <20 <20
Adrenals	DHEA Cortisol	45-320 mcg/dL 4- 22 mcg/dL	84 4
Ovaries- abdomen	FSH LH Estrogen Progesterone Testosterone Sex Hormone Binding	2.5- 10.2 miu/mL 1.9– 12.5miu/mL 50-480 pg/mL pg/mL 20- 76 ng/dL 17-120 nmol/L	4 2.5 35 0.3 <20 <78
Pancreas- abdomen	Insulin Hemoglobin A1c		<2 5.2

So, organ by endocrine organ, the team of patient, mother, and physician organized a medical plan to stabilize and improve each item. The medical plan was to replace all six endocrine hormone systems at the same time and adjust the replacement amounts based on symptomatology and patient compliance. By educating the patient and mother to what was the importance of each system, Dr. Lichten could coordinate all the hormone actions, and monthly visits would be punctuated by frequent telephone calls.

1. C.G. was placed on vitamin D to increase serum levels of vitamin D3, using 1–2 drops (2,000-4,000 IU) each night. She was to take the vitamin D at bedtime and every night. At this dosage, 2,000–4,000 IU per night, Dr. Lichten has not seen side effects.
2. C.G. was placed on human growth hormone and began 1.0 IU per day at night. Because the dosage used for children is much higher than for adults, the dose would be increased to 2 IU per day for the first 30–90 days before titrating down to 1.0 IU/per day. The limiting factor would be side effects of swelling in the hands/carpal tunnel or worsening arthritis. With the IGF-1 levels in normal range and no symptoms, the treatment with hGH for short statue and true hypopituitarism would continue for years.
3. C.G. was placed on Armour Thyroid® 1 grain in the morning. After one month, she still had low basal body temperature, and her thyroid values were still in the normal suppressed range. Therefore, Dr. Lichten added 0.50 mcg of synthetic thyroid. The body temperature did increase 0.5 degrees. There were no further increases in thyroid medication, as the patient could not tolerate additional compounded T3, Armour Thyroid®, or synthetic thyroid.
4. C.G. was placed on DHEA. She developed acne and was offered 7-keto DHEA instead. 7-Keto DHEA was compounded, and the dosage of 25 mg in the morning was too much. She took 10–20 mg in the morning and 10 mg in the afternoon, along with the split dose of thyroid.
5. C.G. was placed on natural cortisol, Cortef® 10 mg. She increased her dosage from 10 mg in the morning and 5 mg in the afternoon to 30–40 mg in the morning and 10 mg as needed in the afternoon. As she had no stimulation to a working adrenal cortex, a form

of central Addison's disease, the patient learned that failure to take her natural cortisol would leave her listless and medically stressed. She adapted herself to this regimen completely and her school days became almost routine.

6. C.G. was placed on oral contraceptives to supply estrogen to prime her body for bone growth and normal pubescent development. In time, she developed breast buds and a true womanly figure.

7. C.G. was placed on lupron acetate to keep the epiphyses (ends of bones) from fusing closed before she had reached optimal height. Under the care of the pediatric endocrinologist, she gained almost eight inches in height.

It was fortunate that the family had sought out Dr. Lichten. As C.G.'s mother would relate, she had seen the chairmen of endocrinology at the local university and had traveled to so many facilities in the United States and Europe, where she had been given no help, yet growth hormone alone had measured so low. C.G.'s mother had heard so many times that "we don't do that" that she was belatedly elated that Dr. Lichten had offered that treatment first.

Follow-up laboratory testing every few months for the next six years found normal levels of these six hormone systems paired with relief from symptoms and a positive response: normal blood levels, relief of symptoms, normal deep sleep, tissue repair, warm hands, no fatigue, no prediabetes, and normal secondary sexual characteristics, except, in this case, no body hair. But Dr. Lichten knew that life had become more normal after C.G. began having regular menstrual periods and her mother reported episodes of PMS. Dr. Lichten discussed this with C.G. who agreed to a change in birth control to a lower-dose pill, one with a mild diuretic, and then three-month packaging without monthly menses. This worked well.

Follow-up laboratory values after six years is as follows. Note that the very high levels for T3, T4, DHEA-sulfate, and cortisol are after ingestion of the hormones that morning. Normal values were seen at half these values after not taking medication for 24 hours.

GLAND- HORMONES	NORMAL RANGE	NORMAL VALUES LABORATORY	LABORATORY / PATIENT'S VALUE
Pineal- hypothalamus	Vitamin D 0,25 OH	20-200 ng/mL	35---> 61
Pituitary- cortex	Insulin like growth factor −1	182-780 ng/mL	114---> 289
Thyroid- neck	TSH T3Free T4 Free: reverse T3: Thyroid antibodies Thyroid Peroxidase ab	0.4- 5.50 miu/L 230-420 pg/dL 0.8-1.8 ng/dL 0.19-0.46 ng/mL <20 iu/mL <35 iu/mL	5.6 --> 0.1 L 245 --> 660 H 1.1 -> 4.8 H 0.25--> 0.83 H <20--> <20 <20--> <20
Adrenals	DHEA Cortisol	45-320 mcg/dL 4- 22 mcg/dL	84--> 702 H 4--> 85 H
Ovaries- abdomen	FSH LH Estrogen Progesterone Testosterone Sex Hormone Binding	2.5- 10.2 miu/mL 1.9– 12.5 miu/mL 50-480 pg/mL pg/mL 20- 76 ng/dL 17-120 nmol/L	4--> 0.7 L 2.5--> 0.2 L 35--> 28 L 0.3 <20--> 60 <78--> 89
Pancreas- abdomen	Insulin Hemoglobin A1c	0-25 miu/mL <6	< 2 5.2--> 5.3

A HAPPY CONTINUING STORY

As Dr. Lichten tells the story, this young lady went on to academic heights never before realized. She graduated from the International Academy in Michigan with seven advanced courses, she went on to the highly ranked University of Michigan to graduate in a little over two years with a degree in biology, and then she entered medical school just before turning 20 years of age. Not once has she ever complained about her fate or her hair, and she is very much the young lady and responsible adult. Not only does she go back to help supervise at the biology/chemistry scientific fraternity, but she organizers special events for children with alopecia throughout the year. Her achievements in medical school, where she is on average five years younger than her classmates, puts her near the top of her class with numerous honors. In fact, she told Dr. Lichten, soon after he became her doctor, that she would be a doctor who would be there to take over Dr. Lichten's mantra: She, too, would treat patients to make them well. And with a deep sense of honor, he says, "I know she will. I couldn't be more proud of her if I were her father." And in a sense, he truly is.

PROLOGUE

And to the age-old question "If a tree falls in the woods and no one is there to hear it, does it make a sound?" Dr. Lichten answers, "Only if you out there to hear it." Medicine and health care can change if you raise your voices over and over again. Medicine can change if you choose to take better care of your bodies and their natural, life-giving hormone systems. Yes, you can live longer and better with proper nutrition. But remember to trust only true science and your best judgment. Advertisers don't care."

BOOK THREE

THE ROLE *of* NATURAL TESTOSTERONE

CHAPTER 11

MALE ANDROPAUSE

"I never thought a man went through men-pause," I would have said at any age before I hit 45. "Men are virile, men are strong, men fight dragons and don't worry about getting old."

But the truth is that men do age, men cannot fight time forever, and every single man will go through a drop in their life-giving hormone *testosterone*. With the state of the world today, the environmental poisons called xenoestrogens and the estrogen-like pellets injected into our food stock, men will fade faster and die earlier.

Historical Perspective

Until the second half of the 20th century, the level of testosterone in the blood was not often measurable. Although testosterone was discovered and synthesized from plant cholesterol by Leopold Ruzicka in Zürich, Switzerland in 1935,[1] testosterone was not a mainstream medication. Of course the Nazis of Germany experimented with testosterone[2] and its derivatives before battle to make over the German soldier as a superman. The allied forces used testosterone to rebuild the wasted concentration camp survivors. Both efforts were incompletely successful, but the myth that testosterone gives a man superior powers and maniacal behavior persists.

Testosterone laboratory tests became available after the Second World War. Once measured, testosterone deficiency was recognized and replacement therapy became common in Europe, albeit rare in the United States. It was not until women learned of hormone replacement and the promise of *Feminine Forever* in the 1960s did the topic really come up about testosterone replacement for men. With the physicians inappropriately blaming testosterone for aggressive behavior, they also sought to have men's lives extended by giving them estrogen. The disastrous results turned off men who could benefit from appropriate physician intervention for more than 50 years.

But just as the 1960s saw large numbers of women leave the home to join the workforce, men of the 21st century are looking to gain more natural energy to compete with younger men in the shrinking employment market. Just as each study of estrogen replacement in women shows an extended and improved overall lifestyle, so men should anticipate a comparable improvement in their own quality of life once given testosterone.

WHAT HAPPENED AFTER WWII?

DDT, dichlorodiphenyltrichloroethane, was invented in WWII[3] and used as a pesticide to clear malaria and typhus and then, after the war, as an agricultural pesticide. With the scientific study by Rachel Carson[4] showing that DDT was concentrating and killing higher life organisms such as birds, it was banned in the 1970s. DDT can still be measured in significant amounts in the tissue of half of the population.[5] DDT is important because, as an organic pesticide, it has estrogenic properties and is thereby called a xenoestrogen.

DDT is an organochloride that has weak estrogenic activity and is chemically similar enough to estrogen to trigger hormonal responses in contaminated animals.[6] TCDD is another organochloride contaminant used with the Agent Orange sprayings in Vietnam. Diethylstilbestrol (DES) is a synthetic estrogen used to treat women extensively from 1940 to 1960 and then used to fatten up livestock. Both synthetic chemicals have hormone-mimicking activity that promotes abnormal gene expression when used in laboratory studies involving mice and rats. We can suppose from what has happened over the past 50 years, that, just like birds, mice, and rats, we humans are being damaged by exposure to these chemical substances that stay in your body for upward of 15 or more years. And the plastic containers we use are also in a related class of xenoestrogens.[7]

Having recognized that there are hormone-like substances in the water, some countries such as Singapore have taken the necessary steps to filter out hormones from their water supply. Other countries have banned adding hormones to oral animal feed and hormone pellets from being injected into animals.[8-10]

No matter what the cause, there is a major problem for men's health. Whether it is too much estrogen, or too much xenoestrogen, or too much synthetic hormone-like substances like TCDD/Agent Orange, the effect is low testosterone levels in men.[11] Taking away testosterone from a man is like taking away not only his reproductive capacity but also his ability to live a long and healthy life.

Personal Perspective

When Dr. Lichten turned 45 years of age, his hormonal levels seemed to have crashed. It seemed like overnight he went from being an enthusiastic, hard working, physically potent man to be a depressed, lethargic, exhausted old man. His symptoms included night sweats so extreme that he had to take two showers each night. His colleagues had no idea what to do—one offered to admit Dr. Lichten to the hospital to get an answer. But, as a physician, Dr. Lichten knew the hospital offered no answers. Rather, the discovery of the cause of his malaise came from the unbiased information offered from his older gynecology patients. Two women told the doctor that their 70-year-old husbands had the same symptoms. So Dr. Lichten ran his established female menopausal laboratory tests on his own blood. Lucky! Dr. Edward Lichten was one of the first recognized "men-pausal" males. With this newfound information, he asked his urologist about testosterone replacement. The urologist told him that no one believed in testosterone for men, it was too dangerous, and the laboratory tests could be best explained by the large number of menopausal women being treated in Dr. Lichten's practice—they had influenced his tests!

So Dr. Lichten searched out the literature, found a doctor who believed in testosterone replacement, and started testosterone replacement under physician supervision in 1995. His life has never been sweeter since he began "drinking from man's bio-identical fountain of youth."

The pictures on Dr. Lichten's Internet webpage show the dramatic changes in his physical appearance. At 42, he was tired, wrinkled, and full-faced— at 51, he was muscular and lean, with a renewed enthusiasm radiating from a healthy body and face! Dr. Lichten reported that his female patients noticed the difference, and since low-dose testosterone replacement has been a mainstay of his treatment of menopausal women, they were intrigued. They asked if Dr. Lichten would treat their husbands: They worried that their husbands' health was being jeopardized, since their husbands had many of the same symptoms as Dr. Lichten.

THE DECLINING TESTOSTERONE LEVELS IN WESTERN SOCIETY

The standard male's blood testosterone measured between 400 and 1,200 ng/dL in the 1950s. The average man's sperm count was 140 million sperm in one cubic centimeter of seminal fluid. The incidence of diabetes in men was 1 million in a population of 150 million in 1950. Today, in a population of 300 million, the incidence of diabetes in men is 10 million, an increase of 500%. The average sperm count has dropped to 30 million, and male infertility has become an epidemic.[12] Studies show that men with sperm counts under 20 million are rarely able to reproduce without medical assistance.

Travison reported that since 1940, men of comparable ages are showing lower levels of total testosterone. She reports a decline of testosterone of an additional 1% or more per year for each year in the past two decades.[13] This equates to a 17% drop every decade of life after age 30.

Men who reached 50 in 1989 had an average total testosterone of 530 ng/dL. Men who reached 55 in 1997 had an average total testosterone of 475 ng/dL, and men who reached 60 in 2004 had an average total testosterone of just 450 ng/dL. That is a 25% drop in average baseline testosterone in just 10 years!

It is normal for the biological hormones to drop with aging: melatonin, human growth hormone, thyroxine, triiodothyronine,

DHEA, estrogen, progesterone, and testosterone. What is alarming is the rapidity in which some environmental factors have wiped out the baseline testosterone levels in just 50 years. Men were programmed for men-pause, but it is coming earlier and earlier and so are the killing diseases: heart disease, stroke, and diabetes.

With a drop in testosterone levels, the question is at what level does the drop become significant. In sperm count, a drop from 140 million to 30 million decreases fertility by 10–20%. But a drop of sperm count from 30 million to 20 million or less would probably drop fertility another 50–75% and truly affect the human race's ability to reproduce.

Recognizing that the drop in testosterone is a real problem and that it correlates to disease in men, what are the steps needed to stem the problem?

RECOGNIZING TESTOSTERONE DEFICIENCY: THE ST. LOUIS ADAM QUESTIONNAIRE

The St. Louis ADAM questionnaire is a good starting point to ask if testosterone deficiency exists. If there is a decrease in sex drive or the erection is less strong, it behooves the male to have appropriate laboratory tests to rule out organic disease (infection, thyroid, anemia, etc.) and differentiate that from true hypogonadism. The drop in testosterone may be temporary during times of peak stress and insomnia; but if it is chronically low, supplementing testosterone will allow him to overcome his performance issues.

1 and 2 or any four answered yes is considered suspect for testosterone deficiency!

1.	Decrease in sex drive	[Yes]	[No]
2.	Erections less strong	[Yes]	[No]
3.	Lack of energy	[Yes]	[No]
4.	Decrease in strength or endurance	[Yes]	[No]
5.	Lost height	[Yes]	[No]
6.	Decreased "enjoyment of life"	[Yes]	[No]
7.	Sad and/or grumpy	[Yes]	[No]
8.	Deterioration in sports ability	[Yes]	[No]
9.	Falling asleep after dinner	[Yes]	[No]
10.	Decreased work performance	[Yes]	[No]

RECOGNIZING TESTOSTERONE DEFICIENCY: THE LABORATORY TESTS

Because there is confusion over what constitutes the correct laboratory test and what measure of testosterone should be considered deficient, the following information will first focus on the laboratory tests that are used to measure total testosterone. The amounts of testosterone that are usable are called bio-available, and this value is measured or calculated as a separate test.

MEASURING TESTOSTERONE

Secondly, testosterone is a hormone that is released to a circadian rhythm. That means that there may be a 10–15% variance between the peak testosterone at 4:00 a.m. and the mid-afternoon testosterone crash. That first peak of testosterone usually correlates to that spontaneous early morning erection. A second peak of testosterone occurs around 8:00 in the morning to ready the man for the workday. The doctor prefers to have the testosterone drawn in the morning for consistency.

Third, measuring testosterone is bundled with the measurement of prostate specific antigen (PSA), which is the screen for prostate cancer. The doctor insists that the male not have sexual intercourse or manual ejaculation for 48-72 hours before the laboratory tests are drawn. Elevated PSA commits the physician and the patient to repeated tests, urologic screening, and potentially an ultrasound and biopsy. (Just avoid sex for two days before the laboratory tests are drawn to avoid a false positive PSA test.)

THE ROLE OF ESTROGEN

Since estrogen and testosterone are the sex hormones, they compete for attachment to the ligand called the sex hormone-binding globulin (SHBG). The coupling of hormone to SHBG is necessary for the hormone to dock against the cell wall, traverse the cell, and enter the nucleus command center. When a hormone enters the command center, specific instructions are sent out to the cells. For the man, these instructions must be manly; he does not need estrogen-making his breasts and abdominal love handles bigger. Measurement of total estradiol in the blood may direct the physician to consider how much of the naturally produced testosterone is being converted to estrogen.

For estrogen and testosterone not only compete for SHBG and entry into the cell, but they both feedback to the pituitary, the master gland. The pituitary releases both follicle stimulating hormone (FSH) and luteinizing hormone (LH) when additional testosterone and estradiol are needed. The presence of excess estrogens in the male reduces the secretion of FSH and LH, thereby reducing the production of testosterone. With increased amounts of aromatized estrogen and xenoestrogens, the physician may find a low level of FSH and LH paired with low levels of testosterone. That is the crux of man's problems: too much bad estrogen and too little good testosterone.

As discussed, the normal evolution of man is to have high total testosterone and high free testosterone (biologically available) during the years of peak reproduction. But by the age of 35–40, the enzymatic conversion of testosterone to estrogen begins in significant amounts.[14] The medical term is aromatization: changing the one molecule on testosterone so it becomes estrogen. An approximation of aromatization activity is the increase in estradiol to testosterone ratio.[15]

THE ROLE OF SHBG

Recognizing that estrogens have a negative effect on man's health is clear. Not only does estrogen compete with testosterone for penetration into the cell; it competes for production from the pituitary stimulating hormones. It also affects the production of the binding protein, sex hormone-binding globulin (SHBG), directly. More than 30 years ago, in 1972, D.C. Anderson in the journal *Nature* showed that estrogen stimulates SHBG production.[16] The highest levels of SHBG are seen during pregnancy, when there are tremendous levels of estrogens produced. Similarly, SHBG is an estrogen amplifier, as SHBG tightly binds testosterone, making it inactive. Bound testosterone is not biologically available, so there is a strong correlation between unbound testosterone with high total testosterone and low SHBG. As seen in young virile males, individuals will have both high values of total serum testosterone concentrations and low levels of SHBG concentration. Anderson proposed the measurement be called the free androgen index (FAI) and that it be calculated as the ratio of total testosterone concentration divided by SHBG concentration. The formula is Total Testosterone/SHBG. Since testosterone is measured as ng/dL and SHBG as nmol/L, the calculation of FAI= $[0.03467 \text{x(TT)}/(\text{SHBG})]\text{x}100$. The 0.03467 is the factor for the conversion of ng/dL to nmol/L. A young male should have a FAI of 0.8 to 1.2; an older male 0.5; and a male diabetic on dialysis may have a FAI of 0.2 or less. This is, in Dr. Lichten's opinion, the primary measurement used to make the diagnosis of testosterone deficiency.

THE NEW FREE INSULIN AND TESTOSTERONE (FIT) TEST

One of the most important concepts that Dr. Lichten has advanced is that high free sex hormone states correlate directly to health and that low free hormone states correlate with disease states like diabetes. What others have documented is that this SHBG molecule, when combined with the proper gender-specific hormone, works with insulin to protect against diabetes.

Male: healthy—high testosterone, low estradiol, low SHBG
Male: unhealthy—low testosterone, high estradiol, high SHBG

Testosterone is good for men and estrogen is good for females. The corollary is also true: Too much of the wrong sex hormone and the wrong amount of SHBG will be found in an individual who is or will be at risk for diabetes and disease.

THE NEW FIT TEST FOR WOMEN

So, to digress for a moment, consider two women. One is shorter, heavier set, has increased facial hair, and a stout body build. We will call her Rosie. Rosie will typically have a "female-not-so-healthy" laboratory profile: high testosterone, low estradiol, low SHBG, and a higher statistical risk of diabetes, obesity, and heart disease. If she is in the reproductive years, the gynecologist may diagnose her with polycystic ovarian disease (PCO). But, what is bad for Rosie is excellent for the majority of men, relatively speaking: high testosterone, low SHBG.

Female: healthy—low testosterone, high estradiol, high SHBG
Female: unhealthy—high testosterone, moderate estradiol, low SHBG

While a healthy woman would have laboratory tests showing low testosterone, high estradiol, and high SHBG, the same results would be indicative of an unhealthy male with testosterone deficiency, diabetes, or heart disease.

The term is "gender-specific medicine." Target the medical treatments to match the hormonal levels ideal or specific to the gender.

While others will argue about the testosterone tests, Dr. Lichten's position is that any abnormal test of testosterone is important, whether you measure total testosterone, the free testosterone, or some aspect of bio-available testosterone. Dr. Lichten has relied on the free androgen index because of its long-term use in Europe and because of the true science behind the measurement. The fallacy of using a non-FAI is that the physician may not realize that SHBG is directly linked to insulin resistance. And that is the key to preventing disease, keeping the insulin resistance low, as showed by G. Phillips.[17] Conditions that elevate the fasting insulin level or increase insulin resistance will increase the risk of every disease, including diabetes, heart disease, and even cancer.

Dr. Lichten and others have determined that an elevated SHBG in a man is paramount in importance to raising the insulin resistance in the afflicted male. Therefore, understanding the prevention of disease or the "antiaging" aspect of medicine in a male is as simple as—

MALE
High testosterone, low SHBG, fasting insulin—low risk of disease
Elevated FAI, low fasting insulin—low risk of disease
Elevated FIT test—low risk of disease

Before Anderson's work on establishing the measurement of bio-available testosterone as a ratio of total testosterone over SHBG, the doctors had to understand what appears on the first line of the box: Men need high levels of testosterone, and it needs to be free, not bound. The free insulin and testosterone ratio (FIT) test goes one step further in incorporating the insulin levels into the calculation. This allows the FIT test to be unique in determining risk of disease.

So if low SHBG is good when coupled with high testosterone, then high SHBG and low testosterone in men implies disease—specifically, diabetes and metabolic syndrome. And as discussed in Chapter 13, both insulin resistance and metabolic syndrome share common components that include obesity, diabetes, heart disease, hypertension, and abnormal cholesterol. Not measuring FAI, TT, E2 and SHBG is not to measure necessary information about the individual's hormonal milieu. Not to measure HgbA1c (glycosylated hemoglobin) and fasting insulin is to not measure the metabolic prediabetic state. These and other laboratory test values in our hands may help predict the prevalence of disease up to 20 years before it is set to develop.

It has been Dr. Lichten's most recent work that ties testosterone levels in men directly to the diabetic state. The FAI fails to consider the role of insulin resistance in causing disease. This has been rectified in the development of the FIT test. By adding both estradiol and insulin lab values to the calculation, the FIT test simplifies the full gambit of information, analyzing automatically the hormonal factors that might warn of diseases yet to develop.

Personal Perspective

T.T. is a 43-year-old male who has been able to stay in very good physical shape by eating right, not smoking, actively lifting weights, and 30 minutes of cardio 3–5 times per week. But T.T. noted that his workouts were flat, that he was unable to get pumped, and that he no longer felt good after a workout. He developed a gut and added 20 pounds around his waist, his sexual performance started to fade, and he had more and more episodes of restless sleep. Exhausted in the morning, he sought out medical assistance from Dr. Lichten.

"Doctor, tell me why I sweat so much at night?" started the discussion. "The sweating is so intense that it wakes my wife. She feels like she is at the water's edge. I have been taking two showers a night but the sweating continues. I'm exhausted and emotionally drained. What am I going to do?"

Dr. Lichten explained that the night sweats are not unusual in men who are going through andropause or male "men-pause." The problem is that the pituitary gland (brain master gland) senses a low level of testosterone, so it puts out a lot of its hormones, FSH and LH. These surges of pituitary hormones, in an attempt to raise testosterone levels, are the direct cause of the change in core temperature and the release of sweat. The only way to stop sweating is to have your hormonal production of testosterone increase and stabilize, then the body will naturally lower the release of FSH and LH.

After suitable laboratory tests confirmed the problem and defined other issues, T.T. and Dr. Lichten discussed testosterone replacement. There are five forms of testosterone available in the United States, five not available in the United States, while all are restricted to prescriptions only by physicians with state and national licensure.

They are:
- testosterone gel Androgel®
- testosterone patch Androderm®
- testosterone injection cypionate
- testosterone pellet Testopel® inject
- testosterone cream compounded
- testosterone capsule Oxandrin®

The European preparations have specific actions that would complement the U.S. products if FDA approval could be secured. Stanozolol®, for example, has complementary and unique antidiabetic and antithrombotic properties that would work well for both men and women in the over-50 population. And Deca-Durabolin®, generically called nandrolone, was removed from production in March 2007. It is the keystone ingredient to any antiaging, antidisease treatment program, especially in men. Whether the male suffers from AIDs or diabetes, heart disease or obesity, poor healing or osteoporosis, early Alzheimer's disease or muscle weakness, the removal of Deca-Durabolin® was a terrible loss to bio-identical health care.

Products Not Available in the United States
- testosterone oral Primobolan
- testosterone oral Anadrol®
- testosterone injection Stanozolol®
- testosterone pellet Organon (three-month)
- discontinued trenbolone

PROBLEMS WITH TESTOSTERONE GEL

In the United States, testosterone gels are most popular, with Androgel® by Solvay Pharmaceuticals reaching sales well over one and a half billion dollars per year. Prescriptions for testosterone were written for 17 million men. These creams and gels have a major problem: The human body is not well equipped to take in hormones through the skin. When estrogen is applied to a woman's skin, it is absorbed and processed as estrogen. The problem with testosterone applied to the skin is that the skin contains so much aromatization potential that it converts testosterone to estrogen in very high amounts. And higher estrogen levels are counterproductive to a man's health.

Estrogen is the first derivative of testosterone. Just by snipping off one extra molecule, life-giving testosterone for men becomes life-giving estrogen for women. But what gives life to women will damage men. Men can circumvent this problem by taking an aromatase-inhibiting drug like Arimidex® (about 1 mg a week works for most men).

THE PROBLEM WITH ESTROGEN IN MEN

For example, it was recognized in the 1950s that women lived longer than men and that the removal of the ovaries from women and their live-giving estrogen would double their rate of heart attack in the next 10 years. So some bright researchers convinced a number of men who had had heart attacks to take Premarin®. By giving these men more estrogen, they were able to kill all the volunteers with heart attacks in the next two years. No—estrogen for men is not just bad, it is deadly.[18-20]

In Europe, estrogen replacement is used in treating some men with prostate cancer. Tivesten recorded in those men on ERT a dramatic thickening of the lining of the carotid arteries, which increases the risk of stroke. The higher doses of estrogen used were correlated directly to more thickening noted in the carotid artery intima.[21]

THE PROBLEM WITH HAVING INSUFFICIENT TESTOSTERONE

Physicians and the general public have missed the magnitude of the problem that results from men developing the syndrome of hypogonadism from insufficient testosterone. The article by M. Shores showing a doubling of deaths for all reasons in the 10 years following identification of low testosterone in a veteran population.[22]

Conclusion #1: Since lack of testosterone results in an increase in unwarranted deaths, add back testosterone to faltering and aging men. The connection that has eluded physicians and the general public to date is that adequate testosterone protects against diabetes. In Dr. Lichten's practice, some men with true diabetes and abnormal glucose tolerance tests revert entirely to normal on testosterone injections alone.

Conclusion #2: Lack of testosterone results in an increased probability of being afflicted with diabetes. Diabetes and insulin resistance are the key risk factors for heart disease. Population studies show that men with low testosterone are 62% more likely to have diabetes than those men with normal testosterone levels.[23]

The treatment and prevention of cardiac disease in men has eluded physicians and general public because of the ignorance about testosterone.

Conclusion #3: Add back testosterone to men suffering with angina, heart attacks, and heart failure. Treat aggressively and treat often.[24,25] Science strongly links lack of testosterone in men to osteoporosis,[26] Alzheimer's disease, and development of chronic muscle wasting.[27]
Prostate cancer is linked to low, not high, levels of testosterone.[28]

TESTOSTERONE AND PROSTATE CANCER

It has been a misconception that testosterone is a harbinger of prostate cancer. Marks[29] established that testosterone by itself was not a cause of prostate cancer when given for replacement to aging males. High doses of testosterone for a half-year failed to induce negative or precancerous changes in the prostate cells.

In a study published by Morgentaler[30] in 2006, a careful prostate examination, ultrasound, and biopsy were performed on men whose total testosterone levels were under 300 ng/dL. The presence of low levels of testosterone, defined as less than 250 ng/dL, identified prostate cancer in 20% and put that male at a twofold or greater risk than the male with a higher total testosterone level.

Conclusion: Prostate cancer is a definite risk of 1:7 in males with testosterone levels less than 300 ng/dL. Yet, once the cancer is removed, the benefits of testosterone replacement outweigh the risk. Testosterone replacement is indicated in the male successfully treated for prostate cancer with physician monitoring.[31]

TESTOSTERONE AND ERECTILE DYSFUNCTION

Since the peak of reproductive capacity is associated with the highest levels of testosterone and biologically free testosterone in the young adult, it is logical to consider erectile dysfunction in the aging male as a sign of testosterone deficiency.[32] Furthermore, the erectile dysfunction (ED) associated even with the use of the most potent PDE-5 inhibitors—Viagra®, Cialis®, and Levitra®—can often be treated by adding back inexpensive androgen therapies.[33]

What is presently known about sexual or erectile dysfunction is that there are three centers that must be functioning normally. The limbic center of the brain must have the "idea" to respond to a sexual stimulus. This is called libido or sexual desire. Secondly, the penis must dilate the arteries leading to the corpora cavernosa and fill the two chambers with blood to become erect. This is possible because of the local release of nitric oxide (NO) sent from brain stimuli and because cGMP causes the local arteries to dilate and quickly fill the penile blood channels. Lastly, there must be a block of the enzymes that cause the penis to deflate. The enzyme that destroys cGMP is called phosphodiesterase (PDE). The PDE-5 inhibitors, such as Viagra®, work only at the last step. The problem with treating erectile dysfunction initially with PDE-5 inhibitors is that the potential cause of the problem, hypogonadism, is not addressed. So, although the literature is filled with references to men with ED having heart disease, diabetes, osteoporosis, strokes, and Alzheimer's disease, no one addresses the simple, safest treatment that offers the greatest overall health potential: Treat with testosterone first!

Urologists generally agree that "screening for hypogonadism in all men with ED is necessary to identify cases of severe hypogonadism and some cases of mild to moderate hypogonadism, who may benefit from testosterone treatment."[34]

So before you reach for that $14 pill in an attempt to maintain your "manly" erection, think how much better off your whole body will be if the manly hormone testosterone is circulating to every organ in your body. In Dr. Lichten's practice, less than 10% of men on testosterone and without cardiac or diabetes disease rely even occasionally on that "little blue pill." The side effects of testosterone include increased muscle mass, clarity of thought, stronger bones, glucose control, and increased heart power and dilation of the coronary arteries—all positives, versus the headaches and vision changes associated with PDE-5 inhibitor therapy.

WHO SHOULD BE TESTED?

Based on the recent analysis of Mohr[35] of the Massachusetts Male Aging Study (MMAS), the normal range of testosterone for 95% of the population will be 251–914 ng/dL for men in their 40s; 216–876 ng/dL for men in their 50s; 196–859 ng/dL for men in their 60s; and 156–818 ng/dL for men in their 70s. What this means is that only 2.5% of the population is expected to have testosterone levels below 200 ng/dL.

Statisticians use this 2.5% number, called two standard deviations below the mean, to define abnormal. However, if one wants to be considered just average, just 50%, then the mean testosterone level would be 580 ng/dL for 40-year-olds, 550 ng/dL for 50-year-olds, 525 ng/dL for 60-year-olds, and 490 ng/dL for 70-year-olds. But more important is recognition of the vast array of symptoms of testosterone deficiency. And treat accordingly.

As Dr. Lichten explains the testosterone threshold, "If testosterone is the breath of life, I want to be at least better than average, over 50%!"

It makes no sense to be less than average, in a medical sense, so Dr. Lichten replaces testosterone levels in all individuals who have symptoms or signs of any disease related to hypogonadism and a total testosterone level less than 450 ng/dL, which is the statistical "average." Furthermore, he tailors the form of testosterone to the individual's body type, as well as estradiol and sex hormone-binding globulin (SHBG) levels. Men with elevated estradiol or SHBG are treated first with Deca-Durabolin®, nandrolone, a bio-identical testosterone that cannot be aromatized to estrogens. Nandrolone lowers serum levels of estrogen and SHBG by suppressing FSH, LH, and biological production of testosterones that can be aromatized. If the estradiol and SHBG levels fail to drop into the normal range, then an aromatization inhibitor such as generic tamoxifen or Arimidex® is used. The key in Dr. Lichten's protocols is to follow the changes in treatment described by the patient with sequential laboratory tests. Natural prostate formulations from over-the-counter supplement houses, with saw palmetto, pygeum, stinging nettles, DIM, and chrysin, are not to be discounted but cannot offer the power of the medical intervention described above.

THE LAST WORD

The trouble with testosterone has been the abuse and overuse by bodybuilders, male and female athletes, and high school and college adults. Normal replacement of an injectable testosterone is 100 to 150 mg per week; these abusive individuals have used upward of 1,000 mg per week to push their blood levels into pharmacological not physiological levels. Whether they cycle on and off makes no difference; once the body senses these high levels, it will work to neutralize them through aromatization. So the bodybuilder at 18 will often look fat, flabby, and diabetic at 30 years of age. Be wary of testosterone replacement except when truly needed and only under the supervision of a doctor who truly understands testosterone's benefits and risks. After everything has been said and done, the most conservative of professors, M.M. Miner,[36] confirms that testosterone replacement "may help" and is "unlikely to pose major health risks."

SAY "YES" TO TESTOSTERONE!

Recent studies have demonstrated that hypogonadism in men may be more prevalent than previously thought, is strongly associated with metabolic syndrome, and may be a risk factor for type 2 diabetes and cardiovascular disease.[37] Clinical studies have shown that testosterone replacement therapy in hypogonadal men improves metabolic syndrome indicators and cardiovascular risk factors. Maintaining testosterone concentrations in the normal range has been shown to contribute to bone health, lean muscle mass, and physical and sexual function, suggesting that testosterone replacement therapy may help to prevent frailty in older men. Based on current knowledge, testosterone replacement therapy is unlikely to pose major health risks in patients without prostate cancer and may offer substantial health benefits. Larger, longer-term randomized studies are needed to establish fully the effects of testosterone replacement therapy.[37]

REFERENCES:

1. Shahidi, N. A Review of the chemistry, biological action and clinical applications of Anabolic-Androgenic Steroids. Clinical Therapeutics. 2001; 22:1355–90.
2. Wade N. Science. June 30, 1972.
3. Available at: http://nobelprize.org/nobel_prizes/medicine/laureates/1948/.
4. Carson R. Silent Spring. Boston: Houghton Mifflin, 1962.
5. Lopez-Espinosa MJ. Organochlorine Pesticides in Placentas from Southern Spain and Some Related Factors. Placenta. 2007 Jul;28(7):631-8. Epub 2006 Nov 15.
6. Warita K, et al. Progression of the dose-related effects of estrogenic endocrine disruptors, an important factor in declining fertility, differs between the hypothalamo-pituitary axis and reproductive organs of male mice. Journal of Veterinary Medicine Science 2006; 68(12):1257–67.
7. Ogawa Y, et al. Estrogenic activities of chemicals related to food contact plastics and rubbers tested by the yeast two-hybrid assay. Food Additives Contaminants 2006; 23(4):422–30.
8. McEvoy JD, McVeigh CE, Currie JW, Kennedy DG, McCaughey WJ. Plasma, urinary and biliary residues in cattle following intramuscular injection of nortestosterone laurate. Vet Res Commun. 1998 Nov;22(7):479-91.
9. Freudenheim M. Beef Dispute: Stakes High in Trade War. *New York Times*. January 1, 1989.
10. Jacobs P. US, Europe Lock Horns in Beef Hormone Debate. *LA Times*. April 9, 1999.
11. Gupta A. Serum dioxin, testosterone, and subsequent risk of benign prostatic hyperplasia: a prospective cohort study of Air Force veterans. *Environmental Health Perspectives* 2006; 114(11):1649–54.
12. Carlsen E, et al. Evidence for Decreasing Quality of Semen during Last 50 years. *British Medical Journal*. 1992; 305:609–13.
13. Travison, TG. et al. A population-level decline in serum testosterone levels in American men. *Journal of Clinical Endocrinology and Metabolism*. 2007; 92:196–202.

14. Gennari L. Longitudinal Association between Sex Hormone Levels, Bone Loss, and Bone Turnover in Elderly Men. *The Journal of Clinical Endocrinology and Metabolism*. 2003; 88(11):5327–33.
15. Vermeulen A, Kaufman JM, Goemaere S, et al. Estradiol in elderly men. *Aging Male*. 2002 Jun;5(2):98-102.
16. Anderson D.C. Sex Hormone Binding Globulin Is an Oestrogen Amplifier. *Nature*. 1972; 240:38–40.
17. Phillips G.B. Relationship between serum sex hormones and the glucose-insulin-lipid defect in men with obesity. *Metabolism*. 1993 Jan; 42(1):116–20.
18. Stamler J, et al. Effectiveness of estrogen for therapy of myocardial infarction in middle age men. *Journal of the American Medical Association*. 1963; 183:632–8.
19. Marmorston J, et al. Effect of premarin on survival in men with myocardial infarction. *Proceedings of the Society of Experimental Biology in Medicine*. 1960; 105:618–20.
20. Myers SM, et al. The effect of treatment with conjugated equine estrogen preparations on estrogen excretion in male subjects with myocardial infarction. *Current Therapeutic Research, Clinical and Experimental*. 1965; 6: 35–49.
21. Tivesten A, et al. Circulating estradiol is an independent predictor of progression of carotid artery intima-media thickness in middle-aged men. *Journal of Clinical Endocrinology and Metabolism*. 2006; 91(11):4433–7.
22. Shores MM. Low serum testosterone and mortality in male veterans. *Archives in Internal Medicine*. 2006; 166(15):1660–5.
23. Barrett-Connor E, Khaw KT, Yen SS. Endogenous sex hormone levels in older adult men with diabetes mellitus. *Am J Epidemiol*. 1990 Nov;132(5):895-901.
24. Malkin CJ, et al. Testosterone therapy in men with moderate severity heart failure: a double-blind randomized placebo controlled trial. *European Heart Journal 2006*; 27(1): 10–2.
25. Steidle CP. New advances in the treatment of hypogonadism in the aging male. *Review Urology*. 2003; 5 Supp 1:S34–40.
26. Beauchet O. Testosterone and cognitive function: current clinical evidence of a relationship. *European J Endocrinology* 2006; 155(6):773–81.
27. Starka L. Testosterone treatment of sarcopenia. *Vnitr Lek*. 2006 Oct;52(10):909-11. Czech.
28. Morgentaler A. Testosterone and Prostate cancer: an historical perspective on a modern myth. *European Urology*. 2006; 50(5):895–7.
29. Marks LS, et al. Effect of testosterone replacement therapy on prostate tissue in men with late-onset hypogonadism: a randomized controlled trial. *Journal of the American Medical Association 2006*; 296(19):2369–71.
30. Morgentaler A, et al. Prevalence of prostate cancer among hypogonadal men with prostate-specific antigen levels of 4.0 ng/mL or less. *Current Therapeutic Research, Clinical and Experimental*. 2006 Dec;68(6):1263–7.
31. Morgentaler A. Testosterone therapy for men at risk for or with history of prostate cancer. *Current Treatment Options in Oncology*. 2006; 7(5):363–9.
32. Saad F, et al. Effects of testosterone on erectile function; implications for the therapy of erectile dysfunction. *British Journal of Urology*. 2007 Feb 15: Epub.
33. Caretta N, et al. Erectile dysfunction in aging men; testosterone role in therapeutic protocols. *Journal Endocrinology Investigation*. 2005; 28(11 Supp):108–11.
34. Mikhail N. Does testosterone have a role in erectile function? *American Journal of Medicine*. 2006; 119(5):373–82.
35. Mohr BA, et al. Normal, bound and nonbound testosterone levels in normally ageing men: results from the Massachusetts Male Aging Study. *Clinical Endocrinology*. (Oxford) 2005; 62(1):64–73.
36. Miner MM, et al. Testosterone and ageing: what have we learned since the institute of medicine report and what lies ahead? *Int J Clin Pract*. 2007 Apr;61(4):622-32. Epub 2007 Mar 2.
37. Braga-Basaria M. Metabolic syndrome in men with prostate cancer undergoing longterm androgen-deprivation therapy. *Journal of Clinical Oncology*. 2006; 24(24):3979–83.

CHAPTER 12

CHOLESTEROL AND HEART DISEASE

HISTORICAL OVERVIEW: UNDERSTANDING CORONARY ARTERY DISEASE

Long before there were prescription medications for cholesterol and as early as the turn of the 20th century, there was little discernible coronary artery disease. People died from infections, whether it was the pandemic flu of 1919 or pneumonia. The first report of deaths from coronary artery disease were originally considered a by-product of chronic infection.[1] By the end of the 21st century, coronary artery disease would become the number one cause of death in Western civilization, killing more than 460,000 Americans in 2001.[2]

Coronary artery disease (CAD) is the partial obstruction of the major arteries that bring blood, oxygen, and nutrients to the heart muscle. It is postulated that deposits of cholesterol form plaques that attach to the arteries. When these plaques break or fall off, they may cause complete obstruction of some part of the coronary artery. The obstruction of blood to the muscle of the heart can cause myocardial infarction, i.e., heart muscle death. If enough of the heart or the electrical system is affected, then the heart is unable to pump blood and the patient dies.

Heart failure is different, in that there are many different disease processes that can weaken the heart enough to cause "failure." Coronary artery disease may progressively destroy more and more heart muscle or infection, or a genetic condition or a metabolic condition may occur that leaves the heart muscle just too weak to pump blood. While coronary heart disease is seen primarily in 40- to 70-year-old men, congestive heart failure occurs in the majority of those living into their 80s.

Cholesterol is the precursor to many of the bio-identical hormones. It is essential for human survival. Since the 1920s, biochemists have used natural and plant-based cholesterol to synthesize pregnenolone, estrogen, testosterone, DHEA, and progesterone. Even vitamin D needs cholesterol to function properly. There are a number of inherited or genetic diseases that result in very high levels of cholesterol-related lipids. They are defined by high levels of various cholesterols, high levels of triglycerides, and abnormal distributions of large and small chylomicrons that hold the fat. As rare lipid diseases are associated with increased cardiac mortality, it was logical to expect researchers to associate abnormal levels of cholesterol with rapid increases in coronary artery disease.

After World War II, Ancel Keys,[3] a physiologist, performed an epidemiologic study of dietary habits and heart disease in countries around the world. He concluded that the cause of heart disease was directly related to the intake of animal fat. His study was flawed, however, in that he selected only six of the 22 countries to "stratify" his study. And as every good mathematician knows, you can prove anything with "stratified" data.

But the doctors and the pharmaceutical companies, in their desire to treat and prevent heart disease, adopted and promoted Ancel Keys' work. Medication after medication has been proposed to block fat and treat/cure coronary artery and heart disease. Over the last 25 years, various medications have been suggested as "cure-alls" for disease, only to be abandoned from use because of unforeseen complications. The list includes:

Atromid-S: Approved in 1975 for the treatment of extremely rare medical conditions where the serum triglycerides rise from a normal of 100–200 to well over 2,000. A large study of 5,000 men for five years of active drug and one year of follow-up showed, under the World Health Organization supervision, a 44% increase in mortality, half from cancer.[4]

Statins: Statins were approved in 1987 to treat abnormal lipids-dyslipidemia. Every one of the statins is reported to have complications of rhabdomyolysis, a sometime fatal breakdown of muscle tissue. This and other side effects of statins are well documented.[5-7] But coenzyme Q10 might help with muscle problems.

Rezulin®: Rezulin® was the first troglitazone used to lower insulin resistance in adults with diabetes mellitus. The complications of this medication included liver toxicity. It was removed within 2–3 years of launch and after sales reached almost a billion dollars per year.[8] Avandia®, a related drug, is also being targeted for removal.

Yet today, with these and their closely related pharmaceutical products still on the market and accounting for billions of dollars of health-care costs, the people of the U.S. and Europe still suffer with some of the highest rates of coronary artery deaths in the world.

Could it be that cholesterol was never the cause of heart disease and that these cholesterol-lowering medications are just one more liver poison? Could statins only artificially suppress lipid profiles, while the real culprit continues to make these cardiac health matters worse?

UNDERSTANDING CHOLESTEROL

Cholesterol is a necessary part of human existence. From cholesterol in the diet and cholesterol manufactured in the liver originates many of the major hormones that fuel the human endocrine system. Cholesterol begets pregnenolone, progesterone, cortisol, DHEA, testosterone, estrone, estradiol, and, during pregnancy, estriol. Understand that cholesterol is necessary for human life.

If the body is stressed and the adrenals are not working properly because of undernutrition or physical exhaustion, cholesterol levels will physiologically increase to attempt to manufacture more DHEA and cortisol. If the thyroid is underperforming, then the cholesterol levels increase to produce more of the other hormones. If a woman has polycystic ovaries with an imbalance of testosterone over estrogen, the cholesterol increases. And if the man is low in testosterone and his testosterone is replaced, his cholesterol decreases.[9]

The point is that hypercholesterolemia is a sign that the body's hormones are not in balance. To treat the symptom, the alleged high cholesterol in the blood, by poisoning the HMG-CoA system, is absolutely ludicrous. Why not understand first the cause of the problem, whether it is dietary fiber[10], omega-3 deficiency[11], or hormones—and address that correctable issue directly?

Total cholesterol levels well over 200 mg/mL were commonly treated with diet,[12] and pharmaceutical-drug intervention was not considered as a first response before the proliferation of pharmaceutical advertising in the 1980s. Dr. Lichten does not prescribe cholesterol-lowering medications except to rare individuals with truly defined classes of hyperlipidemia. Rather, he will first and foremost treat the cause of the cholesterol as a problem of nutrition and a problem of hormone imbalance.

UNDERSTANDING CHOLESTEROL'S ROLE AS A BIO-IDENTICAL PROHORMONE

Cholesterol is necessary for normal human function. Without cholesterol, the following functions do not occur properly:[13]

1. Bile salts are necessary for absorption of essential fats, fat soluble vitamins A, D,E, and K, and minerals. Note that vitamins D is derived from cholesterol.
2. Cholesterol is necessary for vitamin D production.
3. Cholesterol is incorporated into the inner layers of every cell wall.
4. Cholesterol is incorporated into the myelin sheath that insulates every large peripheral nerve cell.
5. Cholesterol is necessary for normal action of circulating T-cells, lymphocytes, and helper B-cells—all part of the immune system.

In the liver, acetyl-CoA, the energy components from the Kreb's cycle, is metabolized to HMG-CoA and into cholesterol. Coenzyme Q_{10} shares a common biosynthetic pathway with cholesterol. Coenzyme Q10 is the very important carrier molecule in the oxidation-phosphorylation cycle within the cell that produces energy that powers the cell. Poisoning the HMG-CoA system can bring down the energy system for the entire body. One of the complications with statins is the loss of adequate levels of coenzyme Q10.

There is no logic in taking a statin drug without massive amounts of coenzyme Q10.

SO, WHY THE "KNOW YOUR CHOLESTEROL LEVEL" HYPE?

In 1985, the National Cholesterol Education Program (NCEP)[14] was created by the National Heart, Lung and Blood Pressure Institute of the Federal Government. The purpose of the NCEP was to raise public cholesterol awareness, including cooperative efforts with the American Heart Association. While everyone now knows their blood cholesterol level, the medical science has yet to prove that "lowering your cholesterol will significantly lower your risk of coronary artery or heart disease."[15]

The reason for this false dichotomy or fuzzy logic is that the pharmaceutical companies and the university- and hospital-based physicians have forgotten the basic rule of science, which was established more than 150 years ago: The only proof of a theorem relies on the completion of five steps. These steps represent the principles of the scientific method[16] upon which science is based. The principles are clear:

Scientific Method
1   Make an observation.
2. Establish a working hypothesis to explain the observations.
3. Make predictions.
4. Test hypothesis.
5. Accept all challenges to your hypothesis. If it withstands all challenges, then the theory is accepted. Results must be reproducible.

But in the last 20 years, a bastard theory called evidence-based medicine has become the teaching point for physicians and the public. Evidence-based medicine makes no proofs; one only has to perform steps 1, 2, and 3. Evidence-based medicine is nothing more than dogma: "My drug is better than your drug" or, more often, "My drug is better than nothing." The true scientist could look at these studies and easily retort, "Neither of your drugs is necessary." The failure that must be considered in present-day health care is that the doctor (1) is too busy to first measure the appropriate hormone laboratory values, and (2) fails to determine what was the cause of the underlying disease. Only with due diligence will he or she be able to answer the advertised "fuzzy logic" studies. Adding fiber and omega-3 fatty acids and replacing the inherently deficient thyroid or testosterone hormones, for example, corrects the patient's underlying medical condition and will often lower cholesterol levels, albeit without statin intervention.

And that is the point. Just because cholesterol levels are elevated in coronary artery disease or heart failure does not mean that high cholesterol was, in any manner, the cause of the malady.

A famous quote is "Statistics do not lie, only statisticians." According to a recent analysis report, randomized controlled trials of head-to-head comparisons of statins with other drugs are more likely to report results and conclusions favoring the sponsor's product compared to the comparator drug. Drug companies may deliberately choose lower dosages for the comparison drug when they carry out "head-to-head" trials; this tactic is likely to result in the company's product doing better in the trial. Also trials which produce unfavorable results are not published, or that unfavorable outcomes are suppressed.[17]

Thus, although the pharmaceutical studies quoted hereafter state there are benefits to statin therapy, they are evidence-based observations not scientifically-based conclusions. A true scientist need only ask these two questions to destroy the statin premise: Was the allegedly high cholesterol treated first with natural therapies of vitamins, minerals, proteins and bio-identical hormones to determine if natural therapies could be therapeutic? Secondly, did the statin intervention save lives? Although intensive-dose statin therapy was associated with a reduced risk for acute coronary syndromes (ACS) or stable coronary artery disease (CAD), it was also associated with an increased risk for statin-induced adverse events. There is an ongoing debate about whether the effects of statins on CoQ10 and cholesterol levels might have a negative impact in patients with chronic heart failure (CHF).[18,19]

The point is that there is no great and overwhelming proof that $50 billion paid to Pfizer for its cholesterol-lowering drugs alone are doing anything to improve the health of the American public. In this chapter is listed peer-reviewed and published medical studies that address bio-identical hormone deficiencies as the cause of heart failure, coronary artery disease and even the carotid intima thickening study on normal people. First, Dr. Lichten states, "Treat the cause." And then, from a scientific and logical standpoint, the pharmaceutical companies are asked to explain how a statin, which lowers cholesterol levels by poisoning the liver, really can make mankind live longer and better. It just does not make sense.

THE TRUTH ABOUT HEART DISEASE

Before there were cholesterol-lowering drugs there was heart disease. As physicians, we need only look back 100 years to see that there was a major problem with heart disease in the form of congestive heart failure causing untold deaths. The term used was dropsy. The cause of death was hypothyroidism.

In a paper presented at the 1997 meeting of the American Thyroid Association, R. Arem showed what every doctor learned in medical school: There exists a strong link between abnormal thyroid function, elevated cholesterol, elevated triglyceride levels, and heart disease. But what physicians knew in the 1890s, that replacement of thyroid medication could prevent and treat "dropsy," has been lost on the physicians in practice today. Dropsy is the end stage of hypothyroid-induced congestive heart failure. There is fluid retention that is seen in the lower legs as edema, in the abdominal cavity as ascites, in the lungs as pulmonary edema, and in and around heart as a pericardial effusion. Low thyroid function can also increase the risk of hypertension and vascular resistance, and contributes to other complications of heart disease. Treatment then and now with appropriate "natural" thyroid replacement that has both the active thyroid molecules will reduce not only (1) heart failure and (2) cholesterol, but also, strikingly, (3) triglyceride levels—sometimes to normal. Arem[20] said so at the American Thyroid Association and in his book, *The Thyroid Solution* (1999).

The history of thyroid disease and medical treatment unfortunately took a wrong turn in 1939. As Broda Barnes, M.D., the leading clinician and researcher in thyroid disease, revealed in his book entitled *Hypothyroidism*,[21] he was approached by the pharmaceutical manufacturers to promote synthetic thyroid, Synthroid®. He allegedly first explained that Synthroid® was an incomplete thyroid, containing only T4, whereas Armour® Thyroid, also a prescription medication, had both thyroxine (T4) and triiodothyronine (T3) from the thyroid glands of pigs or beef cattle. By marketing an incomplete thyroid, Barnes predicted that synthetic thyroid would wreak havoc on the endocrine system. The pharmaceutical company took no heed and proceeded to make synthetic thyroid the drug of choice. Doctors today are taught to be adamant that synthetic is better because they have heard this nonsense hundreds of times. The marketing falsehoods spread about natural or Armour® Thyroid have obviously been important in the shifting of the vast majority of prescription thyroid to Synthroid®; the ratio now favors Synthroid® 15:1; away from Armour® Thyroid.

Yet the medical literature is now replete with the unique functions for the T3 in Armour® Thyroid in treating high cholesterol and heart disease.

To summarize what Barnes and others have stated about normal thyroid function 70 years ago and that remains appropriate and scientifically correct today:

1. Normal thyroid function is necessary for health, life, and normal fertility.
2. Appropriate replacement of thyroid necessitates both T4 and T3 in a balance that re-establishes normal body temperature.
3. Laboratory tests are guidelines, not absolutes, in treating the patients with thyroid disease.

CONCLUSION #1: CHECK HYPOTHYROIDISM AS A CAUSE OF ELEVATED CHOLESTEROL

Thyroid disease is definitely one of the causes of high cholesterol. It goes unrecognized and underdiagnosed in individuals with heart disease. Why worry about lowering cholesterol with some statin when there is an FDA-approved thyroid and appropriate laboratory tests to prove there exists a thyroid deficiency concurrently in the first place? Bio-identical Armour® Thyroid might not only lower cholesterol and lower blood pressure, but there is a 100-year history of it being used to prevent and treat congestive heart failure. Replacing natural thyroid will not only treat those cold hands and feet, increase mental focus, and fix the brittle nails, hair loss, and thinning eyebrows, but might also statistically lower cholesterol. Bio-identical thyroid has scientifically proved to be so much more important in the cholesterol-CAD-heart disease continuum than statin, because thyroid replacement treats the cause. Why then not treat hypothyroidism first, recheck the cholesterol and lipid levels, and follow up with a diet high in fiber, omega-3 fatty acids, appropriate nutraceuticals and instruction to the patient in a change of lifestyle before deciding to add statins or recheck other noncontributory testing parameters?

Is the physician's concern only the allegedly cholesterol-laden plaque in the coronary arteries of 50- and 60 year-old heart attack victims, or the epidemic of heart failure seen in both men and women today?

HEART FAILURE

The incidence of congestive heart failure (CHF) in the United States is increasing, with more than 500,000 new cases per year. While heart failure occurs in 1% of people at age 50, 5% of people at age 75, it occurs in 25% of people aged 85 and older. Congestive heart failure is the most frequent reason for admission to the hospital under Medicare.[22] Could the cause of this increase in admissions be due to misdiagnosed hypothyroidism or the precarious policy of prescribing statins to everyone whose total cholesterol is just over 200 mg/dL?

Statins may be compounding the problem. A study of 20 patients on Lipitor® showed a 66% occurrence of abnormalities of the diastole, or filling stage, of the heart. This is a major component of congestive heart failure.[23] Could statins do more than block production of necessary coenzyme Q10? A search of the literature finds a double-blind study that established clearly that statins do no good for individuals with CHF.[24] There were no demonstrable changes in heart function for those individuals with heart failure placed on high-dose statins. A leading cardiologist[25] states in his book that to treat and prevent heart disease one needs to consider bio-identical nutrient replacement: coenzyme Q10, L-carnitine, and D-ribose. Dr. Lichten has added these products to his everyday vitamin packages and suggests that they are appropriate for almost everyone.

TESTOSTERONE AND HEART FAILURE

Another missed cause of heart failure is the absence of testosterone. As reviewed in the previous chapter, as men age there is both a natural drop in testosterone levels and an increase in SHBG, which binds up more testosterone. To this double whammy is added the increased estrogen poisoning in our food and the xenoestrogens of plastics and DDT. Men continue to experience heart failure at an alarming rate. And modern medication with statins and medical diagnostic equipment tests are missing the connection between low testosterone and heart failure, and low testosterone and coronary artery disease.

The answer to heart failure is right there in every heart cell. The heart is a muscle that must beat billions of times in a lifetime. It never stops to rest. So these heart cells are the most finely tuned energy machines in the entire human body. They are irreplaceable. They are in tune to testosterone. The heart has more testosterone receptors than any other muscle in the body.[26] Actually, the heart has more dihydrotestosterone receptors.[27] Why would it be so sensitive to testosterones if it weren't the most important connection the heart has to the total body's function? Being strong, healthy, and virile is the only way that nature can ensure reproduction of the human race.

We know that testosterone allows a man or woman to run faster. Ben Johnson was a top-notch athlete who became an Olympic gold metal sprinter with supplementary testosterone. Women runners like Florence Griffith Joyner won races at speeds never achieved previously only to die of heart problems, which some people thought secondary to using performance-enhancing steroids.[28] In the cases of athletes and normal people alike, testosterone for men offers improved cardiac function in all measurable cardiac parameters. Testosterone improves heart-muscle-pumping capacity and requires less energy to do so. Testosterone should be of primary importance in treating older men with heart failure.[29,60] And as the following will show, starting testosterone early may prevent the development of other heart problems.

Testosterone is an anabolic steroid. It can make new and bigger muscles, as to what bodybuilders can attest. The same applies to those weak and flabby heart muscles. But to make new muscles, the body needs protein, minerals, vitamins, and essential fats. These are called nutraceuticals.

Note that a number of Dr. Lichten's testosterone-deficient patients both with and without diabetes have recorded a 100-point drop in total cholesterol that persists month after month while on testosterone replacement.

CORONARY ARTERY DISEASE

Coronary artery disease (CAD) refers to plaque-narrowing of the major vessels to the heart. These narrowed channels impair blood flow. When there is a period of stress, the body is supposed to release nitric oxide (NO) into the coronary circulation. This ensures that the vessels will dilate in a fight-or-flight stress mode. The problem with coronary artery disease is that there may be a paroxysmal constriction instead of dilatation in the region with the plague. This spasm can cause the drop in blood flow that may lead to a myocardial infarction.

While cardiologists and pharmaceutical companies have focused on the cholesterol-laden plaque, other researchers have found a way to keep the arteries from contracting—testosterone. Testosterone is lacking in men with CAD.[30]

The testing for coronary artery disease began in 1903. At that time, Einthoven in Holland invented the electro-kardiac-graph (EKG). Recording the normal electrical conduction of the heart, he was able to delineate changes that were consistent with myocardial infarction (MI), enlargement of the heart chambers, congestive heart failure (CHF), and changes predictive of old or new cardiac wall damage. The EKG is a brilliant piece of medical discovery, no doubt, relatively cheap and available in almost every doctor's office. When coupled with the treadmill test, doctors feel that they have a good screening test for heart disease. And to some extent they do, but putting all medical faith in the 100-year-old test leads to too many false assumptions. Half of individuals admitted to the hospital with a diagnosis of myocardial infarction have a normal or nonspecific EKG.[31]

And although cardiologists are using ultrasound imaging to determine if there is abnormal movement of the muscle of the heart, there are simpler and better tests available outside the hospitals. The hospitals of the past 50 years have become home to expensive equipment that serve relatively little purpose in the diagnosis of heart disease. The thallium stress test is still available at a cost of nearly $5,000, yet it shows incomplete information for most heart patients with coronary artery disease. The reason is that these nuclear scans can show only large functional areas of tissue destruction and coronary occlusion, and in many heart patients this information may be discernible clinically. We believe that electron beam tomography (EBT) would be a better initial means of evaluation.

ELECTRON BEAM TOMOGRAPHY

For more than 20 years, the rapid electronic beam tomography (EBT) has been able to pick up calcium scarring in the coronary arteries. This is a test that takes multiple slices of the heart in 30 seconds and re-creates the three-dimensional images in the computer; its image speed is 200 to 400 times faster than the traditional CT scan and 10 times faster than a helical CT scan.[32] The EBT gives a calcium score. The calcium score correlates to arterial-wall deposits of plaque, fibrin, and calcium. In most plaque buildup, the hard calcium represents one-third, the fibrin one-third, and the soft plaque one-third. Young people score well under 20; those at risk score over 100, and those with need for immediate intervention may score 400 or more.

In a study of men screened for chest pain and waiting hospital admission, the EBT was able to exclude emergency admission in 74%.[33]

So, whether you are 35 or 85, this test will tell you to a significant degree whether you are at risk for having coronary artery disease.[34] If you have a low calcium score, why take the statins because you are not at risk? If you have high calcium scores, your cardiologist will put you on statins after attempting to place the surgical stents. In the latter, you would take medication for a definite purpose, because you are "at risk," not just to "lower cholesterol." This is the Rose[35] theorem of separating out low-risk from high-risk populations and focusing medical intervention on high-risk candidates only.

The newest EBT equipment has the ability to take hundreds of cross-sectional pictures of the coronary arteries. Coupled with a radio-opaque dye, EBT-A will give a computer rendition of the three-dimensional appearance of the coronary arteries. Performed as an outpatient procedure for approximately $800 dollars, EBT-A gives pictures almost as clear as they would appear at time of cardiac catheterization. But, again, the health insurance carriers refuse to pay for this EBT-A test but will pay for the $50,000 heart catheterization and thallium tests and coronary artery stents, which have no impact on mortality over the long term.[36]

WHAT TO DO FIRST FOR HEART DISEASE

In a comprehensive review of published medical articles, by cross-referencing the six sets of the key bio-identical hormones discussed in this book against coronary heart disease and heart failure, we find many proofs of the interaction of hormone dysfunction and cardiac disease. Scientifically, vitamin D, human growth hormone, thyroxine, and triiodothyronine, DHEA, and testosterone in men and estradiol in women have strong cardio-protective or therapeutic applications.

To make the case in point, it is good medicine to treat the cause of heart disease. Dr. Lichten suggests supplementing the bio-identical hormones to at least mid-normal physiologic levels first, then concurrently adding the proper nutritional supplements in order to maximize repair of the body, the heart, and coronary disease. Supplements can incidentally also assist in normalizing cholesterol levels, with niacin being a prime example.

THE CASE AGAINST STATINS FOR CHOLESTEROL AND HEART DISEASE

Statins, like all foreign chemicals, will have adverse effects on the human body. Those side effects listed on the package insert appear below:

1. Muscle pain and weakness and joint stiffness are symptoms typical on statins. This is because it blocks the production of coenzyme Q10, whichis necessary for optimal muscle function. If the muscle pain progresses, it may be a sign of rhabdomyolysis, which can lead to a fatal disease of muscle destruction. Physicians need to monitor not only liver but also the muscle enzyme creatine kinase (CK) for this condition.
2. Coenzyme Q 10 deficiency: Concern has been raised that a worsening heart status could occur because of coenzyme Q10 depletion.
3. Brain fog can be a major complaint of patients on statins. This may be due to ultra-low-cholesterol levels.
4. Cancer. The cholesterol drugs formerly and presently on the market, are associated with increased rates of certain cancer.[37]

CONCLUSION

It has been Dr. Lichten's position that treating the laboratory test for cholesterol **by prescribing statins** is fraught with danger for the patient. First, it gives both the patient and physician a false sense of having done something, while in truth the underlying disease process associated with high cholesterol goes untreated. Secondly, using a liver poison to change laboratory values is not only illogical but also dangerous. How it improves survival or reproduction remains unproved.

Many physicians are unsure about what statins are supposed to do anyway. Dr. Lichten reports seeing elderly women with total cholesterols of 220 mg/dL and HDL levels of 80 mg/dL being prescribed this drug. Patients with normal total cholesterol/ HDL ratios are not statin candidates. One of the studies referenced showed no benefit to prescribing cholesterol-lowering drugs to those over age 70.

Dr. Lichten suggests that appropriate laboratory tests listed in the Appendix under LABTESTS be ordered before beginning any course of lipid-lowering drug; that the patient and physician have a face-to-face discussion about hormones; and that a program of high fiber, vitamins, minerals, and omega-3 supplements be taken for a full 2–3 months before repeating the laboratory lipid profile. Then, if the diet and supplement program is successful, no statin need be prescribed. Taking no medications, including statin drugs, is always preferred.

REPLACEMENT OF BIO-IDENTICAL HORMONES TO IMPROVE CARDIAC FUNCTION

The material appearing below appears in referenced medical peer-review publications. These are scientific publications and are included here to reinforce the concept that physicians treat the cause of symptoms, which is often a hormonal deficiency, before treating a symptom, i.e., cholesterol level.

Vitamin D, referenced in Chapter 1 of Book 1, is necessary for the absorption of minerals from the gastrointestinal tract and parathyroid function that regulates calcium metabolism. As salt balance is integral to the energy of the cell, vitamin D deficiencies may directly and indirectly affect heart disease. The genetic marking of alleles finds that the vitamin D allele is located proximal to genetic markers for both coronary artery disease and diabetes.

1. Vitamin D concentrations are low in patients with congestive heart failure.[38] Vitamin D3 is found to increase the speed to peak relaxation of the heart cycle.[39] Heart failure is noted by a prolonged filling stage, therefore, a shorter filling stage is healthier.

2. Zitterman[40] presents results indicating that an insufficient vitamin D status may contribute to the etiology/pathogenesis of CHF. Data include a vitamin D–mediated reduction of elevated blood pressure as well as a vitamin D–mediated prevention of excess parathyroid hormone levels, a pathophysiological state that contributes to cardiovascular disease. Based on population-attributable risks, hypertension and cardiovascular disease have a high impact, accounting for the majority of CHF events.

3. One of the complications of CHF is development of aldosteronism and secondary hyperparathyroidism because of the loss of calcium in the urine. This affects the energy flow of calcium-magnesium in the energy of the cell. Animal studies show that the addition of vitamin D and calcium and magnesium were able to reverse both aldosteronism and secondary hyperparathyroidism.[41]

4. Genetic typing now shows that the allele for vitamin D is associated with development of both CAD and diabetes.[42]

Human growth hormone deficiency is associated with premature heart disease and death in those so afflicted. Not only is growth hormone and low levels of IGF-1 associated with unfavorable risk factors, Fazio[43] used hGH to treat the worst cases of cardiomyopathy, as did Lichten, as explained in Chapter 2.

1. One meta-analysis suggests that hGH treatment improves several relevant cardiovascular parameters in patients with CHF.[44]

2. In those men and women born with growth hormone deficiency (GHD), there is an increased risk of heart disease and a premature death. This data suggest that abnormal lipid, glucose metabolism, and atherosclerotic changes occur frequently in adult patients with GHD.[45]

3. In cross-sectional studies, low IGF-I levels have been associated with unfavorable CVD risk-factor profiles, such as atherosclerosis, abnormal lipoprotein levels,

and hypertension, while in prospective studies, lower IGF-I levels predict future development of ischemic heart disease.[46]

4. Recombinant human growth hormone administered for three months to patients with idiopathic dilated cardiomyopathy increased myocardial mass and reduced the size of the left ventricular chamber, resulting in improvement in hemodynamics, myocardial energy metabolism, and clinical status.[43]

Thyroid hormone has been a recognized cause of heart failure for more than 100 years. With the environmental influx of minerals that displace iodine, there is an ongoing increase in thyroid disease, as noted in Chapter 3. Recent research from Europe is demonstrating that the use of thyroid supplements must contain T3 to be effective.

1. Thyroid hormone metabolic disarray has been identified as a risk factor for the progression of heart disease and the development of heart failure (HF). Both hyper- and hypothyroidism have been associated with a failing myocardium. Poor cardiac contractility and low cardiac output due to hyperthyroidism is a rare occurrence and is mostly seen in patients with preexisting heart disease. Referred to as a "rate related" phenomenon, hyperthyroid-induced sustained sinus tachycardia or atrial fibrillation may further reduce ventricular contractility. Increasingly, the hypothyroid state, and in particular a low triiodothyronine level, has been associated with a reduced cardiac performance and poor prognosis in HF, even in the presence of normal thyroid-stimulating hormone levels. Low thyroid hormone levels alter cardiac gene expression and increase systemic vascular resistance, both resulting in a reduction of cardiac contractility and cardiac output. This review summarizes current data on thyroid dysfunction and HF, as well as the emerging implications of the "low triiodothyronine state."[47]

2. These findings suggest that symptoms of depression in patients with CADare associated with changes in thyroid axis function [T3/ T3r] and with cardiac impairment, especially in men.[48]

3. Subclinical hypothyroidism may be a risk factor for CAD.[49]

The adrenal hormones, specifically the anabolic hormone dehydroepiandrosterone (DHEA), along with T3, testosterone, and IGF-1 are "spark plugs" that trigger energy production. It is logical and scientifically evident that men with congestive heart failure live longest with the highest levels of these anabolic hormones. Not only is DHEA produced in the adrenal glands, but recent discoveries show that DHEA is produced normally in the heart itself. Low levels of DHEA may be associated with coronary artery disease as well.

1. Men with CHF and normal levels of all anabolic hormones had the best three-year survival rate (83%, 95% CI 0.47-0.98) compared with those with deficiencies (74% survival, 95% CI 0.65-0.84), two (55% survival, 95% CI 0.45-0.66), or all three (27% survival rate, 95% CI 0.05-0.49), anabolic endocrine axes (P<0.0001). CONCLUSIONS: In male CHF patients, anabolic hormone depletion is common, and a deficiency of each anabolic hormone is an independent marker of poor prognosis. More anabolic hormone deficiencies identify higher mortality.[50]

2. CYP17 gene expression and production of DHEA were demonstrated in a human control heart. Also, the medical literature who found that cardiac production of DHEA was suppressed in a failing heart. DHEA may exert a cardio-protective action through antihypertrophic effects.[51-52]

3. CONCLUSIONS: The present findings suggest that, in men, low serum levels of DHEA may be associated with coronary heart disease.[53]

INSULIN RESISTANCE AND DIABETES ARE TESTOSTERONE-DEFICIENCY INTERRELATED DISEASES

Diabetes in men is a disease associated with low levels of bio-identical testosterone. The number one cause of death in diabetics is coronary heart disease. To be diagnosed as diabetic raises one's risk of a heart attack to the same status as one who has already had a myocardial infarction (MI). Insulin resistance is an important finding in heart failure.

Congestive Heart Failure (CHF) is a complex metabolic disorder. Metabolic abnormalities include insulin resistance and lack of anabolic hormone activity.[54]

Testosterone has so many cardiac protective properties that space precludes listing them all. Testosterone is a vasodilator that keeps the coronary arteries open, an energy amplifier that strengthens the heart muscle's ability to pump blood, and it has proven antidiabetic properties.

1. Testosterone reduced one direct measurement of insulin resistance called HOMA-IR (-1.9+/-0.8, p=0.03), indicating improved fasting insulin sensitivity, a marker of congestive heart failure (CHF).[53]
2. In clinical trials, testosterone confers symptomatic benefits in patients with coronary heart disease and heart failure, acting as a vasodilator. These observations lend support that testosterone could be a potential treatment for patients with pulmonary artery hypertension (PAH), as vasodilator therapy remains the mainstay of treatment.[55]
3. Beyond sexual function regulation, male steroids are operative in several physiologic homeostatic systems, including the cardiovascular system. By ways of specific androgen receptors, testosterone can mediate cardiomyocyte trophicity in physiologic states as in diseases involving cardiac hypertrophy. Androgenic hormones also regulate pathologic levels of inflammatory cytokines as IL-6 or TNF in advanced

heart failure. They also mediate vascular resistance to improved coronary vasodilatation. Reduced free-testosterone serum levels as seen in age-mediated or in premature coronary artery disease (CAD) promote a plaque-forming lipid profile; a decrease in "good" HDL and an increase of "bad" triglycerides levels. The latter observation has relevant clinical significance for evaluation and treatment of CAD. As most normal and diseased cardiovascular system functions are influenced by androgens, we can foresee an increasing interest for further evaluation of their physiologic implications as well as for large and rigorous studies of their therapeutic potential in two leading disabling pathologies: CAD and heart failure.[56]

4. CONCLUSIONS: Short-term intra-coronary administration of testosterone, at physiological concentrations, induces coronary artery dilatation and increases coronary blood flow in men with established coronary artery disease.[57] Estradiol and heart disease in women is the subject of Chapter 6. The WHI statements must be considered limited to scientific and physiologic studies that show estradiol dilates coronary arteries, which are very positive and cardio-protective effects. Negative aspects of the WHI are mostly restricted to use of MPA (Provera®).

5. CONCLUSIONS: Physiological levels of 17 beta-estradiol acutely and selectively potentiate endothelium-dependent vasodilatation in both large coronary conductance arteries and coronary microvascular resistance arteries of postmenopausal women. This effect may contribute to the reduction in cardiovascular events observed with estrogen replacement therapy.[58]

FINAL CONCLUSIONS

Within this chapter, the material presented has shown a direct correlation between the bio-identical hormone levels and the symptoms and findings of cardiac disease. Other doctors have pointed out the mistake of taking evidence-based data from moderate- to high-risk populations and extrapolating the conclusions to a relatively low-risk population. Lauer made this point this year reviewing the METEOR Study.[59] And these are direct quotes, while brackets [ ] are the author's:

- A number of trials demonstrate that statins prevent cardiovascular events and reduce progression of atherosclerosis; these studies have primarily involved intermediate or high-risk populations.[61-64]

- [But as to make a point] there were only 6 ischemic events, which curiously all occurred in the rosuvastatin group [METEOR study].[65]

- To date there have been no randomized trials showing this particular statin to reduce risk of clinical events.[59]

- Furthermore, epidemiological data have provided overwhelming evidence that low-risk populations are the source of most clinical disease. The METEOR investigators have now provided biological evidence for a plausible but unproved strategy [of giving statins to prevent disease].[65]

A program strategy that is most scientific and logical starts with a change in diet, an increase in fiber, vitamins B, C, D, E, minerals, essential fatty acids (including omega-3), and, most of all, a balance of bio-identical hormones.

Lastly, Lauer went on to state in the prestigious *Journal of the American Medical Association* that "this then raises the question as to whether a medical strategy might be applicable to the low-risk population."[59]

LICHTEN THEORY IN PRACTICE

This is Dr. Lichten's basic medical strategy for treating each patient:

1. Measure the bio-identical hormones
2. Raise, if appropriate for the symptomatology noted, the deficient values above the median value for a healthy 40- to 50-year-old individual.

3. Determine what positive and/or negative effect this intervention has on the primary disease or complaint.

Dr. Lichten reiterates that the evaluation of each patient starts with baseline laboratory measurements to rule out deficiencies of bio-identical hormones. Treat these first and then reevaluate to see if the secondary parameters of cardiovascular risk, lipids, cholesterol, homocysteine, fasting glucose and insulin, and C-reactive protein may return to a more acceptable level!

Bio-Identical Hormonal Parameters as Indices of Disease
1. Vitamin D
2. IGF-1
3. Thyroxine (T4)-free; triiodothyronine (T3)-free
4. DHEA-sulfate, morning cortisol
5. Fasting insulin, hemoglobin A1c
6. Total testosterone, estradiol & sex hormone binding globulin

also
1. Complete blood count, sedimentation rate
2. Metabolic panel, including homocysteine
3. Lipid panel: fasting, including glucose
4. Prostate specific antigen (PSA)

A form to order these tests appears in the Appendix under LAB TESTS, allowing the patient to have access to critical information before meeting with the doctor.

The final point to be made about cholesterol is that it cannot form plaques until it is oxidized. Oxidization is what rust is to metal; oxidation leaves the cholesterol foam cell rough and sticky. Another term for these oxidative changes is an inflammatory response. Inflammatory responses are associated with insulin resistance, diabetes, obesity and atherosclerosis. Therefore, the treatment for all anti-inflammatory processes is to use antioxidant supplements, and for all men, testosterone. Be aware that testosterone is overwhelmingly the most potent antioxidant for men and can offer a profoundly positive improvement in his cardiac, coronary and lipid parameters.[60]

Cholesterol-Lowering Drugs

Niaspan® slo-niacin

Mevacor® lovastatin

Lipitor® atorvastatin

Zocor® simvastatin

Pravachol® pravastatin

Crestor® rosuvastitin

Lescol®fluvastatin

Zetia® ezetimibe

REFERENCES:

1. Jones NW, Rogers AL. The incidence of streptococcal infection in cardiovascular sclerosis. *Ann Intern Med* 1935; 8:834–53.
2. Available at: http://heartdisease.about.com/library/news/blnws01037.htm.
3. Keys A. Atherosclerosis. A problem in the new public health. *Journal of Mt. Sinai Hospital.* 1953; 20:118–39.
4. WHO study: increased deaths from Atromid S. Atromid website.
5. Statin Safety: An Overview and Assessment of the Data—2005. *The American Journal of Cardiology*, Volume 97, Issue 8, Pages S6-S26 H. Bays6.
6. Available at: http://www.fda.gov/cder/drug/infopage/baycol/
7. Request for Crestor to be removed from market. See Crestor Petition to the FDA to remove the cholesterol-lowering drug rosuvastatin (CRESTOR) from the market (HRG Publication #1693).
8. Available at: http://www.fda.gov/bbs/topics/NEWS/NEW00721.html.
9. Kapoor D. Testosterone replacement therapy improves insulin resistance, glycaemic control, visceral adiposity and hypercholesterolaemia in hypogonadal men with type 2 diabetes. *European Journal of Endocrinology.* 2006 June; 154(6):899–906.
10. Available at: http://www.nhlbi.nih.gov/guidelines/cholesterol/atp3xsum.pdf.
11. McKenney JM. Prescription omega-3 fatty acids for the treatment of hypertriglyceridemia. *American Journal of Health System Pharmacy.* 2007; 64(6):595–605.
12. Available at: http://www.cholesterol-and-health.com.
13. Hudson JW. Cholesterol measurement and treatment in community practices. *Journal of Family Practice.* 1990; 31(2):139-44.
14. Available at: http://www.nhlbi.nih.gov/about/ncep/
15. Available at: http://physics.ucr.edu/~wudka/Physics7/Notes_www/node6.html #SECTION 02121000000000000000.
16. Ravnskov U. Statins as the new aspirin. Conclusions from the heart protection study were premature. *British Medical Journal.* 2002 Mar 30;324(7340):789.
17. Bero L, Oostvogel F, Bacchetti P, Lee K. actors associated with findings of published trials of drug-drug comparisons: why some statins appear more efficacious than others. PLoS Med. 2007 Jun;4(6):e184.
18. Silva M, Matthews ML, Jarvis C, Nolan NM, Belliveau P, Malloy M, Gandhi P. Meta-analysis of drug-induced adverse events associated with intensive-dose statin therapy. Clin Ther. 2007 Feb;29(2):253-60.
19. Celik T, Iyisoy A, Yuksel UC, Isik E. The panacea for cardiovascular diseases: The role of statins in the management of heart failure. Int J Cardiol. 2007 Aug 8; [Epub ahead of print]

20. Available at: http://www.suite101.com/article.cfm/womens_thyroid_disease/35085 in patients with chronic systolic heart failure. *Journal Cardiac Failure.* 2007;13(1):1–7.
21. Barnes, Broda. *Hypothyroidism: The Unsuspected Illness.* (1939). Harper-Collins.
22. Krumholz HM. Readmission after hospitalization for congestive heart failure among Medicare beneficiaries. *Archives of Internal Medicine.* 1997;57(1):99–104.
23. Langsjoen PH. Treatment of statin adverse effects with supplemental Coenzyme Q10 and statin drug discontinuation. *BioFactors.* 2005;25:147–52.
24. Krum H, et al. Double-blind, randomized, placebo-controlled study of high-dose HMG CoA reductase inhibitor therapy on ventricular remodeling, pro-inflammatory cytokines and neurohormonal parameters. *Journal of Cardiac Failure.* 2007;13(1):1–7.
25. Sinatra, S. *The Sinatra Solution.* Basic Health, 2005.
26. Shippen E. *The Testosterone Syndrome.* M. Evans & Co., 1999.
27. Sheridan PJ. The heart contains receptors for dihydrotestosterone but not testosterone: Possible role in sex differential in coronary heart disease. *The Anatomical Record.* 1989;223(4):414–9.
28. Available at: http://www.salon.com/news/1998/12/cov_04newsa3.html.
29. Pugh PJ. Testosterone treatment for men with chronic heart failure. *Heart.* 2004;90:446–7.
30. Phillips GB. The association of hypotestosteronemia with coronary artery disease in men. *Arteriosclerosis and Thrombosis.* 1994;14:701–6.
31. Welch RD, et al. Prognostic value of a normal or nonspecific initial electrocardiogram in acute myocardial infarction. *Journal of the American Medical Association.* 2001;286:1977–84.
32. University of Iowa. *Well & Good Issue 1.* 2000.
33. Hoffmann, U. MDCT in early triage of patients with acute chest pain. *American Journal Roentgenol.* 2006;187(5):1240–7.
34. Kondos GT, et al. Electron-beam tomography coronary artery calcium and cardiac events: a 37-month follow-up of 5635 initially asymptomatic low- to intermediate-risk adults. *Circulation.* 2003 May 27;107(20):2571–6.
35. Rose G. *The Strategy of Preventive Medicine.* New York, NY: Oxford University Press, 1992.
36. Merritt R. Coronary Stents Do Not Improve Long-Term Survival. Duke Clinical Research Institute. Nov 7, 2004. http://www.dukemednews.org/news/article.php?id=8249.
37. Newman TB. Carcinogenicity of Lipid lowering drugs. *Journal of the American Medical Association.* 1996;275(1):2755–60.
38. Zittermann A, Schleithoff SS, Tenderich G, et al. Low vitamin D status: a contributing factor in the pathogenesis of congestive heart failure? *J Am Coll Cardiol.* 2003 Jan 1;41(1):105-12.
39. Green JJ, et al. Calcitrol modulation of cardiac contractile performance via protein kinase C. *Journal of Molecular and Cell Cardiology.* 2006;41(2): 350–9.
40. Zittermann A, et al. Vitamin D insufficiency in congestive heart failure: why and what to do about it? *Heart Failure Review.* 2006;11(1):25–33.
41. Goodwin KD, et al. Preventing oxidative stress in rats with aldosteronism by calcitrol and dietary calcium and magnesium supplements. *American Journal Medicine Science.* 2006;332(4):73–8.
42. Ortlepp JR, et al. The vitamin D receptor gene variant is associated with the prevalence of type 2 diabetes mellitus and coronary artery disease. *Diabetic Medicine.* 2001;18(10):842–5.
43. Fazio S, et al. A preliminary study of the use of growth hormone in dilated cardiomyopathy. *New England Journal of Medicine.* 1996;3334(13):809–14.
44. LeCorvoisier P, et al. Cardiac effects of growth hormone treatment in chronic heart failure: A meta-analysis. *Journal of Clinical Endocrinology.* 2007;92(1):180–5.

45. Itoh E, et al. Metabolic disorders in adult growth hormone deficiency: A study of 110 patients sat a single institute in Japan. *Endocrinology Journal*. 2006;53(4):539–45.

46. Ceda GP. Clinical implications of the reduced activity of the GH-IGF-1 axis in older men. *Journal of Endocrinology Investigation*. 2005;28(11 Supp):96–100.

47. Schmidt-Ott UM, et al. Thyroid hormone and heart failure. *Current Heart Failure Reports*. 2006;3(3):114–9.

48. Bunevicius R. Depression and thyroid axis function in coronary artery disease: impact of cardiac impairment and gender. *Clinical Cardiology*. 2006; 29(4):170–4.

49. Walsh JP. Subclinical thyroid dysfunction as a risk factor for cardiovascular disease. *Archives Internal Medicine*. 2005;165(21):2451–2.

50. Jankowska EA. Anabolic deficiency in men with chronic heart failure: prevalence and detrimental impact on survival. *Circulation*. 2006;114(17):1829–37.

51. Nakamura S. Possible association of heart failure status with synthetic balance between aldosterone and dehydroepiandrosterone in human heart. *Circulation*. 2004;110(13):1787–93.

52. Thijs L, et al. Are low dehydroepiandrosterone sulphate levels predictive for cardiovascular diseases? A review of prospective and retrospective studies. *Acta Cardiology*. 2003;58(5):403–10.

53. Lainscak M, et al. Metabolic disturbances in chronic heart failure: a case for the 'macho' approach with testosterone?! *European Journal Heart Failure*. 2007;(1):2–3.

54. Malkin CJ. The effect of testosterone on insulin sensitivity in men with heart failure. *European Journal of Heart Failure*. 2007;(1):44–50.

55. Smith AM. The influence of sex hormones on pulmonary vascular reactivity: possible vasodilator therapies for the treatment of pulmonary hypertension. *Current Vascular Pharmacology*. 2006;4(1):9–15.

56. Smeets L. Heart and Androgens. *Rev Med Liege*. 2004;59(7–8):439–44.

57. Webb CM. Effects of testosterone on coronary vasomotor regulation in men with coronary heart disease. *Circulation*. 1999;100(16):1690–6.

58. Gilligan DM, et al. Effects of physiological levels of estrogen on coronary vasomotor function in postmenopausal women. *Circulation*. 1994;89(6):2545–51.

59. Lauer MS. Primary Prevention of Atherosclerotic Cardiovascular Disease. The High Public Burden of Low Individual Risk. *Journal of the American Medical Association*. 2007;297:1376–8.

60. Barud W. Inverse relationship between total testosterone and anti-oxidized low density lipoprotein antibody levels in ageing males. *Atherosclerosis*. 2002; 164(2):283–8.

61. Roberts CG, Guallar E, Rodriguez A. Efficacy and safety of statin monotherapy in older adults: a meta-analysis. *J Gerontol A Biol Sci Med Sci*. 2007 Aug;62(8):879-87. Review.

62. Doser S, Marz W, Reinecke MF, et al. [Recommendations for statin therapy in the elderly] *Internist (Berl)*. 2004 Sep;45(9):1053-62. Epub 2004 Aug 3. Review. German.

63. LaRosa JC. Understanding risk in hypercholesterolemia. *Clin Cardiol*. 2003 Jan;26(1 Suppl 1):I3-6. Review.

64. Holdaas H, Wanner C, Abletshauser C, et al. The effect of fluvastatin on cardiac outcomes in patients with moderate to severe renal insufficiency: a pooled analysis of double-blind, randomized trials. *Int J Cardiol*. 2007 Apr 12;117(1):64-74. Epub 2006 Aug 4. Review.

65. Crouse JR. Effect of Rosuvastatin on Progression of Carotid Intima-Media Thickness in Low-Risk Individuals With Subclinical Atherosclerosis: The METEOR Trial. *Journal of the American Medical Association*. 2007;297:1344–53.

NOTES

CHAPTER 13

TESTOSTERONE IS THE TREATMENT FOR DIABETES IN MEN

TESTOSTERONE IN MEN WITH DIABETES

The first case of diabetes was recorded on papyrus 3,500 years ago in Egypt, but diabetes must have been a part of mankind for aeons before then. In the first century A.D., Arateus describes diabetes as a "melting down of the flesh" because of the extreme wasting these individuals experienced prior to death. In the Middle Ages, there were urine tasters who diagnosed diabetes from the sweet taste in the urine. However, no treatment was found effective except strict limitation diets until Banting and Best isolated and produced insulin in 1922.

Within four months, Eli Lilly had contracted with them for the mass production of insulin. Oral agents to lower blood glucose, called sulfonylureas, were made available in 1955. In 1959, the differentiation was made between two types of diabetes: type I juvenile insulin-requiring, and type II adult-onset oral-agents requiring. And then it seems the truth about how to treat diabetes got lost in the shuffle for health-care dollars.

The problem with research in diabetes is that there is no true animal model—only the chemically induced streptozotocin rat model.[1] Diabetes only develops spontaneously in humans, and the reasons are still unknown. As previously demonstrated, for any disease to develop there may be both a genetic predisposition and an environmental factor. Recent discoveries show that for type I insulin-requiring diabetes, there are genetic defects, which in some way leave the individual susceptible to specific types of infections. The end result is that these individuals, once infected, are left to become diabetic because of the destruction of the beta islet cells that produce insulin in the pancreas.

Type II diabetes is more a state of beta-islet-cell destruction from overuse. Genetically predisposed individuals may overwhelm their insulin production from first ingesting (1) excessive simple carbohydrates and (2) depositing the glucose stores in the cell wall. These glucose deposits act like molasses on a filter blocking or resisting any further entry of glucose into the cell. The medical term is "insulin resistance," or reduced insulin sensitivity. In the early stage, the body attempts to overpower this blockage, leading to an outpouring of insulin in an attempt to compensate for the cell's inability to efficiently utilize insulin. However, over time, beta cell burn out (dysfunction) and insulin production can no longer compensate for insulin resistance and both fasting and postprandial glucose levels continue to rise, leading to irreversible damage, which we call diabetes, and heart disease, kidney disease, eye damage, gangrene-amputations, and hypertension may also follow if the disease is left untreated. Modern medicine has devised oral medications in an attempt to keep blood sugar controlled, open-heart surgery and stents to keep the coronary arteries open, dialysis machines to keep people with dead kidneys alive, and more oral medication to keep blood pressure below the stroke levels.

But no one has seemed to ask why this was happening at such an increasing rate. How can we put a man on the moon yet watch 20 million Americans and 400 million people worldwide suffer with this disease? The forthcoming answers come from historical reviews, observations, clinical and laboratory studies, and a desire to find a way to prevent the suffering from the number one cause of disease and death—the malady called diabetes.

In the First World War, there is an unsubstantiated report that the testicles from a dead soldier were transplanted into the abdominal wall of a man with gangrene. The story goes that the man recovered and did not need amputation. This story would be considered whimsical if it were not for the work of Jens Moller, M.D.,[2] in Denmark from 1950 to 1984. Moller and 250 other European physicians used injections of bio-identical testosterone to treat diabetes, gangrene, and related heart disease in more than 10,000 men and women. Moller's enthusiasm overshadowed the observation that the dosages of testosterone used significantly increased the incidence of heart disease in treated women.

This led to his public humiliation: a disbanding of the European physicians, and a misconception that testosterone was dangerous.

Personal Experience

Dr. Lichten has personal experience with testosterone deficiency as previously told. It seemed like overnight he went from being an enthusiastic, hard working, physically potent man to be a depressed, lethargic, exhausted old man. His colleagues had no idea what to do—one offered to admit him into the hospital to get an answer. But as a physician, he knew that the hospital offered no answers. Dr. Lichten was one of the first recognized "menopausal" males.

His women patients noticed the difference, and since low-dose testosterone replacement has been a mainstay of Dr. Lichten's treatment of menopausal women, they were intrigued. After questioning, they asked if Dr. Lichten would treat their husbands, not only because of erectile dysfunction and lack of libido, but because they were worried that their husbands' health was being jeopardized. He agreed, and the third man treated was a 295-pound, 5'10" male with adult-onset diabetes.

Joe N., 48, confided that he was worried about whether or not he would see his daughter grow up. Once an active man, he now could not walk up a flight of stairs without becoming short of breath. He knew being diabetic affected his heart as severely as having a heart attack, and he could not lose weight, although he tried. After performing a glucose tolerance test with matching insulin levels,

Dr. Lichten determined Joe to be an early vs. burned-out diabetic. So testosterone injections weekly were begun and his blood sugar was watched. Joe's finger sticks of glucose dropped the first week into the normal range. He felt better and was able to walk up the stairs without difficulty. He lost 20 pounds the first month, allegedly without trying. The second month he joined a gym and lost another 20 pounds. Then, after the third month, he had lost another 10. And at the one-year testosterone-replacement anniversary, Joe weighed in at 215 pounds—80 pounds lighter. And at 18 months, his repeat glucose tolerance test and matching insulin and testosterone hormonal parameters were normal. Able to run on the treadmill for 90 minutes, Joe was, at that point in time, clinically not diabetic. And his wife had returned to Dr. Lichten's office for her biweekly testosterone injection. It seems that the libido-enhancing bio-identical hormonal replacement program with testosterone had proved to be so much more effective than Viagra®.

In the hospital, a 59-year-old insulin-dependent diabetic was scheduled for amputation of his finger. The infection had begun with the repeated glucose testing lancets and had eaten away the tissue to the bone. In the hospital he was listless, unshaven, not eating, and displaying the ominous Q-sign: His tongue was hanging out of the side of his mouth. As a family friend, Dr. Lichten was beseeched to do something, so he offered an injection of short-acting testosterone. The hospital was in an uproar, as this was considered unapproved therapy for diabetes, but his diabetic patient's blood sugar dropped 50 points in the first day—he got out of bed, shaved, and ate his meals. With two more injections that week, his finger started to heal so that the amputation was canceled. He also felt well enough not only to go home but also to make "900-number" calls from the hospital. At home, his wife forbade any more testosterone injections, as she stated his erections had returned after a two-year hiatus. When he died four years later of cardiac disease, he died with his finger healed and every part intact.

Armed with this information, Dr. Lichten approached his colleague James Sowers, M.D., professor and chairman of Endocrinology and Metabolism at Wayne State University in Detroit, Michigan. Dr. Sowers is considered one of the foremost diabetic experts in the United States. Intrigued by Dr. Lichten's observations, he devised a pilot study for up to 100 diabetic men.[3] After baseline studies of their bio-identical sex hormones (testosterone, estradiol, sex hormone-binding globulin), general lab and PSA testing, and a two-hour glucose test with insulin, the volunteer diabetic men would be treated with monthly testosterone implants. The patients would be seen monthly for three months on testosterone and then for four months off testosterone injections. Testing occurred at regular, one-month intervals.

In 1974, R.L. Kraft[4] performed 2,500 glucose tolerance tests of normal and diabetic individuals. The standard glucose tolerance test starts by drawing fasting blood glucose and then drinking a sugary liquid that contains a known amount of glucose, usually 50 or 75 grams. Then the repeat blood samples are drawn at one-half, one, and two hours thereafter. Normal is defined as a fasting glucose under 100 mg/dL; a half-hour and one-hour under 145 mg/dL; and a two-hour below 125 mg/dL. Kraft then added the drawing of insulin levels concurrently. Kraft documented various abnormal patterns of insulin response, predicting the development of diabetes even before the glucose tolerance test became abnormal.

The problem with standard medical care is that the physician rarely performs a glucose tolerance test and almost never performs the corresponding insulin measurements. He first relies on a fasting blood glucose test, but the levels considered abnormal have been decreasing from 124 mg/dL to 105 mg/dL and now less than 100 mg/dL. While a normal glucose tolerance and insulin response appear in the table below, any deviation from this is scientific evidence of metabolic syndrome, prediabetes, and/or insulin resistance. The terminology is irrelevant. The single test is the only definitive test for diabetes: It is called glycosylated hemoglobin or hemoglobin A1c (Hgb-A1c). Levels of hemoglobin A1C greater than 6% indicate a diabetic or prediabetic state.

Normal Glucose Insulin Diabetes Glucose Insulin
Early AODM Insulin-Requiring Juvenile, IDDM, Burnout

0-hour 100 mg/dL 10 0-hour >100 mg/ dL >10 <20
1-hour 145 mg/dL 40 1-hour >145 mg/ dL >40 <20
2-hour 125 mg/dL 20 2-hour >120 mg/ dL >20 <20
3-hour 110 mg/dL   3-hour >120 mg/ dL
AODM: adult-onset-diabetes mellitus

To simplify the diagnosis of normal versus early or insulin-requiring adult-onset diabetes mellitus, Dr. Lichten suggests adding up the zero, one, and two-hour insulin values. He calls this Sum-I. The mathematical formula would look like this: SUM-I= I0+ I1+ I2.

Ergo: The summation insulin= values of 0, 1, and 2 hour insulin values added together.

Normal range of SUM-I: 70–130; Diabetes: ranges >130; hyperinsulinemia < 70 insulin needed.

In the 1997–1999 pilot study,[5] under the auspices of Dr. Sowers, Lichten screened approximately 75 adult men with diabetes who volunteered for treatment. Fifteen men were already on insulin. Ten of them were considered brittle diabetics, as they used 80 to 120 units of insulin per day and were prone to have precipitous drops in blood sugar, called hypoglycemia. A hypoglycemic attack can result in coma and death, and few doctors closely titrate these individuals to achieve a preferred 6% Hgb-A1c blood level. The doctors' fears and the medications previously used bring only a small number under an 8% Hgb-A1c.

The initial evaluation in Lichten's study showed every diabetic man was low in testosterone.[5] Ten years later, E.L. Ding[6] at Harvard would come to the same conclusion. The laboratory measurements relied not only on the absolute number of total testosterone (normal 251–1000 ng/dL) but also on the bioavailable measurement of testosterone. Bioavailable means how much is circulating and can be used. Based on the pioneering work of D.C. Anderson[7] in 1972, published in both *Science* and *Nature*, the "free" testosterone index (FAI) is the ratio of the concentration of total testosterone divided by the concentration of sex hormone-binding globulin. The mathematical formula is: [(0.3467 x total testosterone (ng/dL)) /sex hormone-binding globulin (pmol/L)]x100. Note that the 0.3467 is the conversion factor for the different measurements of ng/dL to pmol/L for testosterone. Only unbound, or "free," testosterone is biologically active.

Anderson showed that a young teenager or adult would have a free androgen index (FAI) of greater than 1.0, and a normal male would remain above 0.7 into his 60s. All the diabetic men in the study had a FAI of less than 0.4, and those experiencing a worsening of the disease (such as insulin-requiring) had lower FAIs, actually closer to 0.3. As the study continued and diabetic men on dialysis

TESTOSTERONE IS THE TREATMENT FOR DIABETES IN MEN

were screened, the ratio dropped to less than 0.2. Less bioavailable testosterone equated to worsening diabetes.

Having no preconceived expectation, the study first followed the insulin-requiring adult diabetics for three months. Most reduced their insulin requirements by half without any change in hemoglobin A1c. Men on 120 units of insulin daily now needed 60 units; men on 80 units needed 40. But the next observation may be destined to change the medical practice of diabetes forever:

THESE MEN ON TESTOSTERONE INJECTIONS HAVE NOT
ONLY BETTER GLYCEMIC CONTROL BUT THEY ALSO HAVE
NO DANGEROUS HYPOGLYCEMIC ATTACKS!!

When Charles came into the office, Dr. Lichten was surprised to see his finger stick glucose at 37 mg/dL. When questioned, he told Dr. Lichten that his internist had called him the night before alarmed at the same low reading from his blood sample sent to the national laboratory. Charles had no symptoms and he knew the symptoms of hypoglycemia and impending coma. He was instructed to reduce his insulin by another 10 units per day. And he agreed to do so. But why didn't he crash?

The medical literature including Tibblin[8] reported testosterone sensitizes the cell in men to more readily admit glucose. This is termed a decrease in insulin resistance. Therefore, whenever insulin is available, it works much more efficiently in the presence of testosterone in men. Of note, estradiol, the female hormone, works counterproductively for the male and worsens insulin resistance.

Dr. Lichten's continuing studies can explain why men on testosterone have much less concern about hypoglycemia and diabetic coma. It is obvious that the second role of testosterone is to accelerate not only the conversion of glucose in the bloodstream to stored cellular glycogen but also to reverse the process when needed: Testosterone accelerates the conversion of stored tissue glycogen to serum glucose. That is the explanation for why diabetic males on testosterone injections are much better protected from hypoglycemic-related coma and death. And with this unique effect of testosterone, tighter control is not only desired, it can be more easily achieved. Dr. Lichten routinely has lowered insulin-requiring diabetic men from an Hgb-A1c of 8%, 9%, 10%, and 11% to between

6% and 7%. Morbidity, mortality, and costs of tighter control statistically may be reduced as much as 35% for every 1% drop in HgB-A1c! Dr. Lichten expects fewer heart attacks, fewer strokes, fewer attacks of blindness, and fewer men tethered to dialysis. Diabetic men can and should live longer and live better!

And then to Dr. Lichten's office came Anthony M., a 50-year-old African-American male without insurance, employment, or regular meals, let alone medication. His fasting glucose was 488 mg/dL and his Hgb-A1c was greater than 18%! (Hgb-A1c of 6% or less is normal.) Dr. Lichten immediately treated Anthony with twice the standard dose of testosterone and followed his blood sugar daily. Over the next four months he titrated Anthony's long-acting insulin from 20 units per day to 90 units and continued a sliding scale of regular insulin at approximately 20 units per day with meals.

What was never expected was the rapidity with which Anthony's intracellular glycogen stores would normalize. His Hgb-A1c dropped in two weeks from 18% to 15.7%, at three months it was 8-9%, and at five months 7.7%! *The Journal of the American Medical Association*[9] reported that in the best of circumstances only 40% of insulin-dependent men could be stabilized at a hemoglobin A1c of 8% or less. And here was a gynecologist driving the worst diabetic from 18% to 7.7%. And he has stabilized there.

	24-hour long-acting insulin use	Glucose (mg/dL)	HbA1c (%)	Testosterone (ng/dL)	Sex Hormone-Binding Globulin (nmol/mL)	Treatment: weet testosteron injections
Date						
7/18/06	14 units	488	>18	643	38	2
7/29/06	30 units	141	15.7	—	—	2
8/06/06	40 units	154	15.2	—	—	1.5
8/12/06	50 units	—	13.5	953	—	1
8/28/06	60 units	161	11.8	493	—	1
9/02/06	70 units	165	11.2	522	—	1
9/15/06	75 units	—	10.1	—	—	1
9/22/06	80 units	308	9.5	894	—	1
10/28/06	75 units	47	8.3	—	—	1
11/14/06	75 units	135	7.9	297	—	1
12/18/06	88 units	175	7.7	—	—	1.5
1/27/07	100 units	65	7.4	792	—	1.5

TESTOSTERONE IMPROVES BLOOD SUGAR, HBA1C IN "ANTHONY," A 50-YEAR-OLD DIABETIC

Anthony had memory lapses originating from the complications of high glucose in his bloodstream and in his brain tissue. This is not unusual for uncontrolled diabetics. One evening he injected 30 units of regular, short-acting insulin instead of his long-acting insulin. During an evening call to Dr. Lichten, Anthony was told to eat his dinner and check his glucose levels every two hours. His glucose testing never showed a value below 129 mg/dL! Another time, he awoke at 4 a.m. and took his regular insulin and went back to bed. Morning glucose was 80–90 mg/dL ranges. No crash, no coma, no severe symptoms!

And, as noted in the table above, no matter how much testosterone was given to Anthony, his total testosterone never exceeded the upper limits of normal for men (1,000–1,200 ng/dL). He never developed polycythemia, which is a high red cell count. This is the only real complication of continuous testosterone injections. And the solution for testosterone-taking patients is to donate blood at the Red Cross every four months. Simple.

Conclusion

For insulin-requiring diabetic men without contraindications, the prescription is to add back testosterone as injections and follow their improved glycemic control while reducing their insulin requirements accordingly. Not only will the improved glycemic control reduce morbidity, but there are positive effects of testosterone replacement on the heart, memory, bone, depression, and sexual performance. Testosterone will reduce the risk of heart attack, Alzheimer's disease, osteoporosis, and the need for Epogen® in dialysis patients. In documented cases, the dose of Epogen® was reduced by 50% or more in men over age 50 on dialysis.[10]

And for the adult-onset diabetic men on diet and oral agents, the results were similarly outstanding. This group of almost 50 men consisted of two groups. The two-hour glucose tolerance test with insulin showed 35 of them to be "early" diabetics with a hypersecretion of insulin and low testosterone. With replacement of the testosterone to normal physiologic levels and a normalization of the FAI, many of these men were able to discontinue their use of oral hypoglycemic agents and show improvement in their

Hgb-A1c while on testosterone injections weekly. For those who could not reach the Hgb-A1c of 6%, the most inexpensive generic hypoglycemic agents were restarted after stabilizing the male diabetic on testosterone injections and watching his insulin requirements fall. And these men on testosterone uniformly were pleased with their reawakened vim and vigor, loss of inches from their waist, and improved workout performance.

But for 15 of these adult-onset diabetic men on oral agents, their personal physicians had not realized that they were, in fact, "burned out." The insulin part of the glucose tolerance test (GTT-I) showed no fourfold increase in insulin value at one or two hours; rather, the numbers were flat and relatively unchanged. Therefore, fully one-third of adult men on oral agents were taking expensive medications that were worthless. Some of these men were able to achieve better control on testosterone alone. And some in time would develop a need for insulin.

Dr. Lichten's goal remains the same as everyone who treats diabetes: a hemoglobin A1c of 6.0% And in Dr. Lichten's office, with time and co-operation from patients, almost all men are stabilized with a hemoglobin A1c in the 6-7% range. Glucose levels below 110 mg/mL are commonplace.

Just last year, D. Kapoor[11] in England published a study of 20 diabetic men reporting improvement in glycosylated hemoglobin (Hgb-A1c), insulin resistance, visceral adiposity, waist circumference, lipids and other parameters that had been referenced 10 years previously in the Lichten-Sowers study. So the naysayers should be ever so humble. Testosterone is a necessary treatment for diabetic men, even more so than insulin. Insulin is applicable to 10% of the male population with diabetes, but testosterone should be useful to almost 100% of men with diabetes (so long as they do not have active prostate cancer). Effective, cheap, safe, and life-saving testosterone is truly man's best adjunct for a long and healthy life, diabetic or not.

COMPLICATIONS AND RISKS

The risk of infection, bleeding, and potential allergy to sesame oil from the testosterone injections is small. The risks, expounded in the literature, are those focusing on prostate and testicular cancer. It is a contraindication to use testosterone in the presence of prostate cancer. Yet Dr. Lichten reports having only one male in the last 10 years develop prostate cancer while on testosterone therapy. In fact, that individual was instructed to go back on testosterone by his doctor at Mayo Clinic after only two years of observation postsurgery.

Rather, Morgantaler[12] showed that testosterone might be protective against prostate cancer. In a large study of men with low levels of testosterone and normal prostate specific antigen (PSA <2; PSA 2–4), a full 15–30% had biopsy-proven prostate cancer. The incidence was almost twice as high for men with total testosterone levels lower than 250 ng/dL. Imagine that not having adequate testosterone levels not only predicts a higher incidence of diabetes, heart disease, osteoporosis, Alzheimer's disease, but also prostate cancer!

So, from a medical and health perspective, every doctor should get the appropriate laboratory tests performed on every male over 35 years of age and especially those with suspected health issues.[13] Without the Hgb-A1c and testosterone measurements, a physician would not suspect that so many men are diabetic and hypogonadal.[14]

AFTERTHOUGHT

Thousands of years ago, man recognized that castration took away a man's manhood both physically and emotionally. The same occurs medically with the use of lupron acetate in men with prostate cancer.[15] In our environment, the use of estrogenic hormone implants in our food stock,[16] the use of xenoestrogen plastics, and DDT-like pesticides is responsible for the dramatic drop in bioavailable testosterone and sperm counts in American men over the past 50 years. In this same time period, the incidence of diabetes and heart disease has increased more than 600%. Without simple, effective, and inexpensive testosterone injections and pellets, not gels that aromatize into estrogen, physicians will continue to be faced by more disease in a younger and younger population.

LOST AND FORGOTTEN RESEARCH

A search of older medical research with testosterone replacement will find two articles from Scotland that document a drop of hemoglobin A1c from 12.3 to 9.5 then 10.8 in 8–12 weeks.[17-18] The significance was not appreciated by the researchers. Similarly, Solvay performed a six-month study with the use of their Androgel® topical cream. Based on Lichten's previous research, it is expected to show an initial drop in the hemoglobin A1c from the 10% to 8% range.[19] The study will probably not be continued for additional lengths of time, however, because, based on past clinical observation, an increased aromatization of testosterone to estrogen with the gel, followed by an increase in SHBG, will show a loss of, and possible reversal of, the gel's beneficial glucose-lowering properties.

TODAY

Today the American Association of Diabetic Educators makes it clear: "Men with diabetes have a two times greater risk of having total testosterone less than 300 ng/dL."[20] The A.A.D.E. October 2006 article states: "Diabetes Education: Screen, test, treat: low testosterone and diabetes." It could not be any more direct than that.

All men must accept the fact that testosterone is their *life hormone* or face premature death and disease unaided by nature's bio-identical protector. *Say yes to testosterone* and we might hold the diseases of diabetes, heart disease, osteoporosis, Alzheimer's disease, and even prostate cancer in abeyance a little longer.

DIALYSIS AND TESTOSTERONE OVERVIEW

As mentioned previously, one of the most devastating and expensive complications of diabetes is end-stage kidney disease. In the kidneys, millions of tiny blood vessels (capillaries) with even tinier holes in them, called glomeruli, act as filters. High blood sugar can damage this filtering system. As a result, the kidneys are unable to filter enough wastes and fluids from the blood, and then the individual is at risk of coma and death. Over the past 50 years, modern medicine has become more efficient at making machines to clear the blood of these waste products. Some individuals have lived for more than seven years tethered two to three times per week to a dialysis machine.

The primary complication of long-term dialysis is that the treatments destroy the body's ability to make red cells. It is well established that anemia will develop in the course of chronic disease, but more so as the red cells are lost through the defects in the kidney membrane. As a result, the body tries to keep up by manufacturing more red blood cells. To do so it produces a protein called erythropoietin. But, in time, the ability to produce erythropoietin is exhausted. That is why patients on dialysis are also treated with pharmaceutical drugs biologically similar to erythropoietin: Epogen®, Procrit®, and now Aranesp®. The standard use of Epogen® for more than 300,000 individuals on dialysis has skyrocketed the parent company, Amgen, to a multibillion-dollar enterprise, with $14.1 billion in sales worldwide and $5.9 billion in profit.

Within a dialysis population, most are diabetic. Within the diabetic dialysis population, more than half are men. What has not been appreciated until the *JAMA* article by Ding[6] is that all diabetic men are low in testosterone. What is key is that treating dialysis diabetic men with testosterone will reduce their need for Epogen® by 50% in some, while others are able to discontinue Epogen® completely for a six-month period.[21]

Personal Perspective

In Dr. Lichten's practice, many different problems present without rhyme or reason. One day, a male patient brought in his father, who had been run over by a tractor and experienced what is called compartment syndrome. The large muscles in the legs had broken down, and the legs had swollen so much that cuts had to be made in the skin to prevent the swelling from destroying the remaining leg muscles. And with the destruction of so much muscle, the kidneys were damaged as the protein tried to filter through. So this elderly man was sitting in Dr. Lichten's office with splits in the skin of both his legs and on renal dialysis three times per week.

Dr. Lichten explained that the first step would be to determine if there was a true testosterone deficiency. Since testosterone is an anabolic hormone, it might be helpful to assist in the healing process. The doctors had not been hopeful that the leg swelling would recede enough for the skin to reclose. Dr. Lichten was firm in stating that the testosterone treatment was not intended to treat either the skin or the kidneys. The father and son decided to try this therapy, as the testosterone level and FAI were well below normal.

The treatment consisted of injections of testosterone cypionate and nandrolone weekly. After the third week, the patient's son stated that he had measured the circumference of the legs, and both legs were 1.5 inches smaller. The elderly man stated that he was feeling better. And then the strangest thing happened: There was a call from the dialysis center. It seems that they had to reduce his Epogen® dose by one-third, as his hemoglobin had increased from the allotted 12 g/dL to almost 14 g/dL. They wanted to know what medication had raised his hemoglobin, because they had never seen this before. Dr. Lichten told them it was testosterone and they said, "Oh."

At that time, Dr. Lichten would routinely discuss with his patients the fact that testosterone-type drugs may raise the hemoglobin in both treated men and women. Because of the low dose used in women, rarely did they find their hemoglobin above 15.5 g/dL (normal 12–14 g/dL). But men will find that their hemoglobin may go above 17.5 g/dL, at which time the treatment is to donate a unit of blood at the Red Cross. Many of Dr. Lichten's patients regularly donate blood every four months.

Now, Dr. Lichten discovered, this side effect of testosterone had a positive effect for men on dialysis: raising the blood count. "And although the business of raising hemoglobin was a multibillion-dollar business, wouldn't it be interesting," Dr. Lichten pondered, "If someone else had tried testosterone for this same purpose?"

Not surprising was the fact that the literature confirmed and documented the common use of the testosterone derivative nandrolone in dialysis patients in both the United States and Europe. In Spain, nandrolone is considered the drug of choice for men over 55 years of age on renal dialysis.

There are key facts in understanding the benefit of nandrolone compared to Epogen® alone. Specifically they are:

1. Nandrolone increased the hemoglobin, along with 6,000 IU per week of Epogen®, and without the 45% incidence of problems with blood pressure.[22]

2. Nandrolone was most effective in treating men over the age of 55. In a study by Teruel,[23] this population of men, over age 55, treated with nandrolone only had a three-fold improvement in hemoglobin compared to men under age 45. The resultant level of hemoglobin was well within the therapeutic target range.

3. Nandrolone increased not only the hemoglobin but also the albumin, and added weight to these men suffering from muscle wasting, even when given after Epogen® was stopped for six months.[21]

4. Nandrolone alone or in combination with Epogen® was most effective and offered the most cost savings.[23]

In contrast, patients receiving androgen in addition to EPO had a significantly greater increase in hematocrit values with treatment. Transfusions were eliminated in both groups of patients.[24] These data show that androgen therapy significantly augments the action of exogenous EPO such that lower doses of EPO are sufficient for an adequate hematopoietic response.[23]

On a personal note, Dr. Lichten reports that his patient showed him, after three months of therapy with testosterone, that the surgeons were able to close the split in the skin of his legs and dialysis was continued at one-third the initial dose of Epogen®. His hemoglobin was above the required 12 g/dL, but the nephrologist would not take him off Epogen®.

On a secondary note, the other multibillion-dollar pharmaceutical product from Amgen is Neulasta®, which is used to raise white blood cell counts. Dr. Lichten knew of a unique combination of herbal and vitamin products that was created by a biochemist to raise the white blood count of a teen who had to undergo extreme chemotherapy and who ultimately survived.

Therefore, it is strongly suggested that before embarking on a course of therapy that may reach $30,000 to $60,000 a year with any of these drugs that a concerted effort be made to determine how effective bio-identical and natural products can be. Bio-identical is always safer, more efficient, and more cost effective than the pharmaceutical medications that are foreign to the body's system.

The Food and Drug Administration has revised the boxed warning for erythropoiesis-stimulating agents in response to six recently completed studies that suggested an increased risk of death, blood clots, strokes, and heart attacks in dialysis patients. It seems that those facilities receiving reimbursement from Medicare were pushing the doses of Aranesp®, Epogen®, and Procrit® above FDA guidelines. This 25% increase in usage resulted in a 25% increase in revenues to both Amgen and the facilities but also an unexpected increase in mortality.

PHARMACEUTICAL PRODUCTS MENTIONED IN THE ARTICLE

Testosterone pellets are bio-identical crystalline testosterone compressed in a matrix that allows for equal release over 4–6 weeks.

Pellet insertion is a three-minute procedure in which the slow-release five-week FDA-approved testosterone pellet, compounded five-week estradiol pellets, or Dr. Lichten's new formulation of three-month pellets are introduced painlessly under local anesthesia in the muscles of the buttock.

Testosterone injections have chemically modified testosterone with a molecule that delays the absorption. That molecule is typically enanthate, propionate, or cypionate. Injections result in rapid peak and dissipation in 4–6 days.

Nandrolone is a naturally occurring anabolic form of testosterone that cannot be aromatized to estrogen. Injections result in rapid peak and dissipation in 4–6 days.

Insulin is available in many forms. They vary from short-acting regular insulin, mixtures of 50/50 to 70/30 of short- to medium-acting insulin, to ultralong insulin. Your physician is best informed to prescribe the ideal form of insulin for your specific needs.

DIRECT REDUCTION IN DRUG COSTS/USAGE WITH TESTOSTERONE THERAPY

Epogen® 25% of $12 billion	$3 billion
Diabetes Medications 25% of insulin and oral agents	$2 billion
Erectile Dysfunction 50% of Viagra®, Cialis®, Levitra®	$1 billion

Erythropoietin-Replacement Drugs
erythropoietin **generic dosage/frequency**
Epogen® 5,000–10,000 IU 3x/wk
Procrit® 5,000–10,000 IU 3x/wk

Aranesp® 400 mcg/wk
pegfilgrastim
Neulasta® 70 mcg every 3 weeks

Diabetic Drugs Delegated to Secondary Status
Medication generic dosage/frequency
Glucophage® metformin 1,000 mg/1–2 day
Sulfonyeureas
Micronase® glyburide 5 mg/1–2x/day
Amaryl® glimepiride 4 mg/1-2x/day
Glucotrol® glipizide 10 mg
Insulin Secretagogue
Starlix® 120 mg
Prandin® 4 mg

Alpha-glucosidase inhibitor:
Glyset® 100 mg
Precose® 100 mg

Thiazolidinediones:
Rezulin® (removed by FDA)
Actos® 45 mg
Avandia® 8 mg

Diabetic Drugs Delegated to Tertiary Status
Incretin mimetic
Byetta® 10 mg 2x/day

Gliptins:
Januvia® 100 mg 2x/day
Galvus®

PPAR-gamma insulin sensitizers:
Muraglitazar
Tesaglitazar

Insulin Products Available
Insulin generic
Humalog® 100 units/mL
Humulin® 100 units/mL
Novalog® 100 units/mL
Novolin® 100 units/mL
Lantus® 100 units/mL
Exubera®

REFERENCES:

1. Lubec B. Aromatical hydroxylation in animal models of diabetes mellitus. *FASEB Journal*. 1998; 12:1581–87.
2. Moller, Jens. Cholesterol. Springer-Verlag. Berlin, 1987. President of the European Organization for the Control of Circulatory Diseases.
3. Lichten EM. Providence Hospital IRB 601–97. http://www.usdoctor.com/research.htm.
4. Kraft RL. In Radioassay: Clinical Concepts. Proceedings from a Symposium On Radioimmunoassay. Held in Washington, D.C. January 28–29, 1974, pp 91–106.
5. Available at: http://www.usdoctor.com/SUMI1.htm and http://www.usdoctor.com/SUMI2.htm.M
6. Ding EL. Sex Differences of Exogenous Sex hormones and Risk of type II Diabetes. *Journal of the American Medical Association* 2006; 295:1288–1299.
7. Anderson DC. Sex Hormone Binding Globulin Is an Oestrogen Amplifier. *Nature*. 1972; 240:38–40
8. Tibblin G, Adlerberth A, Lindstedt G, et al. The pituitary-gonadal axis and health in elderly men: a study of men born in 1913. *Diabetes*. 1996 Nov;45(11):1605-9.
9. Hayward RA, Maning WG, Kaplan SH, Wagner EH, Greenfield S. Starting insulin therapy in patients with type 2 diabetes: effectiveness, complications and resource utilization. *JAMA*. 1997;278:1663–69.
10. Gascan AM, Belvis JJ, et al. Nandrolone decanoate is a good alternative for the treatment of anemia in elderly male patients on hemodialysis. *Geriatric Nephrology & Urology*. 1999; 9(2):67–72.
11. Kapoor D, Goodwin E, et al. Testosterone Replacement Therapy Improves Insulin Resistance, Glycemic Control, Visceral Adiposity & Hypercholesterolemia in Hypogonadal Men with Type 2 Diabetes. *European Journal of Endocrinology*. 2006; 154(6):899–906.
12. Morgantaler A, Rhoden EL. Prevalence of prostate cancer among hypogonadal men with prostate-specific antigen levels of 4.0ng/ml or less. *Urology*. 2006; 68(6):1263–7.
13. American Diabetes Association. Type 2 Diabetes in Children and Adolescents. *Diabetes Care*. 2000; 3:381–389.
14. Cohen PG. Diabetes mellitus is associated with subnormal levels of free testosterone in men. *British Journal of Urology*. 2006; 97(3):652–3.
15. Smith MR, et al. Insulin sensitivity during combined androgen blockade for prostate cancer. *Journal of Clinical Endocrinology and Metabolism*. 2006; 91(4): 1305–8.
16. Swan SH. Semen quality of fertile US males in relation to their mothers' beefconsumption during pregnancy. *Human Reproduction*. 2007; doi:10.1093/humrepdem068.
17. Small M, et al. Metabolic Effects of Stanzolol in type II Diabetes Mellitus. *Hormones Metabolic Research*. 1986; 18:647–8.
18. Small M, et al. The Effects of oral stanozolol on fibrinolysis in type II diabetes mellitus. *Thombosis Research*. 1986; 44:253–9.
19. *Diabetes News*. 13 June 2005. Solvay announces DEMAND (DiabEtes in Men and ANDrogen therapy.
20. Smith L. Diabetes Education: Screen, test, treat: low testosterone and diabetes. AADE Newsletter. October 2006.
21. Gascon AA. Nandrolone decanoate is a good alternative for the treatment of anemia in elderly male patients on hemodialysis. *Geriatric Nephrology and Urology*. 1999; 9(2):67–72.
22. Teruel JL, et al. Androgen versus erythropoietin for the treatment of anemia in hemodialyzed patients: a prospective study. *Journal American Society of Nephrology*. 1996; 7(1):140–4.
23. Teruel JL, et al. Androgen therapy for anaemia of chronic renal failure. Indications in the erythropoietin era. *Scandinavian Journal of Urology and Nephrology*. 1996; 30(5):403–8.
24. Ballal SH, et al. Androgens potentiate the effects of erythropoietin in the treatment of anemia of end-stage renal disease. *American Journal of Kidney Disease*. 1991; 17(1):29–33.

APPENDIX

PROFESSIONAL SERVICES
Executive Health and Wellness Examination

Our comprehensive executive evaluation must include EBT scanning, pulmonary function, laboratory blood tests, EKG, and a comprehensive history and physical examination by a well-trained health professional. The goal of the Lichten Executive Health and Wellness Examination is to identify basic risk factors that may be correctable with supplements and hormonal medication.

Before the initial evaluation, arrangements are made for a comprehensive series of laboratory tests to be drawn at a commercial laboratory, completed, and reviewed by our health professional.

Therefore, the laboratory tests and interpretative results are available at your initial doctor visit. The goal for the physician and the patient is for both to understand the nature of the deficiencies, replace the missing nutrient and hormonal elements, and for the patient to become more involved in his/her own medical care.

THE EXECUTIVE EVALUATION

1. Only a limited number of patients can be scheduled on any single day with Edward Lichten, M.D. The Executive Evaluation can be completed in one day, but most prefer an overnight stay. The requests for Executive Evaluation are recorded by simply calling our office telephone number. Include your name, address, birth date, telephone, fax, and when you wish to be seen by the doctor.
2. Our personnel will record what days and times serve you best. Alternative dates and times will allow us to accommodate your requests.
3. Overnight guests may stay at the 5-Star Townsend Hotel, which is one block from our office. (Rooms are reserved for our patients.)
4. After completing your Executive Evaluation, a comprehensive summary report is generated that includes your history, physical exam, and testing. A copy of *Textbook of Bio-Identical Hormones* by Edward Lichten, M.D., will be given to you.

5. Individuals with computers will receive computer records of their medical file that includes initial history, examination, testing, and laboratory results. Notes and prescription medication can be added.

LICHTEN WELLNESS CENTRE
Birmingham, Michigan 48012-0843
Telephone: 248.593.9999

COSMETIC SERVICES

Cosmetic Medical Services

While our comprehensive medical services are geared to living longer and better, our cosmetic services are directed toward looking better and younger. This is accomplished by a number of skin-defining treatments listed below:

1. Only a limited number of patients can be scheduled on any single day with Edward Lichten, M.D. The Cosmetic Evaluation and Treatment can be completed in one day, but most prefer an overnight stay. The requests for Cosmetic Evaluation are recorded by simply calling our office telephone number. Include your name, address, birth date, telephone, fax, and when you wish to be seen by the doctor.
2. Our personnel will record what days and times serve you best. Alternative dates and times will allow us to accommodate your requests.
3. Overnight guests may stay at the 5-Star Townsend Hotel, which is one block from our office. (Rooms are reserved for our patients.)
4. After completing your Cosmetic Evaluation, a comprehensive summary report is generated that includes your history, physical exam, testing, and before-after photographs. A copy of *Textbook of Bio-Identical Hormones* by Edward Lichten, M.D. will be given to you.

Individuals with computers will receive computer records of their medical file that includes initial history, examination, testing, and photographs. Notes and prescription medication can be added.

Individual Services

1. BOTOX: BOTOX injections can be effective at decreasing movement of active frown lines, raising outer aspects of eyebrows, reducing crow's feet, opening up the smile, and reducing neck lines.
2. FILLERS: Restylane®, Perlane®, Sculptra®, and Radiesse® are used to outline and fill lips, hollow areas in the cheek, raise the facial arch, and straighten the nose and jaw lines.
3. FACIAL PEELS: Peels are applied to remove the top layers of facial skin. The depth can be superficial, moderate, or deep. The deeper the peel, the greater effectiveness at removing the damages that aging brings.
4. LASER PULSED LIGHT: The office is equipped to remove dark red and brown areas, facial and body hair, and perform a skin-smoothing therapy. More than one treatment is usually necessary for appropriate results.
5. After completing your Cosmetic Evaluation and treatment, a comprehensive summary report is generated that includes your history, physical exam, and photographs. A copy of *Textbook of Bio-Identical Hormones* by Edward Lichten, M.D., will be given to you.

GYNECOLOGICAL SERVICES

Gynecological Surgical Services

While our comprehensive medical services are geared to living longer and better, our gynecological services are directed toward the repair of tissue damaged by disease or childbirth. This is accomplished by integration of our experienced university-trained gynecologist and, when indicated, a board-certified plastic surgeon defining treatments listed below:

1. Outpatient laparoscopic surgery includes laser treatments for endometriosis, laparoscopic uterine nerve ablation for pelvic pain, and presacral neurectomy for recurrent chronic midline pain. Only a limited number of patients can be scheduled on any single day with Edward Lichten, M.D. Most out-of-area patients prefer an overnight stay. For those who request

cosmetic surgery coordinated with gynecological procedures, simply call our office telephone number, and our staff will make referrals. Include your name, address, birth date, telephone, fax, and when you wish to be seen by the doctor and for what medical or surgical purpose you are calling.

2. In-patient surgery includes laparoscopic and abdominal total abdominal hysterectomy, bilateral salpingo-oophorectomy, abdominoplasty, hernia repair, and bladder-rectum suspensions. Those requesting cosmetic procedures to correct vaginal weakness, enlarged or distorted labia, and rectal incontinence will require presurgical evaluation by the consulting surgeon.

3. Overnight guests may stay at the 5-Star Townsend Hotel, which is one block from our office. (Rooms are reserved for our patients.)

4. After completing your surgery, a comprehensive summary report is generated that includes your history, physical exam, testing, and before-after photographs and/or videotape of your surgery. A copy of *Textbook of Bio-Identical Hormones* by Edward Lichten, M.D., will be given to you.

Individuals with computers will receive computer records of their medical file that includes initial history, examination, testing, and photographs. Notes and prescription medication can be added.

CONSULTATION SERVICES

Consultation Medical Services
While our comprehensive medical services are geared to providing an in-depth analysis at a face-to-face physician-patient encounter, the consultation is an informal informational-only telephone conversation:

1. Only a limited number of patients can be scheduled on any single day for telephone consultation with Edward Lichten, M.D. The telephone consultation lasts for approximately 20–30 minutes. The requests for a telephone consultation are recorded by simply calling our office telephone number. Include your name, address, birth date, telephone, fax, and when you wish to speak to the doctor.

2. Our personnel will record what evenings and times serve you best. Alternative dates and times will allow us to accommodate your requests.
3. Referring physicians are encouraged to take part in a three-way conversation so that a continuum of care might be established. After completing the telephone consultation, a comprehensive summary report is generated that includes whatever information about your history, physical exam, and laboratory testing was supplied.

Individuals with computers will receive computer records and copies of data supplied to Edward Lichten, M.D, F.A.C.S. in digital format. Included within their medical file may be the supplied initial history, examination, laboratory testing, and photographs. Dr. Lichten will supply the summary.

Professional Services:
Executive Medical Services
Cosmetic Services
Gynecological Surgical Services
Consultation Services

About USDOCTOR
The USDOCTOR Resources Website was organized in 1994 to bring scientific medical information to the Internet for physicians and the general public. All materials are referenced and backed by years of clinical experience.

Edward M. Lichten, M.D., F.A.C.S.
http://www.usdoctor.com

About the Foundation:
FOUNDtheCURE Foundation
http://www.foundthecure.com

LICHTEN WELLNESS CENTRE
Birmingham, Michigan 48012-0843
Telephone: 248.593.9999
CONSULTATION SERVICE

LIST OF SUPPLEMENTARY PRODUCTS

Ordering Procedure

The following cosmetic, vitamin, and supplement providers maintain the highest standards in the industry. Their products are listed below. You may contact this telephone number directly or order at the **www.LifeExtension.com** website to have the products shipped directly to you.

Life Extension Foundation:

All Products: Telephone: 1-800-544-4440, online at **www.LifeExtension.com** or write to:

> Life Extension Foundation Buyers Club
> PO Box 407198
> Ft. Lauderdale, FL 33040-7198

Vitamins: Daily, All purpose

SUPPLEMENT	SUGGESTED DOSE
Two-Per-Day Caplets	One caplet, twice daily
Super Omega-3 Fish Oil	Two softgels, twice daily
Bone Restore	4–5 capsules nightly
Ubiquinol Coenzyme Q10	50 mg 2–3 times daily
Super Booster	One softgel daily
Mitochondrial Energy Optimizer	Four capsules daily

Insomnia Protocol:

SUPPLEMENT	SUGGESTED DOSE
Vitamin D3 capsules (1,000 IU and 5,000 IU)	4,000–5,000 IU nightly
GABA lozenge	125–250 mg sublingual nightly (older individuals may start with just 50 mg each night)
L-Tryptophan capsules (500 mg)	500–1,000 mg nightly (some will benefit by taking an additional 500 mg of L-tryptophan during the day)

Note: If serum measurement of vitamin D status does not exceed 50 ng/mL after taking up to 10,000 IU of vitamin D3 capsules for three months, switch to vitamin D sublingual drops. Two drops each night supply 4,000 IU of vitamin D3.

Hormone supplements:
DHEA 15, 25, 50, and 100 mg capsules
7-keto DHEA 100 mg capsules
DHEA 25 mg/7-keto DHEA 100 mg capsule combination
Sublingual DHEA 25 mg tablet
Pregnenolone 50 and 100 mg capsules
Progesterone cream 2.5%
Melatonin: 300 mcg, 500 mcg, 750 mcg, 1 mg, 3 mg, 10 mg
     capsules; 3 mg sublingual tablets, 3 mg time-released capsules
For men: Ultimate Natural Prostate Formula (one capsule, twice daily)
For women: Breast Health Formula (one capsule, twice daily)

LABORATORY SERVICES

Comprehensive Laboratory Serum and Blood Services

Blood testing is important to do before consulting a qualified physician such as Dr. Lichten. Individuals can obtain the blood tests listed in this appendix by calling 1.888.868.2949 or logging in to www.lef.org/hormonetest

Upon requesting the tests, a requisition form will be sent directly to you with a list of blood-drawing stations that are often located in your neighborhood (throughout the US). You can usually go to one of these blood-draw stations at a convenient time of the day for you (though it is best to go early in the day because 12-hour fasting is usually needed). The results will be sent directly to you to provide to the doctor you have chosen to oversee your comprehensive health restoration program.

Those who wish to use their health care insurance plans need to order tests through their treating physician. Some insurance plans pay for certain tests, while others are not usually covered by insurance.

Based on the discounts available to members of the Life Extension Foundation, it makes sense for anyone ordering these tests to become a member for $75. The savings on the blood tests alone greatly exceed the membership fee.

With the results of your laboratory tests, you can consult with Dr. Lichten by telephone by calling 248.593.9999 or accessing his website www.FOUNDtheCURE.com

COMPREHENSIVE LABORATORY
BLOOD TESTING SERVICES

PANEL 1: DR. LICHTEN COMPREHENSIVE MALE OR FEMALE PANELS

Dr. Lichten Comprehensive Male Panel
Item number: Lichten01M
Retail: $891.66
Life Extension Member: $668.00
12 tests: Profile of all five endocrine glands including IGF-1, FSH, LH, TSH, T4 free, Cortisol, DHEA-S, Estradiol, Testosterone, Fasting Insulin, PSA, Sex Hormone Binding and F.I.T. and F.A.I. ratio. (Free Insulin and Testosterone ratio), Hemoglobin A1c.

Dr. Lichten Comprehensive Female Panel
Item number: Lichten01F
Retail: $891.66
Life Extension Member: $668.00
11 tests: Profile of all five endocrine glands including IGF-1, FSH, LH, TSH, T4 free, Cortisol, DHEA-S, Estradiol, Testosterone, Fasting Insulin, Sex Hormone Binding, calculated F.I.T. and F.A.I ratio. (Free Insulin and Testosterone ratio), Hemoglobin A1c.

Both Male and Female Panels also include CBC, Lipids, Chemistry Panel
40 tests that screen for anemia, infection, lipid abnormality, and normal metabolic function. Hemoglobin A1c screen for diabetes.

PANEL 2: DR. LICHTEN COMPREHENSIVE THYROID PANEL

Item number: Lichten02
Retail: $504.00
Life Extension Member: $378.00
8 tests: TSH, T4, T3 free, Reverse T3, Thyroid antibodies, Thyroid peroxidase antibodies, Red cell Magnesium, vitamin D 25 OH.

PANEL 3: DR. LICHTEN COMPREHENSIVE DIABETES TESTING

Item number: Lichten03
Retail: $323.68
Life Extension Member: $243.00
3-hour Glucose Tolerance Test with 0-, 1-, 2-, and 3-hour insulin and glucose measurements. Hemoglobin A1c. Calculated Sum-I (Summation Insulin).

PANEL 4: DR. LICHTEN HEPATITIS A, B, C PANEL
Item number: Lichten04
Retail: $125.33
Life Extension Member: $94.00
4 tests screen for Hepatitis A antibody; Hepatitis B surface (immunity) antigen (HBsAg); Hepatitis B core antibody (HBcAb); and Hepatitis C antibody.

PANEL 5: DR. LICHTEN CARDIAC RISK FACTORS
Item number: Lichten05
Retail: $260.33
Life Extension Member: $196.00
5 tests: Homocysteine, C-Reactive Protein, Ferritin, Fibrinogen, ABO and Rh blood typing.

Orders for laboratory tests are taken electronically at the website: http://www.lef.org/hormonetest
You can also call 1-888.868.2949 to order these tests (24 hours a day) or ask questions.

INDEX

body temperature, 56, 58-59, 65
bone health (*see also* osteoporosis)
    human growth hormone, 37
Boots Pharmaceuticals, 61
BOTOX, 170
breakfast, 27
breast cancer
    estrogen therapy, 117, 119
    vitamin D, 23
    Women's Health Initiative
        studies, 117-120, 122
British Medical Journal, 186
bromide, 66
Budoff, Penny, M.D., 133
burns, 47

C
Cache County study, 119
caffeine, 77, 91-93, 165
calcitonin, 192
calcium
    heart disease, 239-240
    osteoporosis, 183
calcium scoring, 236-237
cancer (*see also specific cancers*)
    seaweed, 125
    vitamin D, 23
cardiomyopathy, 40
    treatment, 43-45
Carson, Rachel, 208
Casson, Peter, M.D., 85
cellular energy, 40
Cephalgia, 159
cervical cancer
    vitamin D, 23
chamomile tea
    insomnia, 16
chloral hydrate, 16
chloride, 66
cholesterol (*see also* heart disease),
    22, 75, 225-226
    bio-identical hormones,
        239-242, 245-246
    function, 227-229
    hypothyroidism, 230-233

pharmaceutical approach,
    226-227, 247
    statins, 238-239
Cialis, 220
circadian cycles (*see also* sleep), 15,
    17
Climara, 188
cluster headaches
    description, 171
    treatment, 172
codeine, 16
coenzyme Q10, 50
    cardiomyopathy, 45
    increasing cellular energy, 40
    statins, 229, 231, 234, 238
coffee, 27
colitis
    hormone therapy, 45-46
    vitamin D, 22
Collaborative Study of Hormone
    Factors, 119
colon cancer
    estrogen therapy, 115
    vitamin D, 23
compartment syndrome, 263
compounding pharmacies, 127
congestive heart failure (*see also*
    heart disease), 101, 231
    DHEA, 242
    hypothyroidism, 233-234,
        241-242
    testosterone, 234-235
    treatment, 44
    vitamin D, 239-240
Conn's syndrome, 75, 81
coronary artery disease (*see* heart
    disease)
Cortef, 79, 91, 93
cortex, 33
corticosteroids, 40, 64, 76, 80, 190
cortisol, 75-77
    Addison's disease, 80
    deficiency, 90-93, 102
    stress, 83-84
    testing, 88-89

preparations, 128
traditional replacement
therapy, 109-110
types, 113
Women's Health Initiative
studies, 117-118
evidence-based medicine, 230
Evista (*see* raloxifene)
evolution, 15, 33

F
fatigue, 36
adrenal disease, 92
fatty liver disease, 22
Feminine Forever, 109, 208
fibroids, 139
fibromyalgia
description, 38
treatment, 39-42, 48-49 (chart)
fight or flight response, 75
fish (*see also* fish oil), 19
fish oil (*see also* omega-3 acids), 24
Florinef, 81
fluoride, 66
follicle-stimulating hormone (FSH),
33, 113, 132, 213
food
vitamin depletion, 104
Food and Drug Administration
(FDA), 265-266

G
GABA (gamma-aminobutyric acid),
25, 78
cautions, 30
fibromyalgia, 39
insomnia, 26
uses and dosage, 26
gabapentin, 26
gallbladder,
cancer, 23
surgery, 22
gastric cancer
vitamin D, 23
gastrointestinal health
vitamin D, 22

General Adaptation Syndrome, 73,
79, 88, 90
gigantism, 35, 42
glucagon, 103
glucocorticoids, 74
glucose control, 28
adrenal exhaustion, 91
glutathione, 50
goiters (*see also* thyroid hormones),
53, 66
grains, 20
Grave's disease, 63, 67, 92
DHEA, 86
Greenblatt, Robert, 124
growth hormone (*also* human
growth hormone), 28, 33

H
Hashimoto's thyroiditis, 60, 67
Headache, 173
headaches (*see* migraines *and*
cluster headaches)
Headache and other Head Pain, 152
Headache Centre, 159
Health Center, 63
heart disease
andropause, 210-211, 219, 223
coronary artery disease,
225-226, 235-236
DHEA, 242
diagnostic tests, 236
estrogen studies, 119
heart failure, 226
human growth hormone,
43-45, 240-241
hypothyroidism, 54, 231-233
menopause, 114-115
treatment, 237-238
vitamin D, 22, 239-240
Women's Health Initiative
studies, 117
heart failure (*see* heart disease)
Helsinki Heart Study, 23
herpes, 26
H.E.R.S., 119
high blood pressure, 81

Hippocrates, 153
Hodgkin's lymphoma
    vitamin D, 23
hormonal interaction, 34
hot flashes (see also menopause),
    114
human growth hormone (hGH), 36,
    38, 78
        abuse, 37
        complications, 36
        Crohn's disease, 46-47
        fibromyalgia, 40
        function, 35, 42
        heart failure, 43-44, 240-241
        increasing cellular energy, 40
        menopause, 113
        osteoporosis, 183, 191-192
        replacement, 36, 101
Humira, 46
hydrocortisone, 74, 80
hyperthyroidism (see thyroid
    hormones)
Hypothyroidism (book), 232
hypothalamic-pituitary-adrenal axis,
    89, 91, 94
hypothalamus, 33, 35, 89
hypothyroidism (see thyroid
    hormones)
hysterectomy, 137

I
ibuprofen, 133, 149
Imitrex, 157
Imuran, 46
Inderal, 158
infant mortality, 103
infertility, 93
inflammation, 22
        adrenal exhaustion, 79
        bacterial infection theory, 64
        DHEA, 85-86
        glucocorticoids, 75
insomnia, 16-17, 41
        GABA, 26
        L-tryptophan, 25-26
        magnesium, 27

natural cures, 17, 50
stress, 77
sunlight, 17
vitamin D, 25
insulin (see also diabetes), 103, 251,
    266
        testosterone levels, 214-216,
            243-244
insulin-like growth factor-1 (IGF-1),
    35, 36
International Headache Society,
    159, 161, 163
Intrinsa, 189
iodine, 58, 66, 102, 125
Is Your Thyroid Making You Fat?, 58

J, K, L
Jeffries, William, M.D., 88
jet-lag, 18
Johnson, Ben, 235
Journal of Clinical Endocrinology
    and Metabolism, 19, 44
Journal of Reproductive Medicine,
    138
Journal of the American Medical
    Association, 61-62, 245, 258, 263
Joyner, Florence Griffith, 235
kava kava
        insomnia, 16
Kennedy, John F., 80, 161
ketoprofen, 149
ketorolac, 19, 149
Keys, Ancel, 226
kidney disease, 262-263, 266-267
Klonopin, 16
Knoll Pharmaceuticals, 61
Kraft, R.L., 255
LabCorp, 21
LaLanne, Jack, 37
Lancet, The, 125
laparoscopy, 135
laryngeal cancer
        vitamin D, 23
L-carnitine, 50, 234
legumes, 19

prednisone, 46, 71, 190
pregnancy
    vitamin D, 24
Premarin, 109-110, 117-118, 121,
    187, 218
pre-menstrual syndrome (see
    menstrual cycle)
Prempro, 110, 117-118, 185
    negative effects, 119
Primobolan, 218
Procrit, 263
progesterone
    bioidentical versions, 123
    menopause, 112-113
    menstruation, 132
    migraines, 154
    pre-menstrual syndrome,
        141-142, 149
    preparations, 128
    synthetic versions, 118
progestin, 109, 125, 128
prolactin, 33
    function, 34-35
Prometrium, 123
propranolol, 158
prostate cancer
    testosterone, 220, 261
    vitamin D, 23
prostate specific antigen, 212
proteins, 20
Provera, 109, 117-118, 121, 188
pulmonary embolism, 180

Q, R, S

Quest Diagnostic Laboratories, 21,
    35
raloxifene, 126
rectal cancer
    vitamin D, 23
Regelson, William, M.D.,
    Melatonin Miracle, 18
Reid, Robert, M.D., 145
Reid-Rowell, 159
Remicade, 46
renal cancer
    vitamin D, 23

reproduction, 99-100
Rezulin, 227
rheumatoid arthritis, 67, 80, 93
    DHEA, 84-85
rickets, 18, 100
Rudman, Donald, M.D., 36
RUTH trial, 126
Seaman, Barbara, 110
seaweed, 125
Science, 256
scientific method
    testing DHEA, 85-86
seasonal affective disorder (SAD), 17
seizure disorders, 26
selective estrogen receptor
    modulators (SERMS), 125-126,
    128
selenium, 58, 102
Selye, Hans, 73-74
serotonin, 18, 25, 28
sex, 35, 212
sex hormone binding globulin,
    212-216
Sherwin, Barbara, Ph.D., 147
silica, 39, 50
skin cancer, 29
skin tone
    vitamin D, 22-23, 29
sleep (see also insomnia), 15
    fibromyalgia, 38-39
    prescriptions, 16-17
Sleep-Aid Formula, 26 (chart), 27-28
small stature, 35, 43
smoking, 22
Society for Gynecologic
    Investigation, 120
Solu-Cortef, 89-90, 92-93, 95
Solvay Pharmaceuticals, 159, 218
somatostatin, 35
Sommerville, B.W., M.D., 154
Sonata, 16
Sowers, James, M.D., 254
spironolactone, 78, 81-82, 149
Stadol, 134
Stanozolol, 217-218
statins, 227, 230-231, 234, 237-239, 245

Stein-Leventhal syndrome, 82
Sterling-Winthrop Laboratories, 156
steroid hormones, 74
stress, 22, 73-77, 88
    DHEA and cortisol, 83
stroke, 100-101
    andropause, 210-211
    estrogen therapy, 115
    Women's Health Initiative
        studies, 117
sulfasalazine, 46
sumatriptan (*see also* Imitrex), 157,
    159
sun damage, 24
sunlight, 29
    vitamin D, 18
Synarel, 138
synthetic hormones, 72-73
Synthroid, 58-59, 61, 66, 232

T, U, V
tamoxifen, 125-126, 222
Technische Hochschule Zurich, 35
teeth, 18
testicular cancer, 261
Testim, 127
Testopel, 217
testosterone, 35-36, 93, 103
    abuse, 222
    aldosterone, 82
    andropause, 207-211
    bound versus free, 213-214,
        256-257
    cardiomyopathy, 45
    coronary artery disease,
        235-236
    cluster headaches, 172-173
    Crohn's disease, 46
    depression, 147
    DHEA, 82
    diabetes, 243-244, 253-260, 262
    erectile dysfunction, 220-221
    gels, 218
    increasing cellular energy, 40
    insomnia, 16
    kidney disease, 262-264

    measuring, 211-212, 214-216,
        221-222
    menopause, 111-112
    menstrual irregularity, 78
    osteoporosis, 183-184, 186-191
    replacement, 128, 217-219,
        223, 261, 266
    risks, 261
tetracycline, 64
    fibromyalgia, 41
thallium stress test, 236
thiocyanate, 66
thyroid gland, 28
    blood tests, 56-57 (chart)
    DHEA, 86
    dietary issues, 66
    fibromyalgia, 41
    function, 54
    heart disease, 231-233,
        234-235, 241-242
    hypothyroidism, 53-56, 67-68,
        231
    hyperthyroidism, 63-64, 68
    insomnia, 16
    menopause, 113
    prostate cancer, 220
    replacement hormones, 50,
        57-60, 66, 78, 101-102
    resistant syndrome, 65
    resistant to therapy, 65-66
Thyroid Solution, The, 232
thyroid stimulating hormone (TSH),
    33, 54
Toradol, 134, 149, 158
Travell, Janet, M.D., 161
trazodone, 16
trenbolone, 218
trigger points, 148, 162, 167-168
tuberculosis, 80
tumor necrosis factor (TNF), 22
ultrasound, 236
United Kingdom General Practice
    Research Database
        estrogen/progestin studies, 120
University of California, San
    Francisco, 61

University of Paisley, 35
University of Parma, 159
University of Pennsylvania, 120
Upjohn, 109, 118
uterine cancer
    estrogen therapy, 115
    vitamin D, 23
Utian, Wolf, M.D., 121
vaccination, 198
valerian root
    insomnia, 16
Valium, 16
vasopressin, 33
    function, 34
Viagra, 220-221
Vicodin, 134
vitamins
    intravenous injection, 51
    thyroid conditions, 58
vitamin A
    thyroid conditions, 58
vitamin B group, 50
vitamin B12
    adrenal exhaustion, 90
    bioavailability, 19
    Crohn's disease, 46
    thyroid conditions, 58
vitamin C, 45
    adrenal exhaustion, 78, 88, 90,
        102
    thyroid conditions, 58
vitamin D
    benefits, 21-24
    fibromyalgia, 39
    insomnia, 18, 25, 41
    description, 19-20
    dosage, 20-21, 24-25, 29
    heart disease, 239-240
    optimal ranges, 21, 24
    osteoporosis, 183-184
    overdose, 25
    reproductive value, 100-101
vitamin K, 190
Vivelle, 188

W, X, Y, Z

warfarin, 190
Wayne State University, 254
weight gain, 77
    corticosteroids, 40
wheat, 20
Wilson, Robert, M.D., 109
Wolff, Harold, M.D., 152
*Women and the Crisis in Sex
    Hormones*, 110
Women's Health Initiative, 157, 183,
    187-188
    estrogen studies, 110, 112,
        117-121
Wyeth-Ayerst, 121
Xanax, 16
xenoestrogens, 35, 208-209, 261
yeast, 19
yoga, 169
zinc, 58, 102
Zuspan, Frederick, M.D., 155-156

George Balanchine

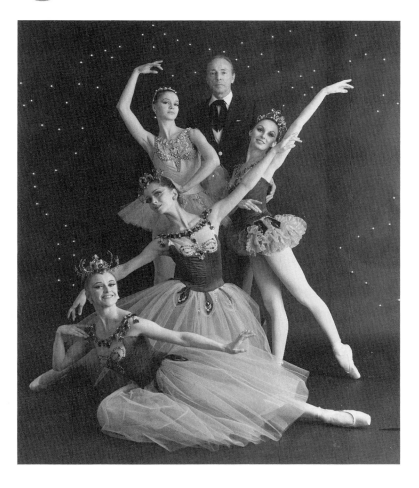

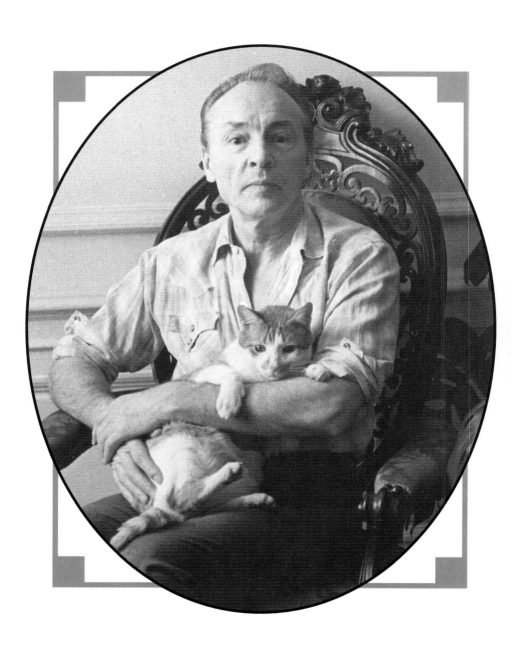

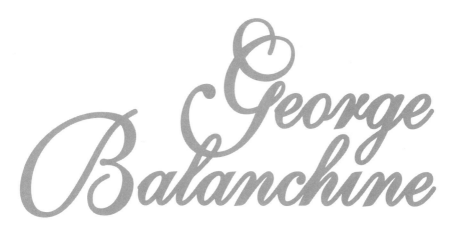

George Balanchine

AMERICAN BALLET MASTER

DAVIDA KRISTY

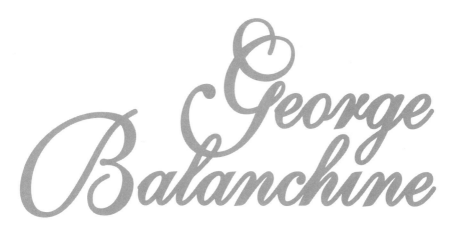

LERNER PUBLICATIONS COMPANY • MINNEAPOLIS

To Brickton, Martine, and Apryll

The author acknowledges with gratitude the generosity, cooperation, and encouragement of the following people: Balanchine's biographer, Bernard Taper, for the use of quotations from his book; Barbara Horgan of the Balanchine Trust; Madeleine M. Nichols, Curator, New York Public Library for the Performing Arts; and Barbara King, Ann Alper, Joanne Burch, and Joan Prestine.

Library of Congress Cataloging-in-Publication Data

Kristy, Davida.
    George Balanchine : American Ballet Master / Davida Kristy.
        p. cm.
    Includes bibliographical references and index.
    Summary: A biography of the Russian-born choreographer largely responsible for popularizing and developing ballet in the United States.
    ISBN 0-8225-4951-4 (alk. paper)
    1. Balanchine, George—Juvenile literature. 2. Choreographers—Biography—Juvenile literature. [1. Balanchine, George. 2. Choreographers.] I. Title.
GV1785.B32K75   1996
792.8'2'092—dc20
[B]   95-46075

Manufactured in the United States of America
1 2 3 4 5 6 – JR – 01 00 99 98 97 96

Contents

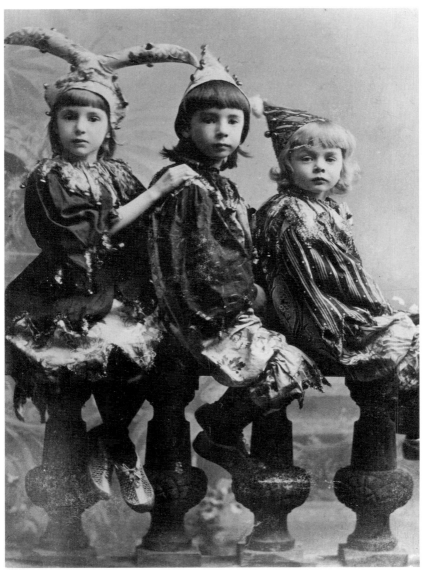

Gyorgy Balanchivadze, center, *poses in costume with his older sister, Tamara, and his younger brother, Andrei, for a family portrait.*

ONE

Prisoner on Theater Street

1904–1913

*S*tand straight. Walk. Run. Sit. Kneel.

The ballet teacher barked orders to Gyorgy as if he were a dog. But his mama was watching, so Gyorgy did as he was told. At least no one expected him to dance. He *hated* dancing. When his brother Andrei hopped around at family Christmas parties, stealing all the attention, Gyorgy refused to join him. Ballet? He had never even seen one. What's more, he didn't want to.

So why was he here, auditioning for Russia's Imperial School of Ballet with all the other nine-year-olds? Only to keep his sister Tamara company. When the audition was over, he would go home to the country and study with his tutor for another year. By then there would be openings at the Imperial Naval Academy. Gyorgy liked the idea of becoming an officer on a Russian ship.

When Gyorgy's turn was over, he sat with Mama and Tamara until the director called the names of the chosen children. He listened for his sister's name and was shocked—no, *horrified*—to hear his own.

Gyorgy Balanchivadze stood in line with about 20 other boys and girls. He looked toward his mama with pleading eyes, but her face was fixed in an encouraging smile. He knew she was happy that he would get a good education, and that there would be nothing to pay. Stay here, Gyorgy, her eyes told him. Here you will be clothed and fed and taught.

The line of new ballet students moved through the doors to the private rooms of the ballet school. Gyorgy moved with them into his new life.

Gyorgy's childhood had been a happy one. He was born on January 22, 1904. His father's name was Melton Balanchivadze. According to Russian custom, Gyorgy's middle name was Meltonovich—the son of Melton. Their last name, Balanchivadze, meant that their ancestors had probably been jesters or roving minstrels.

Melton Balanchivadze was a musician and a composer. He was from Georgia, a province of Russia near the country of Turkey and the Black Sea. Georgian people had the reputation of being carefree and generous. Melton was a real Georgian. He didn't make much money, but he was a happy man with many friends.

Melton often traveled to remote parts of Russia where people remembered ancient folk songs and hymns. He taught these songs to a choir. The choral performances and the sale of music, some of which Melton composed himself, gave the family their income.

Gyorgy lived with his father, his mother, Maria, his older sister, Tamara, and his younger brother, Andrei, in a tiny apartment in St. Petersburg.

When Gyorgy was three or four years old, the family

won a lot of money in a lottery. Melton bought a larger city apartment and a country house in Lounatiokki, a town about three hours north of St. Petersburg by train, in what was then Finland.

Soon the apartment and the country house were all that was left of the lottery money—the rest was gone. Melton had given the money away to friends and lost it in bad business ventures. His creditors put Melton in debtors' prison. Maria took the children to live in Finland and told them Melton was in the mountains collecting folk songs. When Melton was released, he gave up thoughts of business and returned to his songs and his choir.

Without money for the apartment in St. Petersburg, the Balanchivadze family lived in their log house in Lounatiokki. Gyorgy played outdoors when the weather was fine. He liked to roam through the woods and gather mushrooms. He had a pet pig and a small garden patch.

From the time Gyorgy was five or six, a tutor taught him arithmetic, grammar, penmanship, the Bible, and a little history. His mother, Maria, was a talented musician and taught him piano.

Gyorgy hated piano lessons. He hated practicing scales and chords and what he thought were stupid little songs about butterflies and dancing moonbeams. But his mother knew he had talent. She felt he would do better with a teacher who could demand more of him, so she hired a piano teacher. This woman rewarded him with a piece of chocolate from her purse if he did well at a lesson. Gyorgy thought the chocolates tasted like face powder.

One day Gyorgy was practicing the piano. The notes were correct and so was the tempo. But suddenly, he understood that the notes could be different, could be more. If he played softer, sweeter, lighter, or slower, the notes became *music,* and the music became beautiful. He recognized that music was a way to express feelings without words. After that, music was Gyorgy's greatest pleasure. He developed an extraordinary talent as a pianist.

Music helped Gyorgy deal with his feelings. Unlike his father, Gyorgy was reserved and shy. Rather than show his feelings and risk being scolded or laughed at, Gyorgy played music of sorrow or frustration or pounded out his anger on the piano. He could just as easily play his joy and excitement. Away from the piano, if Gyorgy had to cry, he hid from his family and kept his hurt to himself.

Religion was also important to Gyorgy. He truly believed in Russian Orthodoxy, a religion similar to Roman Catholicism. He loved to stand in church on a Sunday or a holiday to see the priests' gorgeous robes and feel the thrill of the choir's chants.

When he was nine years old and money was scarce, Maria took Gyorgy and Tamara to St. Petersburg for the day. She hoped to get Gyorgy into the Imperial Naval Academy and Tamara into the Imperial School of Ballet. Tuition at both schools was free. This trip did not work out quite as Maria had planned—the Imperial School of Ballet chose Gyorgy.

Gyorgy was terrified when his mother left him at the school on Theater Street. He wasn't ready for such a big change in his life. No one had prepared him for the idea of sleeping at school, and no one told him when—or if—he would see his family again. That same evening, he ran away to the apartment of his mother's cousin Nadia. Aunt Nadia gave him supper, but she took him right back to Theater Street and begged the director not to expel Gyorgy for running away.

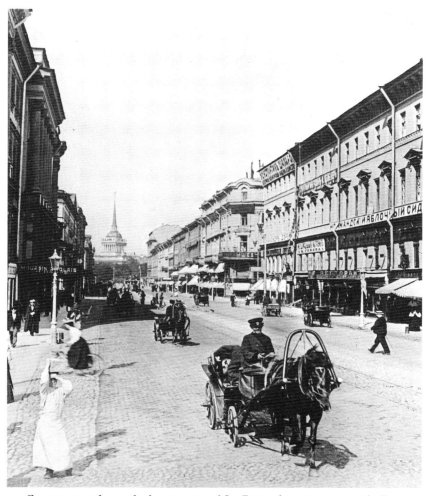

Gyorgy ran through the streets of St. Petersburg to escape ballet school.

The director was a compassionate person and didn't punish Gyorgy. But Gyorgy felt punished by being forced to stay at the school. For him, the Imperial School of Ballet was a jail.

Gyorgy began his sentence.

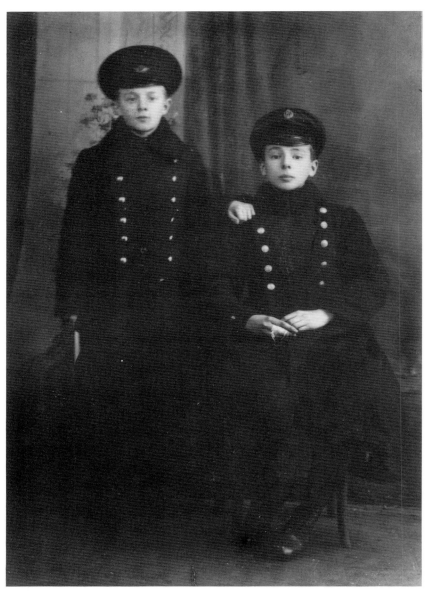

Dressed in his ballet-school uniform, Gyorgy, right, *sits next to his brother, Andrei.*

TWO

Young Ballet Master

1913–1923

*W*hen Gyorgy entered the Imperial School of Ballet in 1913, he became a dancer in the service of Tsar Nicholas II, the Russian emperor. Russia entered World War I in 1914 under Tsar Nicholas's leadership. Gyorgy was learning his first ballet steps when the country went to war.

Outside the school, life became difficult. Trains that used to bring food from the farms to the cities now carried troops instead. Farmers had to leave their lands to join the army. Soon food was scarce and very expensive.

The pupils at the Imperial School of Ballet were still under the tsar's protection. They dressed warmly and well in dark blue uniforms with velvet collars and ate nourishing food so they would have energy to dance. They hardly knew a war was being fought.

Gyorgy slept in a huge room with 29 other boys. Maids made their beds and took care of their clothing. Each morning, the boys marched to the ballet classrooms below the dormitories and went through what Gyorgy thought were torturous exercises.

By this time, ballet had grown to be a highly specialized and rigorous form of theatrical dancing. Ballet originated in

13

Europe in the 1500s, where dancing in royal courts and castles gradually became elaborate and stylized. Kings, queens, and members of their courts performed for each other in spectacular dance productions. They learned to dance from their fencing masters who knew how to train the body for grace and agility. The masters adopted the basic posture of the fencer, with feet and legs turned out, as the basic position for dancers. From this pose, a dancer could move quickly and easily in any direction.

In 1738 Russian Tsarina Anna established the Imperial School of Ballet in St. Petersburg. She ordered a Frenchman, Jean-Baptiste Landet, to direct the school and devise a demanding teaching method to train dancers for royal performances. This was the same curriculum that later trained Gyorgy.

Ballet classes were based on the idea that muscles can be used properly and safely only after they have been carefully warmed up. Gyorgy and the other ballet students began each lesson with muscle-warming exercises, which they performed while holding onto a wooden rail or *barre.* These exercises at the barre began with slow movements, repeated many times. Gradually the dancers' bodies became warm and flexible. Then the dancers could do faster, more difficult movements.

From the barre, students moved to the center of the room to practice the leaping, spinning, and traveling steps that were used in ballet performances. In addition to classical ballet steps and exercises, Gyorgy and his classmates learned to perform national folk dances, such as the mazurka and the polonaise. After about eight years of training, the students would become part of the ballet company at the Maryinsky Theater.

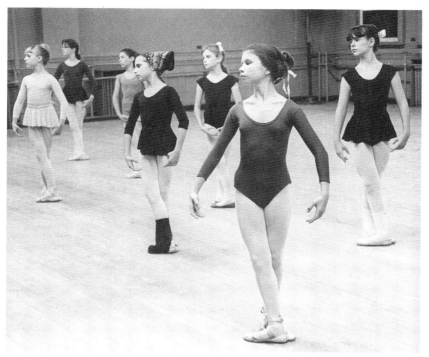

Ballet students move to the center of the room after warming up at the barre.

The men who taught the boys' classes were respected dancers. They were generally kind but demanding. They often pushed the boys' bodies into the proper position. One teacher wore heavy rings on his fingers and used to hit the boys to position their legs and arms correctly. The bruises his rings made were a common sight in the dormitory.

In Russia, French was the language of cultured people. Only peasants spoke Russian all the time. French was also the language of ballet, and Gyorgy had to speak French in his ballet classes and learn French grammar. He got used to being called Georges, the French form of Gyorgy.

Georges and his schoolmates studied academic subjects in the afternoon. Georges got high marks in religion and music—the subjects he liked. He did fair or poor work in arithmetic, French, and Russian grammar and literature.

Georges enjoyed reading. Some of his favorite books came from other countries. He liked Jules Verne's *Twenty Thousand Leagues Under the Sea,* the Sherlock Holmes mysteries, and "dime novels"—cheap, cardboard-bound serials— mostly about Nick Carter, an American detective.

Usually Georges kept to himself, playing the piano or standing for hours in the school chapel on Sunday. For as long as he could remember, he had a funny habit of sniffing and twitching his upper lip at the same time. This tic exposed his front teeth, so cruel classmates called him "Rat." The boys also teased him and played tricks on him. One boy was particularly determined to aggravate Georges, and he finally succeeded. In a rare display of temper, Georges attacked him and broke the boy's collarbone.

At the end of the year, Georges found he had passed his final examination and would continue to study ballet at the Imperial School. His future was more firmly fixed than ever. And he still hated dancing.

Georges's teachers believed that young students should perform before an audience as part of their training. In his second year of school, Georges's class appeared in Tchaikovsky's ballet *The Sleeping Beauty* at the Maryinsky Theater. He played a little monster, the slave of the wicked fairy. In the second act, he played a page and held one end of a garland during Princess Aurora's solo.

Night after night, Georges watched the ballet in amazement from backstage. He saw how all the elements of the production came together to make something beautiful. The soloists transformed Georges's dreary, painful exercises into joyous leaps or graceful bends. Music added emotion to the movements. Scenery, costumes, and makeup all made an illusion of beauty that thrilled and excited him.

Just as one moment had changed boring piano exercises to music, the weeks of watching *The Sleeping Beauty* changed ballet lessons into artistic preparation. Georges no longer thought of himself as a prisoner on Theater Street.

Also in Georges's second year at the Imperial School of Ballet, he attended classes in music theory, composition, and piano at the Conservatory of Music. When a senior ballet student chose him to play piano for a dance recital, he gained status and respect in the eyes of his classmates.

Had they known that another girl from the class ahead of Georges had a crush on him, he would have commanded even more respect. Alexandra Danilova, called Choura by her friends, thought Georges was "distinctive and mysterious."

By 1917, the third year of World War I, the tsar could no longer protect the school from conditions outside its walls. The Russian army was forced to declare a cease-fire with its enemies. Revolutionaries threatened to topple the tsar from his throne. Food was almost impossible to find, and in March, fighting broke out in the streets between starving soldiers and police who were trying to protect the citizens. At last the news came—the revolutionaries had forced the tsar from his throne and taken control of Russia.

Georges's secure, secluded world burst wide apart. His family, who had been living in Finland, moved back to St. Petersburg, now named Petrograd by the new government. The ballet school was shut down, and 13-year-old Georges was finally reunited with his loved ones.

For almost a year, the Balanchivadze family struggled as

everyone else struggled. The revolutionary government sent Melton to Georgia as its minister of culture. Food seemed more plentiful in Georgia, so he sent for the family. Georges stayed behind. He hoped the school would reopen, and he wanted to be there if it did. Also, he wanted to look after Aunt Nadia, the woman who had taken Georges back to school when he ran away.

Georges found a job as an assistant to a saddle maker, who paid him with coffee grounds and potato peelings. He also played the piano for silent films in a run-down movie theater. When he could, he stole food. There were no pets left in Petrograd. Georges knew why—starving Russians had eaten them.

Every day, Georges went to Theater Street to see if the school was open. Georges met other 14-year-old students on the same errand. He became less self-conscious and re-served. The real-world problems Georges faced left no time for hiding in a book or at a piano.

At last the commissar of education persuaded the revo-lutionaries that the new Russia would benefit from well-trained artists. The ballet school reopened and the students reassembled. They were now the servants of the state, not the tsar. The state had no money for fixing pipes, for heating fuel, or even for food. The students made new shirts for themselves out of the tsar's leftover velvet drapes. They burned the floorboards of the school's attic for fuel.

The ballet students shared their living quarters and classrooms with students from the School of Russian Drama. Georges liked these new classmates. He preferred character roles in ballets because they required acting along with danc-ing. He befriended the drama students and learned their act-ing secrets.

Dancing lessons went on as before, and Georges made progress as a classical dancer. He understood that the techniques he had learned were the foundations of all dance, but these techniques might be more flexible than his teachers believed. He thought of emotions and music he'd like to express by using traditional ballet movement with a fresh, new style.

When Georges was 16, the director allowed him to arrange a dance for a school performance. He chose a piece of music by Anton Rubenstein called *La Nuit (The Night)*, made up a dance, and rehearsed it carefully with a girl from his class. This was Georges's first choreography, his first dance composition.

For this dance, Georges was the ballet master, the person in charge of a ballet company. He had to establish his authority. He did this by being firm but extremely courteous, and by pretending he knew exactly what he was doing. His partner responded well.

In *La Nuit,* Georges tried to show a man conquering a woman with love. At the end, as she stood on one toe-point, he lifted her with one arm held straight in the air and ran off the stage with her. He gave the impression of a man carrying off a prize.

This ending movement so shocked one member of the school staff that he demanded that the school expel Georges. Fortunately, Georges's choreography impressed the school director, who not only insisted that Georges stay but told other students that they should imitate Balanchivadze's enterprise and artistry.

Georges graduated from the school in 1921 at the age of 17 and joined the company of the State Theater of Opera and Ballet. At 5'7" tall, he was really too short to be a classic *danseur noble,* the strong, elegant partner to a ballerina. He

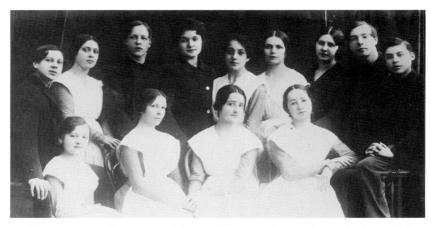

Georges, standing second from right, *graduates from the Imperial School of Ballet in 1921.*

was good-looking and slim, and he wore his dark hair slicked straight back from his forehead with a single lock drooping over one eye. He still had the facial twitch that wrinkled his nose and exposed his teeth, but by now people who knew him were used to it.

Georges had amazing stamina. He once danced a *pas de deux,* or duet, after chasing a train, missing it, and riding 16 miles on a bicycle. Despite this energy, Georges began to show signs of tuberculosis, a serious lung disease. In the days before antibiotics, many people died from tuberculosis. One of the cures was high-protein, fatty foods, which Georges could not obtain.

The State Theater did not pay their dancers enough for them to buy food at Petrograd's inflated prices. The dancers earned extra money—and sometimes food—by offering entertainment for social and political occasions. Georges was especially good at arranging dances for these performances, and his group of friends had many engagements.

Georges liked dancing his character roles at the State Theater. But he was always thinking of new movements to try, variations on existing dances, and whole new ballets. The State Theater didn't care much for experiments, so Georges planned a series of "Evenings of Young Ballet" with his friends, Choura Danilova among them.

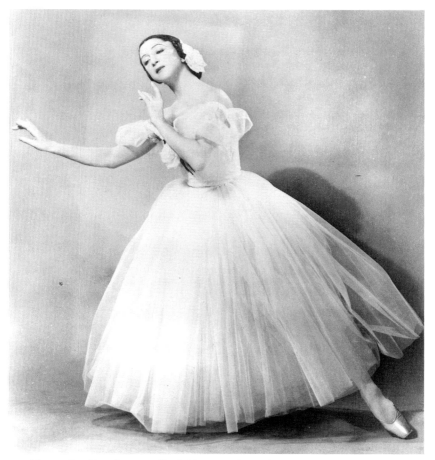

Alexandra Danilova, called Choura, thought Georges was "distinctive and mysterious."

After the revolution, the State Theater added evening classes to make ballet training available to more people. These students didn't have the technique of the Maryinsky dancers, but some were quite good and could be easily re-taught. Among these night school pupils was 15-year-old Tamara Zheverzheyeva. Georges invited Tamara to perform his choreography to Anton Rubenstein's *Romance.* They worked well together, his friends liked her, and Georges included her in the cast for his "Evenings of Young Ballet."

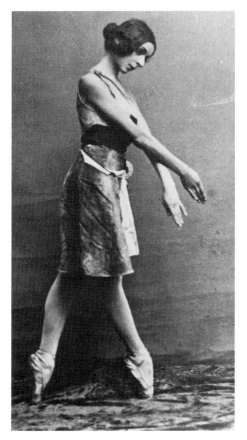
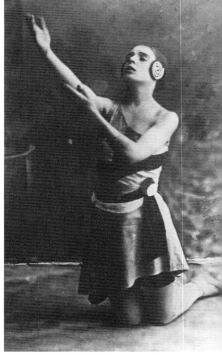

Two dancers perform in Georges's "Evenings of Young Ballet."

After his workday at the State Theater ended, Georges and Tamara rehearsed their new dances. They also found work in small nightclubs, where she sang and he played the piano for her.

The first of the "Evenings of Young Ballet" was scheduled for June 1, 1923, in a hall that had formerly housed the Petrograd City Council. The cast couldn't afford publicity, but people packed the large hall anyway. The audience loved the show, but the next day, a newspaper carried a terrible review by a critic who hated anything new or innovative.

The bad review didn't matter to Georges. He believed that reviewers and the public had to be educated to look at inventive works. The more they saw, the more they would understand. Since this was Georges's first presentation, he didn't expect immediate acceptance.

Tamara's father, who had been a wealthy cloth manufacturer before the 1917 revolution, became quite fond of 19-year-old Georges. Georges rented a room from them, and a few months later, he married Tamara in the chapel at the ballet school.

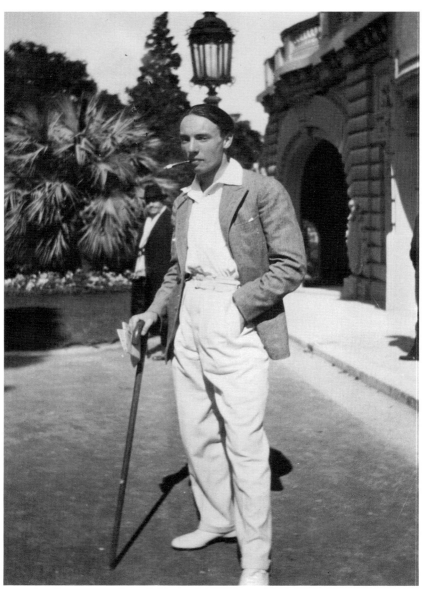

In Monte Carlo, Georges created ballets for the influential producer Serge Diaghilev, standing in the background.

THREE

Europe at His Feet

1923–1926

The young married couple did not get along with Tamara's mother. She continued to treat Tamara like a child, so Georges and Tamara found a dingy little place of their own.

Georges didn't care where he lived. The fact that his salary barely covered the cost of food and rent did not bother him, but he needed satisfying work. Now that he had staged several short ballets, Georges had ideas for many more. The directors of the State Theater gave him some small assignments for charity performances or in summer theaters. Georges himself found more places to work outside the State Theater, where he had freedom to try new choreographic ideas and innovations. Youthful audiences applauded his ideas.

In 1923 the Mihailovsky Opera Theater, the main opera company in Petrograd, hired Georges to arrange dances and processions. The opera directors expected Georges to learn the way things were done and to do them in the same way. He completed several acceptable projects for the company, but then he staged a procession for Rimsky-Korsakov's opera *Le Coq d'Or (The Golden Cockerel)* and had the nerve to use his own ideas. Georges was in trouble again.

When Georges produced a second "Evening of Young Ballet," the State Theater directors announced that they would fire anyone who danced in Georges's future productions without special permission. No one could get special permission.

Vladimir Dmitriev, a man about 40 years old, came to Georges with an interesting idea. Dmitriev was an opera singer whose voice had failed. At the time he approached Georges, he was earning good money in a state-run gambling casino. He obtained permission from the government to take a small group of dancers and other artists to Europe to demonstrate the wonders of art in the Soviet Union. He had money. He could get exit permits. Did Georges want to go with him?

Georges did.

Dmitriev assembled a small group of dancers—including Georges, Tamara, and Choura—for a brief tour of Europe. The dancers knew in their hearts they would never be part of life in Russia again.

They left Russia in April 1924 and traveled across the Baltic Sea by steamer on their way to Germany. Georges described the first night in the steamer's dining room: "It was such a beautiful sight—all that beautiful bread just sitting there like that, so casually, with no one guarding it—I almost wept."

The group ate well on the boat, and when they got to Berlin, they shopped. Berlin was a shabby city in the 1920s, but to the Russians, who dressed in made-over draperies, the city looked like the height of style. After Berlin, Dmitriev arranged performances at resorts along the Rhine River, so the dancers had money coming in until autumn.

Their next job was a four-week booking in a London vaudeville theater as one short act in a long program of singers, jugglers, and animal acts. The theater manager fired the dancers after 10 days because their costume changes took too long.

The performers did not want to go back to Russia. Life was so much better in the West. At home they faced years of dancing in old-fashioned ballets for tiny salaries. Georges especially didn't want to go back to a place where new ideas were squelched.

The troupe's London work permit expired. They traveled to Paris, where they received an invitation to meet the producer of the *Ballets Russes,* or the Russian Ballet.

At this meeting, the dancers saw a tall imposing man with a large head. He wore a monocle in one eye, and his black hair was streaked skunklike with white from front to back. This man was Serge Diaghilev.

Diaghilev himself was not a dancer or an artist, but he had a genius for recognizing the gifts of others and combining their talents in exciting ways. Diaghilev moved in the highest society and charmed people into helping to pay such modern artists as Pablo Picasso and Georges Braque to design sets and costumes for the Ballets Russes. Wealthy patrons helped pay Igor Stravinsky and Erik Satie to compose music for the ballets.

Diaghilev's ballet company was a success until World War I broke out in 1914. Then the company fell on hard times and lost its biggest stars. Without these attractions, audiences and revenue dwindled.

Diaghilev made an agreement with the Monte Carlo Opera in Monaco. The dancers could rehearse and perform new ballets in the opera house. In exchange, they had to perform in the operas. Diaghilev now needed a choreographer to arrange the opera ballets.

Most choreographers wouldn't do opera ballets. They considered it beneath their talent. Opera directors didn't really want ballets in their productions. They put up with them because operas often called for waltzes in ballroom scenes, wedding dances, or folk dances at village fairs. Dancers hated to work on a stage crowded with singers and fought with opera conductors about the timing of music for dance.

Georges didn't know all of this. He was not intimidated by the great Diaghilev either. All Georges wanted was a job.

Diaghilev asked Georges if he could choreograph opera ballets very fast, and Georges, who had never choreographed a complete opera ballet, answered with a confident "Yes."

Then Diaghilev asked Choura to dance for him. She said, "Dance for you? What do you mean?"

Diaghilev explained politely that this was an audition.

Choura was indignant. "Do you know that I come from the Maryinsky Theater?" she asked. "If I am good enough for the Maryinsky Theater, I am good enough for you."

She danced anyway, and all went well until Diaghilev asked how much she weighed. "Are you buying a horse?" she asked. "Maybe you want to see my teeth!"

Diaghilev seemed pleased with the audition. He had Choura, Georges, and Tamara sign contracts and directed them to his winter headquarters in Monte Carlo.

With their contracts signed, Diaghilev took up the matter of names. Tamara Zheverzheyeva? Georges Balanchivadze? Too complicated. The Parisians, the English, and the Spaniards would never be able to say those names. The pair became Tamara Geva and Georges Balanchine. Choura's name, Alexandra Danilova, was just fine.

Once they joined Diaghilev's company, Georges began to understand that this was not a mere job. This was also a

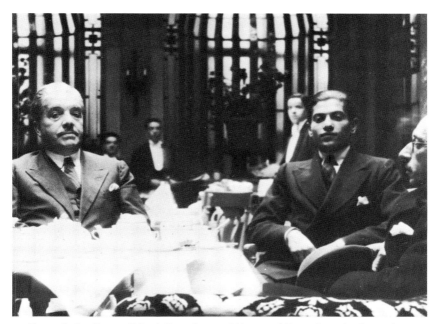

From left, *Serge Diaghilev, Serge Lifar, and Igor Stravinsky enjoy tea at the Savoy in London.*

connection with the most exciting cultural exchange attempted up to that time.

Diaghilev's regular choreographer left soon after Georges was hired. Diaghilev was preparing a dancer named Serge Lifar to become a choreographer. While they toured Europe, Diaghilev took Lifar to museums, talked about literature and music, and tried to make him more worldly and sophisticated. Since Diaghilev did not feel Lifar was ready to choreograph yet, the producer began to train both Lifar and Balanchine. He helped the young men to think and to see things the way *he* thought and saw things. Georges later said that it was Diaghilev who established his outlook and defined his taste.

Georges was traveling throughout Europe and meeting people who spoke neither Russian nor French. By using pantomime, Georges could generally make himself understood. Once when he wanted a glass of milk, he produced a sad-eyed look for a waiter and voiced some pathetic "moos." The waiter nodded, smiled, and brought him a steak!

Georges choreographed new dances quickly and well, to please his new boss. The company found him easygoing, amusing, and invariably courteous. He gained their full confidence, and within five months, had choreographed 16 short opera ballets and directed a whole opera, Ravel's *L'Enfant et les Sortileges (The Spellbound Child)*. This brief opera was Georges's first success and one of his favorite works.

Balanchine's first original ballet for Diaghilev, *Barabau* to music by Vittorio Rieti, was a comic piece, full of bawdy slapstick. The ballet featured four men who sang onstage. *Barabau* might have become a hit, but Diaghilev did not want the extra expense of paying singers. After its first season, he took it off the schedule.

Another ballet Georges choreographed was Stravinsky's *Le Chant du Rossignol (The Song of the Nightingale),* based on a Chinese fairy tale. Tiny 14-year-old Alicia Markova played the nightingale. One night, Alicia was sick and Georges was the only one who knew her steps. He squeezed himself into a fluttery costume and then into the cage in which Alicia usually made her entrance. He later said that while Markova looked like a delicate bird in the cage, he "looked like a gorilla." He danced the role with a self-mockery that had the audience laughing—with him—almost convulsively.

In Monte Carlo, Georges and Tamara rented a room in a boardinghouse where a few other Diaghilev dancers lived. After evening performances, Georges and Tamara often gave parties. Georges was a lively host. He played piano and guitar and sang funny parodies of Russian folk songs in a sad voice. With no instruction in cooking and hardly any money, he prepared wonderful late-night suppers.

Georges made very little money working for Diaghilev, but he was a happy man. He had a secure job doing creative work. In 1926 Georges created three complete ballets, several restagings of older works, and many opera ballets and dance scenes. He also performed regularly. He loved the work and the interesting people he met. But he no longer loved Tamara.

Tamara herself was only 19. She felt tied down by her marriage and wanted some fun, some excitement. She felt that Georges was too wrapped up in his work.

The couple talked about the situation and agreed to part, though Tamara stayed with the company for a while. The two remained friends.

Before long, Georges and Choura fell in love, but Georges could not divorce Tamara. He had left his marriage papers in Russia. With no proof of marriage, there could be no divorce.

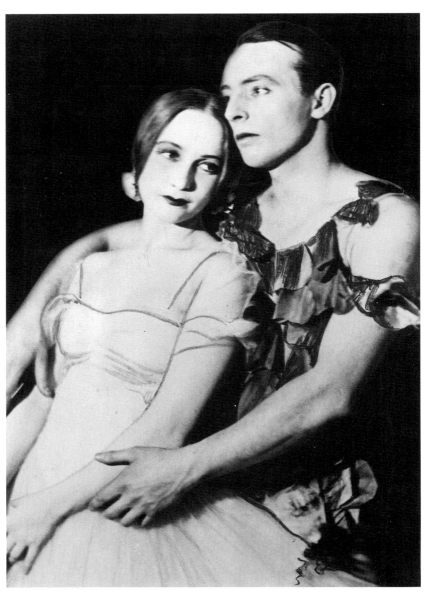

Ballerinas enjoyed dancing with Georges, who was a considerate partner to them.

FOUR

Dancing for Diaghilev

1926–1929

*R*ussia's Imperial School of Ballet had trained Georges to be a classical dancer. He had learned to partner a ballerina, lifting and supporting her but doing little else. Women liked to dance classical roles with Georges. He was careful and considerate of them, and his good looks made it easy to pretend to be in love with him.

Georges still preferred character roles, where he could do exciting leaps and spins. As the villain magician, the clown with the big bottom, or the peasant waving his legs and feet instead of his arms and hands, he loved to improvise. He made his characters funnier and more outlandish than the original choreography called for. During one performance, Diaghilev's stage manager got angry and fined Georges for a particularly outrageous improvisation. But Georges was enjoying himself.

In 1926, while rehearsing a difficult dance step in *The Triumph of Neptune,* Georges twisted his knee and probably tore cartilage. This knee had not been strong since early in his career at the Maryinsky Theater. There, in the role of a warrior, he had hit himself in the knee with a knife he carried. The knee had not healed well.

This new injury was serious. Doctors operated, and Georges wore a cast on his knee for a month. When the cast came off, Georges found he could not rely on the knee for strength or fully bend and straighten it.

Georges reacted to his disability with a laugh, "Good! Now I won't have to work so hard." The fact that he had never liked dancing as much as he liked choreography helped him face the end of his performing career at the age of 22. Because he choreographed successful ballets for Diaghilev, Georges knew that his job with the Ballets Russes was secure and that he could still be part of the ballet world.

In 1928 Georges's new ballet, *Apollon Musagète (Apollo, Leader of the Muses),* was an artistic and popular success. Igor Stravinsky, Diaghilev's friend and collaborator, wrote the music for *Apollo,* as it was later called.

Stravinsky had composed music with irregular rhythms and unlovely sounds that shocked audiences in the early 1900s. When his ballet *Le Sacre du Printemps (Rite of Spring)* was performed for the first time, the audience booed, threw things at the dancers, and started fistfights. Diaghilev had to cancel the rest of the ballet's performances. Years later, audiences grew used to the sounds and rhythms in Stravinsky's music, and the company once again performed the ballet.

Stravinsky and Balanchine liked each other instantly. The composer felt that in Georges, he had found a choreographer who understood his language—music. In Stravinsky, inventive Georges found a mentor and teacher.

Stravinsky wanted *Apollo* to be a classical ballet. He saw the choreography as strictly traditional, with the muses in the long white fluffy skirts of classical ballerinas. These concepts were not for Diaghilev, who wanted everything he presented to be new. Georges pleased both these demanding

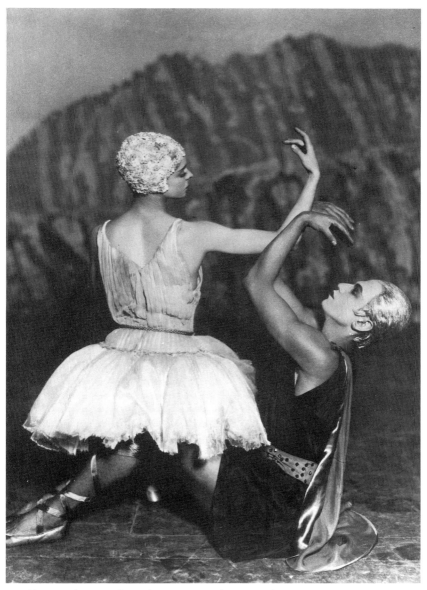

Choura dances the role of Terpsichore, and Serge Lifar appears as Apollo in Stravinsky's Apollon Musagète.

men by creating a dance that was "neoclassical." The movements were cleanly done on a grand scale, the steps were balletic and not acrobatic, but the style was fresh and adventurous. Stravinsky did not get his long fluffy skirts for the ballerinas.

Music inspired Balanchine, but *Apollo* taught him to select from all the ideas he imagined. Stravinsky's music had discipline and restraint, and so should the movement. Balanchine wrote, "I began to see how I could clarify, by limiting, by reducing what seemed to be myriad possibilities [of dance patterns] to the one possibility that is inevitable." He remembered this lesson well and let it guide his work.

Apollo featured Serge Lifar as Apollo, the Greek god of artists. In Greek mythology, the muses were nine sisters believed to inspire artists. In his ballet, Georges used only three

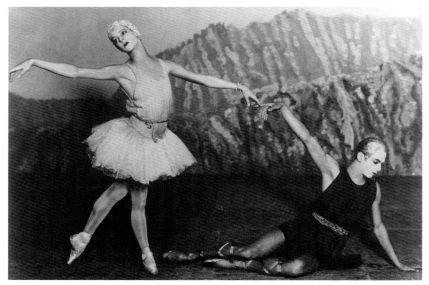

In Apollo, *Terpsichore's inspiring touch evokes Michelangelo's painting of the Creation.*

muses to represent the arts of dance, epic poetry, and pantomime. Choura portrayed Terpsichore, the Muse of Dance.

Balanchine designed the role of Terpsichore with a special woman, Choura, in mind. In later years, other dancers inspired Georges to create roles for them. They were his muses. He never made better dances than those he choreographed for women he loved.

Apollo established Balanchine as a success with the Diaghilev company and ballet audiences. Dance critic Edwin Denby later described the ballet as "an homage to the academic ballet tradition—and the first work in the contemporary classic style. . . . And it leaves at the end, despite its innumerable incidental inventions, a sense of bold, open, effortless and limpid grandeur."

Though they traveled almost constantly with the company, Georges and Choura wanted to buy an apartment in Paris—but they had no money. Georges was generous when other dancers needed money and he had any to lend. Now he tried to collect on some debts. Like his father, Georges found it hard to ask for money and easy to believe the excuses and hard-luck stories of his debtors. Finally, Diaghilev lent Georges and Choura 4,000 francs and an apartment was theirs.

In his next assignment, Rieti's *Le Bal (The Ball)*, Georges found a new way to present the *adagio,* the slow section of a pas de deux. Until then, an adagio had been a dance for a ballerina as she was supported, balanced, or lifted by her partner. The man was little more than something for the ballerina to hold onto. In *Le Bal,* Georges insisted that the adagio be a true dance for two people. The steps for the male as well as the female dancer should be as interesting as he could make them. And the movements had to follow the slow, drawn-out rhythms of the music. Georges tried to display these qualities in all his later adagios.

In 1929 Balanchine based the ballet *Le Fils Prodigue (The Prodigal Son)* composed by Serge Prokofiev on a story from the New Testament. Because it had a plot and characters, *The Prodigal Son* differed from Balanchine's previous work. For the first time, Georges had to make the audience care about the characters. Otherwise the final scene, in which the father forgives his wayward son, would not be poignant. Diaghilev had taught Serge Lifar, who danced the role of the

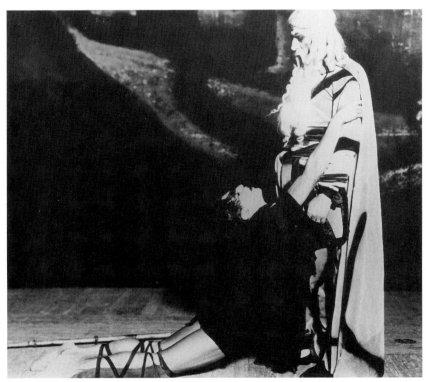

Prokofiev's The Prodigal Son *was one of the few story ballets Georges ever choreographed.*

son, that emotions were not part of dancing. Now Balanchine demanded that Lifar dance emotions as well as movement. When Lifar complained to Diaghilev, the producer told him to obey Balanchine.

On opening night, when the audience wept at the touching final scene, Lifar bragged that his acting had made the ballet a hit. Georges generously agreed with him. But Diaghilev was proud of Georges and praised his work in the *London Times*.

Balanchine's biographer, Bernard Taper, wrote, "There are very few modern works, in any art form, that can match this ballet's horrifying sense of degradation or the tenderness and wonder that the scene of redemption and forgiveness at the end achieves."

When the company broke up for the summer holiday, Diaghilev assured everyone that the next season would hold more success and profit for all. He had bookings in Spain as well as in Monte Carlo, Paris, and London. Everything indicated that the Diaghilev company could produce fresh, interesting ballets that would entertain Europe indefinitely.

Georges and Choura took separate vacations that year. Choura went to Nice on the French Riviera. Georges went to London to choreograph a short dance for England's first sound motion picture, *Dark Red Roses*.

One afternoon on the soundstage, Georges sat with two other dancers to wait for the movie director to film their dance. Time went slowly, and everyone was bored. Someone picked up a newspaper. The headline read "SERGE DIAGHILEV DEAD IN VENICE."

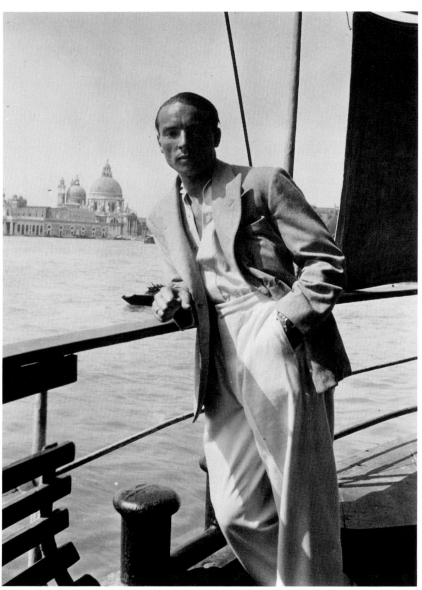

Georges traveled, danced, and choreographed in many European cities.

FIVE

Choreographer on Call
1929–1933

$\mathcal{G}$eorges was 25 years old and out of a job. Diaghilev's death shocked and saddened him. He admired the man who had been his mentor and benefactor. But Georges's life was ahead of him, and he had to decide what to do next.

He did not have to worry for long. His talent had attracted attention, and by October 1929, Georges had a job staging the ballet *Les Créatures de Prométhée (The Creatures of Prometheus)* at the Paris Opéra. The Paris Opéra Ballet was not a very good company. Its director wanted Georges, employed as resident ballet master, to stage the ballet and rebuild the company's reputation.

Georges worked hard on the ballet, but when he was about half finished, he fell ill with pneumonia. In those years before antibiotics, pneumonia was not easy to cure. The director asked when Georges would be back to work.

Georges was too sick to even consider finishing the job. He had to tell him to get someone else to finish the ballet and suggested Serge Lifar. Diaghilev had educated Lifar just as he had educated Georges. With half the ballet done, Lifar could use the ideas Georges noted in the musical score for the rest.

Lifar was not sure he could do the work. His one try at choreography for Diaghilev had failed. "Do you think I can do it, Georges?" he kept asking.

For a week, Lifar bombarded Georges with questions about every movement. Designers ran in and out of Georges's hospital room with fabric samples and drawings. Musicians came with questions of tempo and phrasing. Georges became more exhausted and sicker than ever. His pneumonia sparked the tuberculosis he had been harboring for years, and his doctor finally banned all visitors. Georges's illness became so serious that the doctor sent him to a Swiss sanitarium, a medical facility for tuberculosis patients.

Choura went with Georges to Switzerland, where for three months he ran a high fever. He did nothing but rest in the sun, wrapped to his neck in blankets in the cold Swiss winter. He was supposed to eat protein-rich food, but he had no appetite.

When his doctors wanted to operate, perhaps to remove the bad part of his lung, Georges remembered the disastrous operation on his knee. He had just enough strength to refuse. He never wanted surgeons to cut into him again.

Somehow, complete rest was effective. In time, Georges was able to get up, to dress, to walk about the sanitarium and then the grounds. By January 1930, he was well enough to leave.

Georges was not really cured, however. For many years, he had symptoms that told him he carried the infection in his body. X rays showed permanent damage in both lungs, and late in 1930, one lung collapsed completely.

Georges didn't have enough breathing capacity to dance. His energy was gone by early afternoon. But his head was full of new dances. He knew that if he heard the right music, these dances would spring to life. All he needed was a stage and some dancers.

When he returned to Paris, Georges thought he might resume his work at the Paris Opéra. He talked to Lifar about it, and Lifar convinced him not to return. Georges knew that if he really wanted the job, he could have gone to the director and fought for it. He didn't have to listen to Lifar, who was not as talented or experienced as Georges.

But Georges's illness had sapped his confidence. He didn't understand theatrical jealousy, and he didn't care about personal fame. He had been very ill and was still weak. When Lifar advised him not to work at the Paris Opéra, Georges passively agreed. He would find some other place to work.

A few weeks later, the Paris Opéra Ballet announced that its new ballet master would be Serge Lifar.

In 1930 one of Georges's old friends from Diaghilev's ballet company—Vera Nemchinova—asked him to choreograph a short ballet for her. Vera's faith in Georges's ability bolstered his self-confidence. His skills were as sharp as ever, and he found reserves of energy for work. He choreographed the ballet with his usual speed and ingenuity. He could move well enough to teach her the dances. Since he believed that "to teach you must be able to show," this success made him feel whole and capable again.

Georges went to London for his next job as choreographer for a theatrical "revue," an evening of brief skits, songs, and dances. The revue was popular with audiences, and Georges was paid well at last. After sending a share of money to Dmitriev, who had rescued him from Russia, Georges followed an impulse to treat himself well. He had not known luxury since his childhood, and now he ordered some clothes from fine tailors in London.

When his money was almost gone, Georges heard from Choura, who was still living in the Paris apartment that she and Georges had bought. She was not working and wrote to Georges for money. But he had taken a job in Copenhagen as the guest ballet master for the Royal Danish Ballet and wouldn't be back in Paris for at least five months.

The Danes wanted Georges to reproduce exact copies of Diaghilev's most popular ballets. Georges never liked to simply restage anything this way. He always found something new in the music or the action. Even when he restaged his own works, he couldn't resist tinkering with the choreography.

The Danes, however, wanted the original choreography. This was difficult, since the dancers weren't trained in Russian technique. To highlight the strengths of the Danish dancers, Balanchine choreographed ballets that featured mime and dramatic emotion rather than the complicated turns, lifts, and jumps of the Russian style. The company's administrators were not pleased. They had all seen the original ballets, and they wouldn't believe their dancers couldn't do exactly what Diaghilev's dancers could do. At the end of the five months, the company did not ask Georges to stay. He was not surprised.

Georges did earn quite a bit of money in Copenhagen, however. He bought an American car and took it to London when he returned. He loved to dress in his stylish London clothes and drive pretty young girls through the countryside. The best work he could get in London was vaudeville, but the pay was good. Georges enjoyed this situation while it lasted and spent money freely.

Unfortunately, during the early 1930s, most of the world was experiencing the Great Depression. People had very little money, and theater of any kind became a luxury. Even vaudeville audiences dwindled. Soon Georges was out of a job again, and unemployed foreigners could not stay in England. Georges spent time and money trying to get permits to stay, but failing in the end, he headed for Paris.

Georges drove his car onto a ferryboat and crossed the English Channel. When he got to France, he couldn't afford to pay the import fee for the car, so he simply handed the keys to a stranger he saw on the dock and caught a train for Paris. This action was typical of Georges. Possessions meant nothing to him. He couldn't pay the fee for the car, so he gave it away. One day he would get another car.

Choura might have been looking forward to that car and to Georges's return, but now he had no job, no money, and no car. Choura wanted security. Besides, Georges had the nerve to bring her a gift of cologne from England—cologne for Choura, who lived in a city full of French perfume!

Choura took a job in London and angrily wrote Georges a letter suggesting that they part, since their careers seemed to take them on opposite paths. Yet, when Georges wrote back that she should do what she thought best, Choura realized she did not really want to break with Georges. She loved him and missed him very much.

Georges's luck changed again and a job came to him. Two ballet producers, René Blum and Colonel de Basil, were reorganizing the Diaghilev ballet company under the new name of *Les Ballets Russes de Monte Carlo*. They recruited some of Diaghilev's collaborators for the company, and Georges decided to join them. He wanted to participate in the planning so he could choose his own projects.

Georges was eager to work with very young dancers. He had an idea for a new kind of movement, and a young amateur would be more open to fresh ideas than a professional.

He visited classes taught by former Russian ballerinas and found three teenage girls who fit his mental picture of the dancer needed for his new movements. They were tall and slender with long legs and arms. When the lanky young

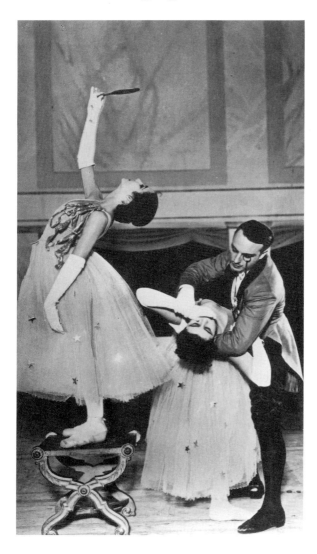

People who witnessed the haunting Cotillon *in 1932 considered it Georges's best work.*

dancers began to dance in public, people nicknamed them "the baby ballerinas."

The first full season of Les Ballets Russes de Monte Carlo opened in March 1932. Balanchine created several new ballets for the company. *Cotillon,* to music by Emmanuel Chabrier, was first performed on April 12 and may be the best work Balanchine ever did. It didn't have much of a story—only a girl at a party, a fortune-teller, and lots of party guests in costumes—but a haunting sadness dominated the gaiety of the occasion. Most people who saw the ballet never forgot it.

After this first successful season, Colonel de Basil forced his partner, René Blum, out of the company and decided not to include Georges in the next season's plans. Georges wasn't the only artist de Basil let go. Many of the dancers looked to Georges, their former ballet master, for leadership.

Soon Balanchine had a company of his own, which was called *Les Ballets.* He had dancers but no money to pay them, to rent a theater, or to hire musicians. Les Ballets limped along on donations. Then, like an angel from heaven, a rich Englishman named Edward James gave them money for new dance productions.

Les Ballets received poor reviews. In addition, Colonel de Basil came to Paris boasting of how his own company had improved since he had ousted Georges Balanchine. The struggling company didn't have a chance.

Georges was 29 years old. Since Diaghilev had died, the young artist had choreographed 20 ballets and innumerable opera dances, most of them largely forgotten. He had been ill. He had gone from job to job without much rest and little security. He was deeply discouraged, but some ballet lovers still saw him as an important part of the ballet scene.

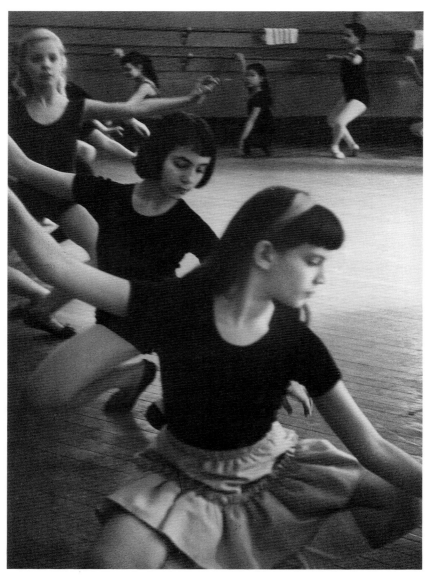

The School of American Ballet (S.A.B.) has trained young dancers since it was founded by Lincoln Kirstein and George Balanchine in 1934.

SIX

An American Ballet

1933–1934

$\mathscr{L}$es Ballets gave its last few performances during the de Basil company's most popular year, 1933. One night Georges substituted for an injured dancer. Performing left him exhausted. He could barely be polite to the tall young man from the United States who came to his dressing room. Georges received his compliments through a haze of fatigue.

Lincoln Kirstein was 6'3" tall and husky without appearing heavy. He wore wire-rimmed glasses, and his dark hair was slicked straight back from his forehead.

The night they first met, Kirstein realized that Georges was too tired for an important conversation, so he waited four days before making a second contact. Balanchine, who vaguely remembered Kirstein's backstage visit, agreed to an appointment on July 9, 1933. They had to speak French, their only common language, but both spoke that language well. Kirstein told Balanchine about himself and his ideas for developing ballet as an American art form.

Ballet was Kirstein's first and best love. He continually talked and wrote of Americans as a great potential audience for dance. He had taken ballet lessons from one of Diaghilev's choreographers, who scoffed, "He can't get

49

his feet off the floor." Lincoln knew he was no dancer. He just wanted to feel what dancing was like and to understand how ballet should be taught.

Kirstein could have imported a European ballet company to New York. But he really wanted only a few people who would help him find and train American dancers. In his search for a teacher-choreographer, he had traveled around Europe to see the work of people from Diaghilev's company. When he spoke with these people, he often heard high praise for Georges Balanchine. Indeed, one of the "baby ballerinas" told him she didn't want to work for any other ballet master.

At their meeting on July 9, Kirstein and Balanchine also talked about the state of ballet and the future of the art form. Now Kirstein let Georges do most of the talking. He wanted to know whether their personalities would allow them to work well together. Then he proposed that Balanchine join him in the United States to create a new ballet company— one that would define ballet for the future.

Balanchine sized up this earnest 26-year-old man and decided to trust him. Things were not going well in Europe, and a change would be good. Balanchine quickly let Kirstein persuade him to move to the United States because, "I always wanted to have a start, with really clean, beautifully taught ballet people who could dance the way I want." Kirstein heard Balanchine promise that "with twenty girls and five men he could do wonders" toward building an American ballet company.

Kirstein arranged to establish a ballet school in Hartford, Connecticut. The Wadsworth Athenæum, a Hartford museum, would sponsor the school and furnish classroom space and a theater. Kirstein arranged all this through his friend Chick Austin, the Athenæum director.

Kirstein secured entry permits and booked passage for Balanchine and Dmitriev. Georges would not leave Europe without his old friend. Ever since Dmitriev had brought him out of Russia, Balanchine had shown his gratitude by paying Dmitriev part of anything he earned. In return, Dmitriev acted as Balanchine's agent, handling business details Balanchine disliked. Balanchine wanted Dmitriev to manage the new school.

Balanchine and Dmitriev sailed for New York in September 1933. Kirstein met them there at the dock on October 17. Kirstein's friend and partner Edward Warburg wrote his first impressions of Balanchine as "a remarkable little man. He looked ill, which he was. He was also shy, gentle, and very precise."

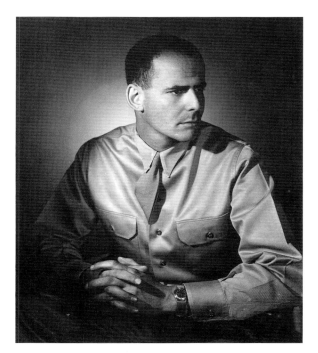

Lincoln Kirstein

Balanchine asked Kirstein and Warburg not to show him any cathedrals and to help him learn American slang. He also asked for help in finding his first wife, Tamara Geva, whom he had heard lived in New York with her new husband. When they met, Tamara gave Georges a warm welcome.

After a few days of New York sightseeing, Kirstein took Balanchine and Dmitriev to Hartford and showed them the facilities at the Athenæum. But Balanchine hadn't left the capitals of Europe to work in a sleepy Connecticut town. He inspected the hard floors of the studio and the small stage of the theater and said, "Look, Lincoln, let's go, because first of all it's too small. Let's go to New York." Hartford, Georges thought, was "a very little place and nobody wanted us there, and there were, you know, already three teachers there that were against us. And the reporters immediately came, you know, and began writing things like 'Why did he come here to spoil our life?' "

Kirstein knew if he insisted on staying in Hartford, Georges would leave the project. But if he told Chick Austin the deal was off, he would lose an important friend. He decided to keep Balanchine happy and end things with Austin as tactfully as he could. Then he looked for a museum in New York that might give them classrooms and a theater. But word had spread in the artistic community. Kirstein's enterprise was tarnished because he'd backed out of his deal with the Athenæum. Every New York museum he approached turned him down.

By the time they abandoned Hartford, Georges had become truly ill, probably with a full recurrence of tuberculosis. A doctor prescribed six months of complete rest and warned Georges that he could not expect to live longer than 10 years. But with the help of a friend who fed him rich, fatty food and tended to him carefully, Georges was ready to work in a month.

By appealing to his wealthy friends for money, Kirstein leased a studio for a school on the fourth floor of a building on New York City's Madison Avenue. The ground floor housed Sammy's Delicatessen, which quickly became the ballet students' hangout. The second floor was the Tuxedo Ballroom, where people danced fox-trots and tangos every evening. On the third floor, a tailor ran his sewing machine to the rhythms of the student dancers bouncing above his head. And then, one floor below a painter's loft, was Kirstein's School of American Ballet, which came to be called by its initials, "S.A.B."

The School of American Ballet had no financial backing other than what Kirstein and the wealthy Warburg could provide themselves or wangle from their friends and relatives. To open the school, Kirstein needed money to buy mirrors and pianos for the studio, and lockers and plumbing for the dressing rooms. Dmitriev needed a desk, a chair, and a file cabinet.

Kirstein hired three teachers and advertised for students. He and Balanchine wanted pupils in their teens and early 20s who had some ballet training, who could benefit from lessons, but who could also perform. Later they would start teaching younger children.

Pupils began to audition. Warburg called them "field hockey girls" because most of them were shorter, stockier, and more robust than Balanchine's ideal dancer. The first classes began on New Year's Day 1934, just six weeks after George landed in New York, with 32 students.

From January to June, S.A.B. was "organized chaos." Dmitriev seemed to enjoy each crisis. If everything was going well, he would create a problem. When Dmitriev couldn't have his way, he would threaten: He'd quit! He'd call a strike! He'd take Georges back to Europe! Kirstein and Warburg gave in to him. Dmitriev seemed to despise the wealthy young men, and he enjoyed finding menial work for them. The classroom mirrors didn't hang straight. There would be no classes until they were right again. That would keep the two Americans busy for a while! Kirstein did everything from lecturing students on the history and art of dance, to sound-proofing the ceiling, to handling immigration problems for the Russians.

Balanchine, who had now Americanized his name to George, seemed unaware of the trouble Dmitriev stirred up. Classes usually went on unaffected by the crises around them.

George taught very few classes. After only a few months, when he was stronger, he began to choreograph. The school could earn money with performances, and students needed to understand how their ballet classes applied to real danc-ing—on a stage, in costume, and before an audience.

Balanchine's first American ballet was *Serenade* to music by Tchaikovsky. As was his custom, he tailored the ballet to the abilities of his dancers. The American students had strong legs and feet, but they were slow. So Balanchine made a slow dance for them. He found combinations of steps that appeared elegant, but cleverly disguised his dancers' lack of professional technique. During one rehearsal, a dancer ran in late. Another fell and burst into tears. Balanchine used these events as episodes in *Serenade*. Over the years, he restaged this ballet several times, changing it to suit the increasing abilities of his dancers.

Although critics did not care for *Serenade* at first, they soon realized that Balanchine had accomplished something

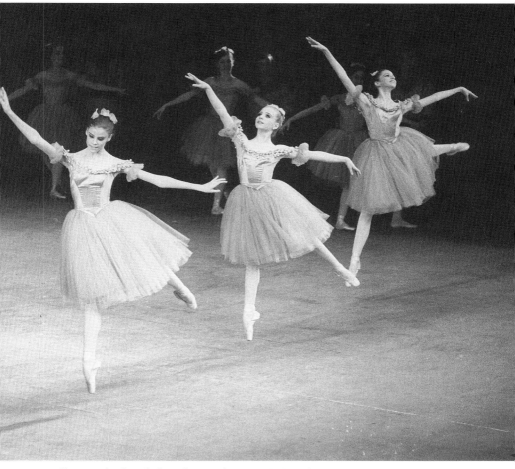

George insisted that the students at S.A.B. become comfortable performing in front of an audience.

extraordinary with this ballet. By giving his untrained dancers simple movements to perform in absolute unison, he emphasized teamwork. Rather than being dazzled by complicated or athletic solos that European dancers performed, audiences watching *Serenade* saw the incredible beauty and

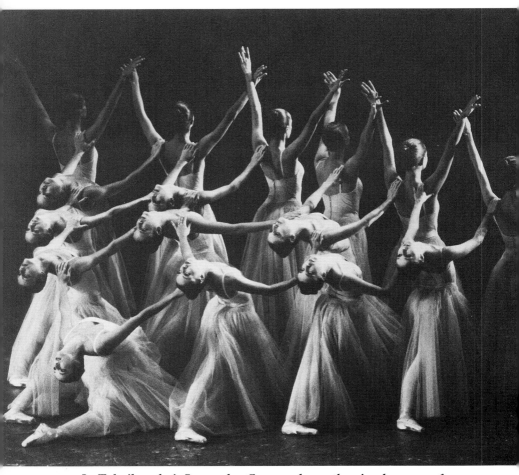

In Tchaikovsky's Serenade, *George shows the simple grace of the human form and the eloquence of bodies moving in unison.*

emotional power of pure, unadorned human movement. In this way, Balanchine produced a new, entirely American classical ballet style.

By June 1934, the American Ballet, a company of the most advanced S.A.B. students, was ready to perform four short ballets. But the company had no money to rent a theater or pay musicians.

Warburg wrote, "Suddenly it was decided that what I wanted more than anything else for my upcoming birthday was a performance by this company of ballet dancers at the family place in White Plains, New York." The wealthy, accommodating Warburgs put up an outdoor platform, hid a piano in the bushes, and had enough food prepared to feed the audience of about 200 people. "The dancers stood with their arms raised to the moon and the heavens, and the heavens responded with heavy rain." Without asking the Warburgs, Lincoln Kirstein called out from the stage to invite the guests back the following evening. Mrs. Warburg was upset at having to give the same party twice and wondered where she would get food on a Sunday. She certainly couldn't count on Saturday's leftovers—the dancers were eating everything in sight!

Yet food was arranged, and the Sunday night performance impressed everyone who attended. The summer break from school routine began on an upbeat note.

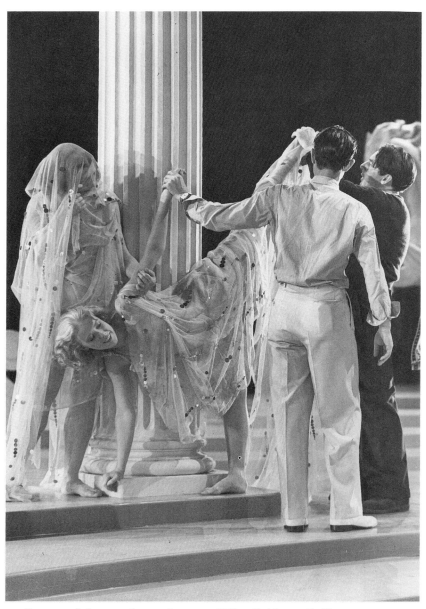

George, right, *works on the set of* The Goldwyn Follies.

SEVEN

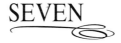

From Broadway to Hollywood

1934–1939

George Balanchine was happy in 1934. The United States was in the middle of an economic depression, but George was not easily depressed. He had work, he had some money, and he had New York City, where he felt at home. He liked its easy, informal atmosphere. He enjoyed watching Americans. They moved with an uninhibited, athletic looseness that would find its way into his dances.

In New York, George adopted a friendly, outgoing personality. Without looking back with nostalgia for the old days, he became friends with many Russian dancers, artists, and musicians who lived in New York.

But no matter how many friends he made, George remained reserved. He was kind and sympathetic, but he rarely shared his emotions. As a compliment, Kirstein called him "sinister," possibly because Kirstein was never really sure what George thought or felt.

At first Balanchine's limited English may have made him seem distant. Over the years, Balanchine learned to use English colorfully and to express himself almost poetically. He loved puns and jokes with double meanings. But he never lost the Russian way of constructing sentences. He might say something like "Step is like Charleston" or "I know can do this dance." Balanchine didn't want the world to think that he couldn't master English. He asked reporters to quote him in correct English. He told wonderful stories and loved to talk about his life, science, politics, and movies.

In his first years in New York, George lived alone in a series of small apartments close to S.A.B. He would furnish one apartment and then move to another a few months later.

He saw a car he liked and bought it on the spot. No shopping, no comparing, no analysis of engines or prices. A friend said, "I spend more time buying a *tie* than you just did buying a car." George filled the car with friends and students and drove out to the countryside to find a restaurant that served Russian tea.

When classes started again at S.A.B. in September 1934, the advanced students resumed their dual roles as pupils and performers. They presented a program of ballet in Hartford that suffered from horrible costumes, squeaky toe-shoes, a tiny stage, and inept stagehands. But the dancing attracted a theatrical agent who thought the troupe should have a professional engagement.

The agent booked the American Ballet into the Adelphi Theater in New York City. Balanchine persuaded Tamara Geva and a few other experienced dancers to join the company. They performed before nearly empty seats for at least a week.

Edward Johnson, the manager of the Metropolitan Opera Company, was one of the few people who saw their show. He approached Balanchine about joining forces to produce opera ballets. Balanchine had done hundreds of these in

Monte Carlo. He knew the lowly position of dance in an opera company where everyone felt that music came first. But faced with an opportunity to put his company to work professionally, he chose to believe Johnson, who said he wanted "freshness, youth, and novelty" in ballets. The Metropolitan Opera, called the Met by opera fans, would be George's new cradle of creativity.

One look at the dancers' damp, cramped, dingy dressing area should have told Balanchine all he needed to know about working at the Met. The dancers were not simply second-class, but fourth-class citizens at the opera. The management scolded them for wearing out too many dancing shoes. Conductors changed the music without telling Balanchine. Worst of all, Edward Johnson, who wanted "freshness, youth, and novelty" in ballet, accused Balanchine of having no respect for tradition. Balanchine answered, "Of course not. The tradition of the ballet at the Met is bad ballet." Balanchine's free-spirited movement and the Met's traditional, rigid performance style caused many conflicts, but they worked together through the 1937–1938 opera season.

Balanchine had one success at the Met. An opera season always includes certain gala evenings. Balanchine and Kirstein talked Edward Johnson into producing a Stravinsky Gala. George restaged *Apollo* and created two ballets to new music by Stravinsky, *Le Baiser de la Fée (The Fairy's Kiss)* and *Card Game: A Ballet in Three Deals*. Stravinsky, George's good friend since his Diaghilev days, conducted the orchestra. Edward Warburg financed these dance productions. Audiences received the ballets so enthusiastically that the ballets almost paid for themselves—to Warburg's great relief.

The Stravinsky Gala marked the end of the association between the American Ballet and the Met. George could not resist taking verbal revenge as he left. He told the newspapers that "the Met is a heap of ruins, and every night the stagehands put it together and make it look a little like an opera."

Balanchine might have been more upset by the experience with the Met if this had been his only work. But he had been working on several Broadway shows at the same time that he was involved with the Met. While the opera management resisted Balanchine's ideas, the Broadway musical theater embraced them. Broadway producers invited him to choreograph their musical shows, and George enjoyed this new artistic outlet.

Vladimir Dukelsky was a Russian composer and an old friend of Balanchine. He knew Ira and George Gershwin, who wrote the scores for many Broadway musicals. The Gershwin brothers changed Dukelsky's name to Vernon Duke and asked him to write music for the *Ziegfeld Follies* of 1936. In turn, Duke got his friend Balanchine a job as the show's choreographer.

Although his dances for the *Follies* were not great, the experience helped George learn the English words he needed to teach Broadway dancers his choreography. Ballet and Broadway dance steps are related but different, and George couldn't name them in French and expect Broadway dancers to understand.

When his next Broadway opportunity came, Balanchine was ready. *On Your Toes,* with music by Richard Rodgers, told the story of a Broadway tap dancer who got involved with a Russian ballet company very much like Diaghilev's. Tamara Geva acted the part of the Russian ballerina. Ray Bolger—best known as the Scarecrow in the movie *The Wizard of Oz*—played the tap dancer. Balanchine had no experience with tap, so someone else choreographed those sequences under Balanchine's supervision.

On Your Toes was the hit of the 1936 Broadway season, and the dances played an important part in its success. The high point of the show was "Slaughter on Tenth Avenue." In the ballet, a gangster tries to shoot a tap dancer, who must dance madly until the police arrive. Balanchine allowed Ray Bolger to improvise this final dance. Bolger was supposed to be dancing to save his life, and it seemed more real to the audience when he made it up as he went along.

The show's credits originally read "Dances by George Balanchine." Broadway billed all choreographers this way. George asked his producer if the credits could read *"Choreography* by George Balanchine" instead. The producer thought about it and decided, why not? As a matter of fact, that line had class. From then on, all Broadway musicals had choreographers. Balanchine gained respect for his craft and for other choreographers who followed him.

Broadway producers eagerly asked Balanchine to choreograph their shows in the late 1930s and early 1940s. Balanchine worked on *The Boys from Syracuse, Where's Charlie?,* and *Babes in Arms.* Producers and directors found Balanchine easy to work with. "Un-temperamental, logical, objective," Richard Rodgers said. When he was told a choreographic segment wouldn't work, "Balanchine would just take it in his stride and cheerfully produce on the spot any number of perfectly brilliant ideas to take the place of what came out."

Rodgers once told him, "I will write anything. What do you want? Do you want something special?"

Balanchine replied, "No, you write. I do."

Movie producer Samuel Goldwyn invited Balanchine to choreograph dances for a 1938 film called *The Goldwyn Follies.*

He was eager to try this new medium. The movie had no plot, just a group of unrelated sequences, one or two of which would be ballets. Balanchine had seen enough movies to know that the camera could enhance a story, and he thought he knew exactly how to use it creatively with dance.

He talked the project over with Lincoln Kirstein. Kirstein still wanted to build S.A.B. and to create a strong American ballet company for American audiences. The two finally agreed that Kirstein would continue to provide performances with a company called Ballet Caravan. Balanchine would take some of the advanced dancers to California with him to work on films.

Goldwyn hired 19-year-old Brigitta Hartwig, a pretty blonde whose stage name was Vera Zorina, to join Balanchine's cast at the Goldwyn Studios. Brigitta had stud- ied ballet with many different teachers for short periods of time. She could dance well, but she lacked the focus that a single training method might have given her. She wasn't Balanchine's ideal tall, long-legged, willow-slim dancer. Nev- ertheless, George included her in his circle of friends. The group met frequently to cook huge Russian meals, devour caviar, and argue late into the night.

As Balanchine worked to prepare Brigitta to dance in the film, he taught her to use her hands and feet his way. He helped her change her center of gravity, which gave her better balance. In other words, he tried to remake Brigitta into a "Balanchine dancer"—the perfect interpreter of his choreography.

His working methods amazed Brigitta. "He played a piece [of music] over and over again on the piano until it was entirely in his head. He had no scraps of paper, no diagrams with choreographic notes, but would begin choreographing

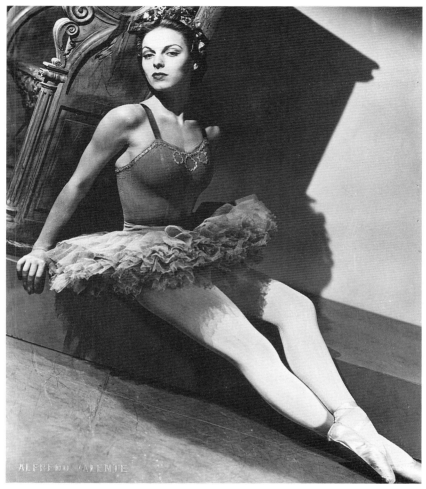

Brigitta Hartwig, known as Vera Zorina, became George's next muse.

by lightly touching a dancer's hand and telling him or her how or where to move. He was certain what he wanted but sometimes stood still as if listening to inner music and visualizing dance movements."

Goldwyn was not sure Balanchine knew what he was doing. When George finally allowed him to see one ballet, Goldwyn discovered that George had ordered many small sets to be built on the soundstage. He, the great Sam Goldwyn, had to *move* every five or six minutes when the ballet moved to a new set. Balanchine asked Goldwyn to crouch or to lie down to watch—to pretend to be the camera. Goldwyn, not known for tact or open-mindedness, told Balanchine to cancel the whole ballet. Make a dance that a person could look at sitting in a chair, Goldwyn directed. And not so much ballet—it should look *modern.*

Balanchine responded by taking a group of friends, including Brigitta, to the San Bernardino Mountains. After long walks and several good talks—and despite the 13 years' difference in their ages—George fell in love with Brigitta. But she was not ready for love or marriage. She asked him to wait until she was older and more sure of what she wanted from life. He agreed.

After two weeks, Goldwyn realized that he couldn't finish his movie without Balanchine and begged him to come back. Balanchine obliged and invented a modern tap-ballet dance for the movie.

One dance sequence for *The Goldwyn Follies* probably resulted from Balanchine's fascination with Hollywood production tricks. Wind machines, elevators, lights, and mirrors gave him ideas. Brigitta, dressed as a sea nymph, emerged headfirst from the center of a pool of water (by standing on a tiny elevator platform) and danced on the surface of the water, which was now glass. In one sequence, Balanchine had the wind machine blow off most of Brigitta's clothes.

When they finished filming, George and Brigitta returned to New York so that she could star in the Broadway

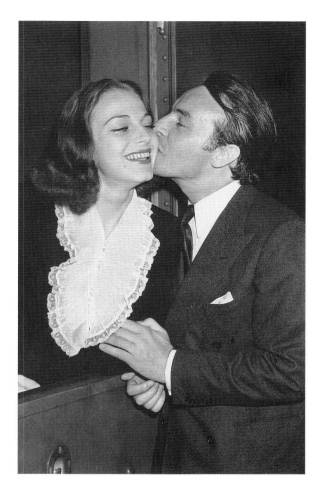

George kisses his new bride, Brigitta.

play *I Married an Angel*. Balanchine did the choreography for her and then worked on two other shows. He was blissfully in love, and now he had a lot of money. He bought an apartment facing Central Park, a fancy car, and a house on Long Island. He gave Brigitta extravagant gifts, and on Christmas Eve 1938, she agreed to be his wife. They ferried to Staten Island and were married by a judge that same night.

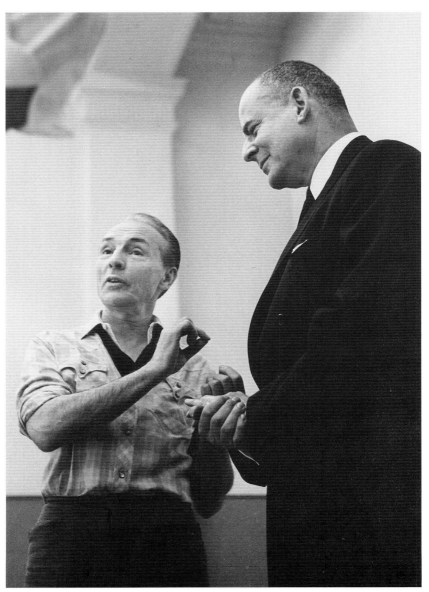

Lincoln Kirstein, right, *brought George to the United States and American audiences to the ballet.*

EIGHT

"Give Me Three Years!"

1939–1948

From 1937 to 1945, the School of American Ballet flourished. Lincoln Kirstein bought out Dmitriev's shares, and when Dmitriev left the school, the atmosphere at S.A.B. changed. Everyone was happier and more optimistic. New teachers and administrators made the training even better.

But Kirstein had a hard time getting professional engagements for Ballet Caravan. A rival company called Ballet Theatre had formed in New York, and the two groups competed for the same small audience.

George's marriage to Brigitta did not work well. The 13-year age difference between them was a huge gap. Brigitta loved him and respected him with her mind but was not in love with him in her heart. She seemed angry that she wasn't free to take full advantage of her fame and often insisted on living separately, even when they were both in the same city. Gossip columnists in New York and Hollywood wrote that Brigitta was having a romance outside their marriage.

George was deeply in love with Brigitta and tried to save the marriage. He bought Brigitta presents he could not afford. Sometimes, when they were living apart, George hung around outside Brigitta's apartment and wretchedly

waited for a glimpse of her. Kirstein called him "a lost man"—
he had lost Brigitta and he had lost his connection to classical ballet. Kirstein knew instinctively that George belonged
in the ballet world.

George himself created one of the worst stresses on the
marriage. He liked female dancers to look light and slim.
Brigitta was a naturally sturdy woman, though she was never
fat, and she had married a great cook. George would tempt
her with some delicious dish and then remind her to watch
her weight. In her confusion, Brigitta developed an eating
disorder called bulimia, which meant that she would overeat
and then vomit to lose weight.

The marriage worked best when George created dances
for Brigitta. She appreciated his attention and his skill, and
he presented her to the public in her best light. He gave her
sound advice about her career.

George became a U.S. citizen in 1940 at the age of 36.
When the United States entered World War II in 1941,
George could not serve in the military because he was past
the draft age, married, and had a defective knee and tuber-
cular lungs. Kirstein was drafted, and though S.A.B. continued to function well, no one on the staff took charge to find
bookings for Ballet Caravan.

In 1941, while Brigitta worked in Hollywood and went on
tour to entertain troops, Balanchine took Kirstein's Ballet
Caravan to Argentina for a four-month tour. After all the time
working in Hollywood and on Broadway, he enjoyed being
back in a true ballet atmosphere with well-trained dancers.
The dancers were thrilled to have him with them. They
began to call him "Mr. B." as a term of respect and affection.

On tour, Balanchine completed two new ballets,
Tchaikovsky's *Ballet Imperial* and Bach's *Concerto Barocco,*

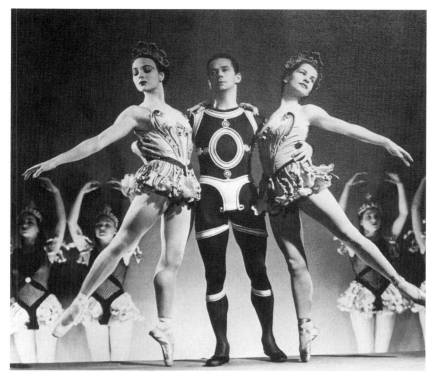

George choreographed Bach's Concerto Barocco *on Ballet Caravan's Argentina tour.*

now considered classic examples of his work. *Ballet Imperial* was the first work in which Balanchine discovered how to use the chorus, called the *corps de ballet,* as an important part of the dance and not as background for soloists. This device, hinted at in *Serenade,* became part of the Balanchine style. Future members of the corps had to be as good as the soloists, because their roles were just as difficult and demanding.

In 1942 Balanchine cooperated with the Ringling Brothers Circus to produce a ballet for 50 women and 50 elephants. He called his good friend Igor Stravinsky.

"I wonder if you'd like to do a little ballet with me," Balanchine said.

"For whom?"

"For some elephants."

"How old?" Stravinsky asked.

"Very young," Balanchine assured him.

There was a pause. Then Stravinsky said gravely, "All right. If they are very young elephants, I will do it."

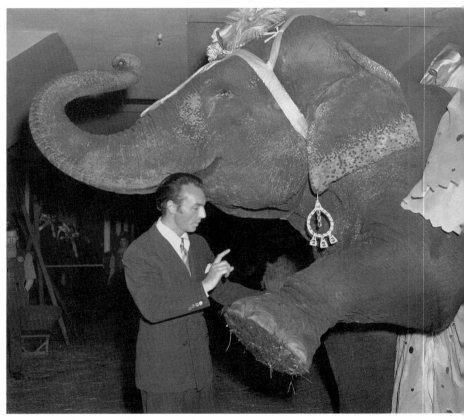

George instructs Modoc, a Ringling Brothers elephant, for Stravinsky's Circus Polka.

Stravinsky's dedication on the score of *Circus Polka* read "For a young elephant."

Not surprisingly, Balanchine had a hard time teaching his steps to the elephants. They stubbornly insisted on doing the same routine they had done for years. So the costumer dressed them in tutus, tiaras, and long earrings, and Balanchine concentrated on training the 50 young women. He exhibited his famous patience with a dancer who repeatedly fell off her elephant. "You must learn to land on the balls of your feet, my dear," he told her quietly.

Brigitta was eager to dance with an elephant. She appeared at the New York opening of the circus and had the thrill of dancing with and riding on the lead elephant, Modoc. Few husbands could give their wives such a gift.

During the war years—1941 to 1945—Balanchine took whatever work came his way. When Ballet Theatre invited him to create a ballet for Brigitta, he cast her as Helen of Troy, the legendary beauty, thus paying her an elegant compliment.

In 1944 Balanchine accepted work with the Ballet Russe de Monte Carlo—the company founded 12 years earlier by Colonel de Basil, who had fired Balanchine after a single season. De Basil was gone, and now the company offered George a difficult job. The Ballet Russe dancers had learned different techniques at different schools in different parts of the world. George had to make them dance as though they belonged together. He managed amazingly well and the dancers quickly learned his technique.

One of the stars in this company was George's old friend and companion, Choura. By then the past was behind them and they were good friends.

The Ballet Russe de Monte Carlo had no home base. The company toured the United States for many months, but Balanchine was not always with them. He didn't want to form a permanent tie with a touring company. Touring was hard on dancers, and audiences demanded lots of tricky acrobatics. Making those kinds of dances didn't satisfy Balanchine. He would leave to work for another company and then come back.

In 1944 Balanchine did another Broadway show, *Song of Norway,* and persuaded the producers to use the Ballet Russe as the chorus of the show. The show was a great success, but then Balanchine was off to his next project. He worked frantically during 1944 and 1945, possibly to avoid thinking about his unhappy marriage.

Brigitta finally made George face the idea of divorce. She had fallen in love with someone else and wanted to remarry. George admitted to himself that he couldn't force the marriage to work, but he regretted its end.

Since divorce was inevitable, George began to look at women differently. Instead of friends or dancers, women became potential sweethearts. One Ballet Russe dancer who caught his eye was Maria Tallchief. George had designed dances for her in *Song of Norway,* and she had understudied Choura's solo. George courted Maria the way he had courted Tamara, Choura, and Brigitta—by choreographing dances for her.

When Balanchine began working with the Ballet Russe, 19-year-old Maria was still in the corps de ballet. She had danced professionally for some famous choreographers, and most agreed that she had a bright future. Maria recalled that when she started to dance for Balanchine, she had to learn to dance all over again. Balanchine liked working with her because she could do anything he asked of her. She had the strength, technique, and musicality to be a Balanchine dancer.

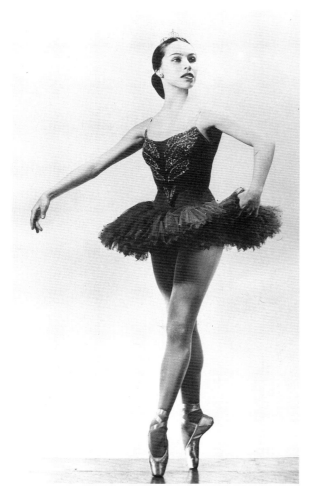

The talented Maria Tallchief attracted George's attention.

George's divorce from Brigitta was final in January 1946. He and Maria married the following August, when George was 42 and Maria was 21.

When the company danced in Oklahoma, George met part of Maria's family. He bought himself a western wardrobe. For the rest of his life, he favored cowboy shirts and string

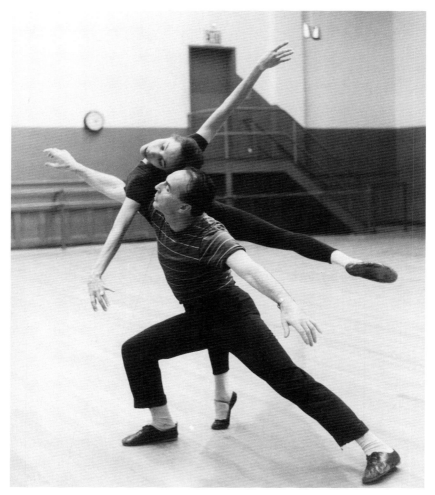

George rehearses with Maria, the embodiment of a Balanchine dancer.

ties. He also acquired a distinctive silver and turquoise bracelet that he wore constantly, even with a tuxedo.

In 1946 Lincoln Kirstein came back from the war. In the army, Corporal Kirstein had served as an interpreter and a courier. He realized that the military had a lot in common with ballet companies. Both required organization and unquestioned authority. His experience in the army had made him a better ballet administrator.

The School of American Ballet was now financially independent and operated well as a nonprofit educational institution. Professional dancers from many New York companies liked to take morning class there, so the inexperienced students learned from their classmates as well as their teachers. When Mr. B. had time, he would teach. The students were always excited on those special occasions.

Kirstein inherited $250,000, which he decided to spend on his dream of making an American ballet company. Kirstein and Balanchine formed a new performing company. To avoid competing with Ballet Theatre and the Ballet Russe, they asked New Yorkers to subscribe to the Ballet Society, a series of evenings of dance, lectures, and opera. Eight hundred people subscribed at a price of $15 each. With this working capital of $12,000 and Kirstein's contribution, their budget was tight. Kirstein didn't care if the Ballet Society made money as long as it was an artistic success. Once, when a booking agent offered friendly advice, Kirstein stressed, "Sir, I am not in ballet to make money."

The first Ballet Society performance took place in an uncomfortable high school auditorium. The two works on the program had elaborate and expensive costumes and scenery. *L'Enfant et les Sortileges,* the same one-act opera Balanchine had done in Monte Carlo, was first on the program. *The Four Temperaments,* a pure ballet with music by Paul Hindemith, featured a new soloist, a 16-year-old S.A.B. student named Tanaquil LeClercq. She danced with quick, flashing movements that contributed to the success of the evening.

The Paris Opéra invited Balanchine to work with them again in 1947. Serge Lifar had been the director there ever since he had taken over during Balanchine's bout with tuberculosis. The Opéra directors had suspended Lifar for sympathizing with the Nazis during the war. They now needed someone to revitalize the company. Balanchine probably hoped to be named their permanent director. The Paris Opéra Ballet was a well-established company with good dancers, constantly in need of new ballets. The Ballet Society was not turning into a permanent company. He could fulfill his commitment to the Ballet Society on a part-time basis.

Balanchine stayed in Paris only five months. The dancers were so loyal to Lifar that they would hardly cooperate with Balanchine. He created only one new ballet, Bizet's *Symphony in C.* He used 48 dancers for the plotless ballet, the largest group of dancers he'd ever assembled. Whenever the colorful, lyrical ballet appeared on the program, audiences were delighted to see it.

The Paris Opéra Ballet reinstated Lifar at the end of the season.

Back in New York, Balanchine and Stravinsky collaborated on a new version of *Orpheus* featuring Maria Tallchief. When the ballet was presented in 1948, the audience stamped and shouted their approval. But the production was too expensive for the Ballet Society. The scenery builders refused to deliver the set because the society didn't pay its bill. When Kirstein couldn't raise the $1,000 needed for a silk curtain, Balanchine suddenly appeared with $500 in each hand. He wouldn't say where he got the money, but he promised that he had not robbed a bank.

Kirstein faced reality. The Ballet Society had sold only enough subscriptions to pay for a single performance of each ballet. But they couldn't spend large sums on scenery and costumes for a ballet that was only performed once. Hoping to earn enough to keep the society going, Kirstein rented the New York City Center, a run-down auditorium on West 55th Street, and sold some tickets for a program that included *Orpheus*. The chairman of the City Center finance committee, Morton Baum, dropped in to see who'd rented the place. He was immensely impressed with what he saw. To help this struggling company, he proposed that the directors of the City Center offer them a home.

The finance committee was against it. Committee member Gerald Warburg warned, "You play around with Balanchine and Kirstein and you'll lose your shirt." He remembered his brother Edward's expensive experiences in the 1930s.

Baum visited Kirstein and later wrote

> It was the strangest meeting. Kirstein was belligerent, almost hostile to me, [bitter] against the entire ballet field, its policies, managers, repertoire. He seemed not to believe in the sincerity of my call and was suspicious of everything I said. He told me that the funds of Ballet Society were exhausted and that it might have to fold, but that he would carry on in his struggle to create an American ballet.

When Baum was finally able to get a word in, he offered the use of City Center, rent free several weeks a year for three years, and the right to call the company the New York City Ballet. The company would still have to cover their production costs, but if Kirstein were clever, they could survive.

Kirstein was stunned. Then he swore, "If you do that for us, I will give you in three years the finest ballet company in America."

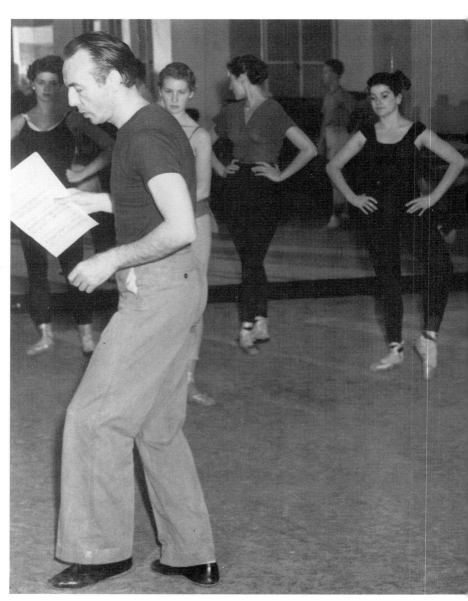

George refers to a copy of the score as he works out new movements for a dance.

NINE

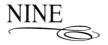

Birth of the
New York City Ballet

1948–1957

*T*he agreement with City Center solved the company's biggest problems. They had a free theater for about 12 weeks a year and space for rehearsal. Touring ballet companies could no longer rent the City Center, which helped Kirstein by limiting the competition.

But the dancers needed to earn a paycheck for more than just 12 weeks a year. Kirstein struggled to keep the company together and well trained. They toured a little, but traveling all night and dancing all day undermined the quality of the dancing.

During the nine years the New York City Ballet (NYC Ballet) was housed at City Center, neither Balanchine nor Kirstein drew a cent in salary. When Balanchine needed money, he staged a ballet for another company or found work on Broadway. He earned a lot of money for a television version of Prokofiev's *Cinderella*.

Morton Baum suggested that the NYC Ballet dance for the New York City Opera, which was also housed at City Center. This was not the Metropolitan Opera Company, where Balanchine had had so much trouble in the 1930s. The plan was worth a try, so Balanchine found himself back where he had started, staging waltzes for *La Traviata* and grand marches for *Aida*.

The NYC Ballet attracted experienced people from other schools and companies. Melissa Hayden and Nora Kaye, famous Ballet Theatre dancers, joined Balanchine's company. Jerome Robbins, a Broadway and Ballet Theatre choreographer, wanted to work with the NYC Ballet. Within a year, he became Balanchine's associate artistic director.

Balanchine and Robbins had completely different ways of working. The Russian's dances seemed to come from inspiration and improvisation. He would take someone's hand, pause a moment, maybe twitch his nose once or twice, and then begin dancing and teaching the dance at the same time. The American's ballets were carefully planned. Robbins wrote everything down and didn't allow the dancers to modify a step. Ironically, audiences saw Robbins's work as spontaneous and emotional and Balanchine's as mechanical and cold.

Dancers said that working with Robbins was like working with a tough athletic coach. They looked forward to the relaxing influence of Mr. B. to balance Robbins' strict discipline.

The company controlled costs wherever it could. They kept dancers' salaries consistently low. Other ballet companies offered high salaries to famous dancers. Balanchine opposed this star system, which he felt hurt morale and created a barrier between stars and lower-paid dancers. Kirstein knew high salaries could drain a company's finances and leave nothing for production costs.

Then Balanchine heard that the sets and costumes from an old Diaghilev ballet called *The Firebird* were being sold for only $2,500. It was a good deal.

Stravinsky's *The Firebird* was one of Diaghilev's earliest story ballets. Balanchine generally disliked ballets that had

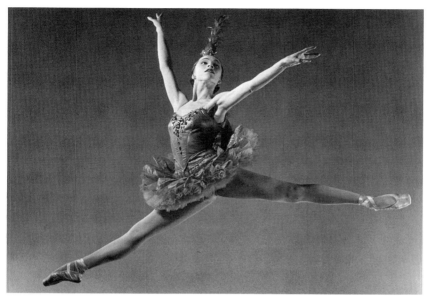

Maria inspired George to create what became her trademark role in The Firebird.

stories. He believed ballets should be about music, bodies, and movement, not princes or goddesses and their love stories. But George could see Maria Tallchief as the magic bird who repaid a debt to a prince and broke a sorcerer's spell. The story formed a background for her dashing, technically brilliant dancing.

Balanchine couldn't just restage an old ballet. He choreographed a whole new *Firebird* as a gift to Maria, and the role became her trademark.

The NYC Ballet toured many European cities and enjoyed great success. In Florence, Italy, the company was so popular that the theater management begged them to make their home there. Balanchine seriously considered the offer because he could not always get what he needed at the City

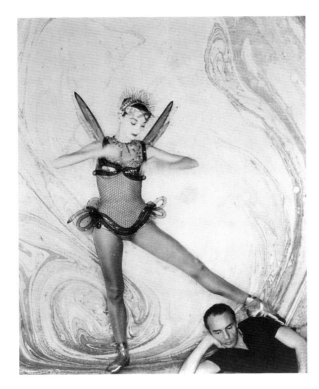

Tanny LeClercq, in costume for Metamorphoses, *poses with George.*

Center. But at last he decided that the NYC Ballet was an American company and an important part of the cultural life of New York. He was now an American.

Maria was a star in Europe, but so was "Tanny" LeClercq, who was living as a guest in the Balanchines' apartment. Maria and George were seldom alone together. Their marriage was in trouble.

George's second wife, Brigitta, said that George wanted to idolize and worship a woman. He wanted his wife to be a beautiful muse to inspire him. "It can become oppressive to be adored too much—even suffocating," she wrote. And once a woman showed signs of being human, George lost interest.

Maria spoke her mind, liked to play poker, and enjoyed keeping their home clean and tidy. George did *not* want to live with a housewife! Maria also wanted a baby.

"Any woman can become a mother," George said, "but not any woman can become a ballerina." The marriage was annulled in 1952.

George's ex-wives all remained George's good friends. Tamara, Brigitta, and Maria continued to take class at S.A.B. and were as friendly and affectionate with George as when their marriages were fresh.

By the end of 1952, Balanchine was married for the fourth time—to Tanaquil LeClercq. He was 48 years old. She was 23.

Tanny was the only one of Balanchine's wives who was a product of his training from her childhood. When she had come to S.A.B. on a scholarship in September 1940, Tanny had been a skinny, solemn 11-year-old who thought Mr. B. was a dull teacher and an old fogy. But she had not closed her mind to him and made good progress as a dancer. She was intelligent and developed a sense of humor. After five years of training, she could perform almost any role.

In 1953 the City Center management grew anxious about the huge expense of the ballet productions and canceled the fall and winter seasons for the NYC Ballet. Each dancer's earnings were cut in half. Kirstein arranged another European tour, but everyone was angry and upset. Rumors reached the City Center management that the dancers and their choreographer might find themselves another theater. Frightened, they promised Balanchine six to eight weeks of ballet performances, four times a year. This gave George a sense of his power at City Center. The NYC Ballet had become an asset to New York City.

Around this time, S.A.B. moved to a new studio at 82nd Street and Broadway. With a new studio and a new deal with City Center, Balanchine and Kirstein decided to try to make some money with their company.

Most ballets Balanchine created for the NYC Ballet were short—about eight to thirty minutes long. Balanchine called them "hors d'oeuvres," or little tastes of dance, like party sandwiches. Now he wanted to make a full-length story ballet in several acts that would last a whole evening.

He chose Tchaikovsky's *The Nutcracker,* which was first danced in Russia in 1892. Balanchine knew the old choreography because he had danced the role of the child prince at the Maryinsky Theater. But he wanted all his ballets for the NYC Ballet to bear his signature style, to look like Balanchine ballets. So George re-created the ballet from his memories of the old Russian masterpiece and added his new inventions. *The Nutcracker* offered a chance for many children to perform. Stage experience was part of the training at the Russian school, and George wanted it to be part of the training at S.A.B. too.

Audiences loved *The Nutcracker.* Box office money filled the company treasury. Balanchine shared his choreography for the ballet with companies all over the world. For the right to perform *The Nutcracker*—or any of his ballets—companies paid Balanchine royalties. *The Nutcracker* earned more royalties than any of his other ballets, enabling him to live quite comfortably from then on.

From 1953 to 1956, Tanny inspired Balanchine. He designed the finale of Hershy Kay's *Western Symphony,* full of difficult steps and flirtatious smiles, especially for her.

The company set out for another tour of Europe in 1956. They had excellent dancers and dozens of short ballets in

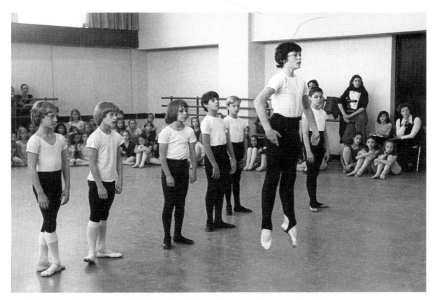

Young dancers audition for The Nutcracker *at S.A.B.*

their repertoire. But in Copenhagen, Tanny was stricken with polio. George was frantic. Once the diagnosis was definite, he arranged for every possible cure and therapy.

George, Tanny, and Tanny's mother stayed in Copenhagen for five months. George did some work for the Royal Danish Ballet, but he was too distracted to do his best. In March 1957, he brought Tanny back to New York.

Tanny had to learn how to live with her condition, and George devoted himself to helping her for another six months. Tanny was depressed at first, and George was not used to dealing with emotions. "I can stand any amount of work," he said. "I can work endlessly. But I can't cope with human relationships, difficult relationships."

Tanaquil LeClercq was permanently paralyzed from the waist down. At the age of 27, her career was over.

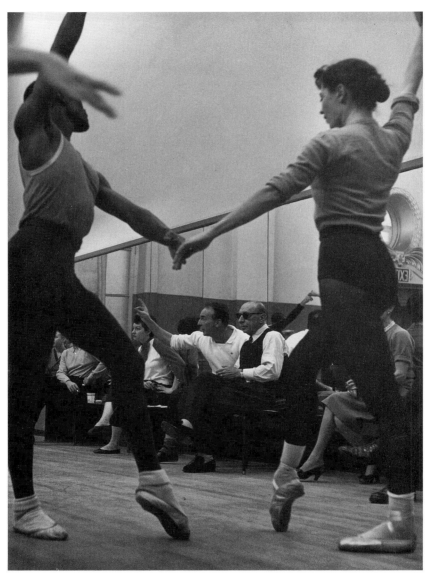

Balanchine and Stravinsky, center, *collaborate on the creation of*
Agon. *Dancers Arthur Mitchell and Diana Adams appear in the
foreground.*

TEN

The Balanchine Style

1957–1962

During the break in his career caused by Tanny's illness, George changed his whole style of living. He focused his attention on their home in New York, an apartment on 79th Street near Broadway, which he decorated in western style. George once said, "If you were to say to me, 'What's the best thing in America, artistically the best thing?' I would reply, 'Cowboys! Westerns!' When I see on the screen that wonderful Nevada or Arizona space and horses galloping beautifully across it, I am instantly satisfied. I find no fault in it at all."

George and Tanny owned an eight-acre property in Weston, Connecticut. Tanny enjoyed planning the landscaping, and George seemed happy doing the digging. Rumors circulated that he was going to retire.

In November 1957, Balanchine went back to work at S.A.B. and the City Center. He had been away for almost a year, and Tanny would not get any better. Perhaps she realized how important work was to him and urged him to return.

His renewed interest in the NYC Ballet was obvious. He choreographed four ballets within the next five months. They were *Square Dance* to music by Corelli and Vivaldi, *Gounod Symphony,* Stravinsky's *Agon,* and Sousa's *Stars and Stripes.*

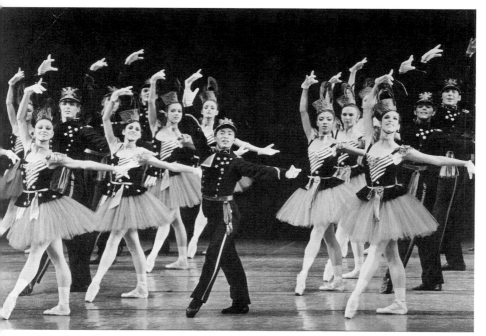

George called Stars and Stripes *an "applause machine" because it was so popular with audiences.*

The NYC Ballet could at last be called a success. The critics offered praise, and audiences offered profits.

After this sensational season, the company went on a tour of Japan, Australia, and the Philippines. Balanchine stayed in New York to think and plan.

In 1957 the Ford Foundation offered a few scholarships to S.A.B. on an experimental basis. Mr. B. and dancer Diana Adams made a short tour of ballet schools and established some guidelines for Adams to use to select future scholarship winners.

Adams wrote, "It was fascinating what Balanchine could see. It was never just the proportion or the physical gift. It

was a whole quality. He could just see talent . . . before the
students could do anything, what the possibilities were."

Balanchine gave 15-year-old Suzanne Farrell a private
audition at S.A.B. and awarded her one of the first scholarships. He did not tell Suzanne what he saw in her, but if his
perceptions were as sharp as Adams maintained, he knew
there was greatness in this young girl.

Balanchine's style of choreography was well established
by this time. Two of its most obvious elements were balance
and speed. His dancers often seemed to be off balance, with
their bodies angled out as if they had been flung. They had
to move fast at this angle to keep from falling. English

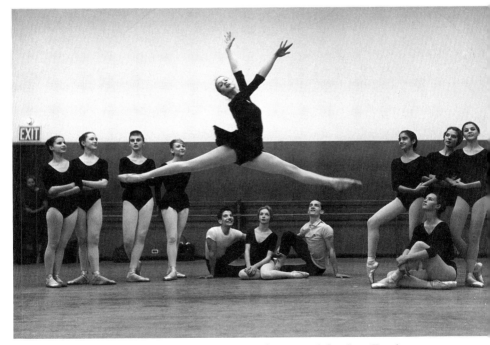

*Suzanne Farrell demonstrates a leap as the rest of the first Ford
Foundation scholarship winners pose.*

dancer Moira Shearer learned the style when Balanchine visited her company in the early 1950s. "Everything was *off*," she wrote. "It had to look dangerous. . . . He expected [you to be able to do] it, and you just couldn't let that man down—you just couldn't."

Balanchine loved flashing feet doing technically difficult steps at unbelievable speed. He once arranged a tarantella, a dance with a fast, steady beat. A tarantella has no rests for the orchestra or for the dancers. The first time Edward Villella danced the duet from beginning to end, he said that by the halfway point, "I felt as if I were going to collapse. I had never been so desperately exhausted in all of my career."

Balanchine's style didn't portray emotions, it evoked them. Audience members, not dancers, were the ones who felt emotions such as wonder, awe, amazement, sadness, loss, or excitement. Balanchine told dancers not to analyze. "Just dance, dear." If the movements were done properly, they would arouse emotion in the audience.

Once Balanchine was asked what the difference was between the Russian style of ballet and the style he created. "The Russians divide the dancer's body horizontally—heads, bodies and legs," he answered. "I divide it vertically," and he sliced downward with his hand, making a line from his head to his crotch.

This strong vertical line meant that in an *arabesque,* where the dancer stands on one foot, the other leg extends very high. Sometimes it can look like a gymnastic split, done standing up. Before Balanchine, people thought a high extension was vulgar. Most dancers didn't raise their legs very much above their waists. But Balanchine thought stopping the rising leg at any point other than at its ultimate, natural stopping place made the movement stiff and mechanical. He gave his dancers exercises to help them raise their legs higher, and after a while, young women competed with one another for the highest extension in class.

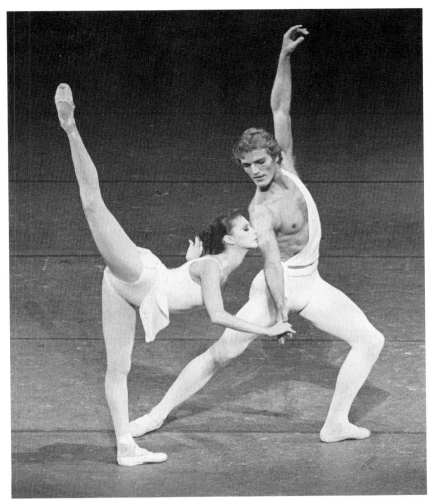

Supported by Peter Martins in Apollo, *Suzanne Farrell performs a fully extended arabesque, a movement that became part of the Balanchine style.*

Balanchine favored tall, slim girls. When people criticized him for discriminating, he said, "First of all, this is my company. . . . If somebody doesn't like it, he doesn't have to come and look at it. . . . I like tall people. I'll tell you why I like tall people. It's because you can *see* more." Lincoln Kirstein supported Balanchine's preference. He said that a long piece of string was needed for an elaborate knot.

Though young dancers couldn't make themselves taller, many tried to make themselves thinner. They could see that the slim girls got the attention and the chances to perform in school concerts. At a point when young bodies are maturing, many dancers found themselves dealing with anorexia nervosa, an eating disorder in which a person compulsively refuses to eat. Other girls suffered bulimia, as Brigitta did. Balanchine never advocated dieting to starvation, but many believed his attitude fostered the disorder in his students.

Through the years, Balanchine developed his own style of teaching. He didn't like to spend too much time on warm-up exercises at the barre. Some dancers could go from short barres to body-jarring jumps. Others need longer warm-ups. Students joked that they needed to take class from someone else to warm up before they took class from Balanchine.

After a short barre, his class would often focus on one step to perfect it or to work out a choreographic problem. Do the step over and over, then double the step, do it on toe-point, do it flat-footed, do it jumping. When a dancer performed well or overcame a bad habit, Balanchine would give high praise by saying, "Thaaaat's right!"

When he saw a consistent problem with the way students performed a step or position, he would analyze it carefully and find a better way to teach it. When he thought students' ankles needed strengthening, he would tell their teachers to keep them on their toes for whole classes and not allow them to put their heels down. Teachers and students would grumble, curse, and fall, but eventually the improvement Balanchine foresaw would come about.

Much of the time, he didn't use the traditional French names for arm positions and steps. He would describe movements. "Open wide the French windows. . . . Now step over the sill into the beautiful garden. . . . Look around at the flowers."

In 1958 the state of New York funded Lincoln Center. They planned space for the Metropolitan Opera, two theaters for plays, and City Center tenants, including the NYC Ballet.

Balanchine was eager for this theater to become a permanent, comfortable home. He worked hard with the architect to make it perfect. He single-handedly stopped construction when he realized the orchestra pit would hold only 35 musicians. He made such a scene that construction workers brought in jackhammers to remove the already-poured concrete and double the space.

The new theater was important, but George wasn't doing much of the work he did best—choreography. Though he created roles for many dancers, George seemed to be waiting for a special, real-life muse to inspire him.

Lincoln Center was still under construction when the U.S. State Department asked the NYC Ballet to tour the Soviet Union. George Balanchine had not seen his Russian homeland for 38 years.

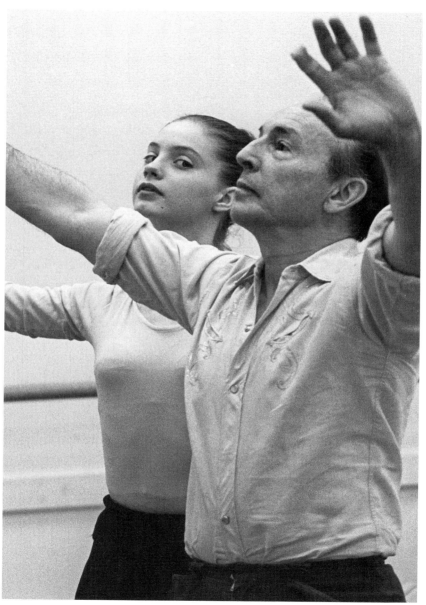

Suzanne Farrell watches George closely during a rehearsal.

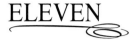

ELEVEN

The Final Muse

1962–1969

George Balanchine was not happy or comfortable on his return to the Soviet Union in 1962. His father had died in 1937, after refusing to have a badly infected leg amputated. George's mother had died just a few years before his visit. He had written to her often over the years, and when he was allowed, had sent her boxes of food. His sister Tamara had been killed in a bombing raid during World War II. Andrei, George's brother, was the only family member left to meet him at the airport in Moscow when the NYC Ballet arrived.

George had seen the Bolshoi Ballet in New York in 1959, so he knew what was popular in the Soviet Union—the same sorts of ballets that had been done for the tsar in the 1800s. There were new dances, but no new steps, no new concepts, no experiments. Balanchine knew Russian audiences would not easily understand his work.

Balanchine arranged a special rehearsal-performance so the Bolshoi dancers could see *Agon, Symphony in C,* and *Serenade.* After the performance, the Bolshoi's choreographer smiled broadly and told Balanchine that in the Soviet Union such works would be condemned as "formal" and "inhuman." Smiling in return, Balanchine replied that he wasn't interested in making a beautiful dance "as a caption for some silly story."

"Ah, well," the Russian responded jovially, "some day you'll come around to our way of doing things."

"What do you mean, 'come around?' " Balanchine asked pleasantly. "I went through all that and left it behind me long ago—35 years ago, to be exact."

Balanchine refused to be treated as a Russian returning to his homeland. He wanted to be thought of as an American citizen who voted Republican and wore a Native American turquoise bracelet. He still carried bitter memories of starving during the revolution and of being restricted by the State Theater.

At first, Russian audiences didn't know what to make of Balanchine's abstract ballets. By the end of the performance series, ballet fans—who attended every performance—grew to understand what they were seeing and to like his ballets more and more.

The company was in Moscow on October 18, 1962, when the U.S. government found out that the Soviet Union was building missiles in Cuba and aiming them at targets in the United States. President John Kennedy warned the Soviet Union to remove its missiles from Cuban bases or face nuclear war.

But Russian audiences didn't mix art and politics. They continued to attend and to enjoy the American ballet company's performances. By October 28, the Soviets moved their missiles. Television audiences enjoyed the last performances of the NYC Ballet in Moscow. The live audience applauded almost continuously, and there were countless curtain calls.

After a nostalgic visit to his old home in Leningrad, Balanchine felt depressed and a bit paranoid. He thought that someone was following and spying on him, that maybe the Russians wouldn't let him leave the Soviet Union. To reassure himself, he flew back to New York. A week later, he returned to his company for the last week of the tour.

The dancers were now in Tbilisi, in the republic of Georgia. Tbilisi was the Balanchivadze ancestral home and the city where George's family had lived while he studied in St. Petersburg. Tbilisi welcomed Balanchine as a long-lost son, with daily ceremonies, banquets, and parties.

The travel-weary company returned to New York for its last season at City Center. On April 23, 1964, they moved into their new home at Lincoln Center. The Lincoln Center theater had large wings, or spaces on either side of the stage. Dancers could line up in the wings or take a running start to

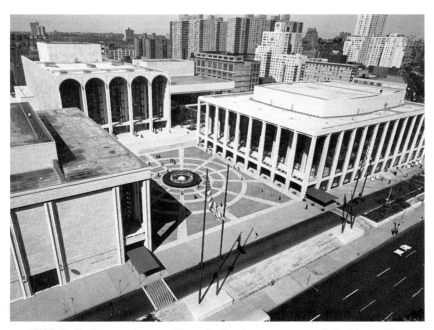

NYC Ballet's new home, Lincoln Center, was completed in 1966.

make a fast, leaping entrance. The City Center theater had had only three feet of wing space.

Balanchine had to restage some of his works for the larger theater. The stage was so much bigger that dancers had to move like lightning just to get to their positions on the stage. Company classes began to focus on large gestures rather than on details. Small details didn't show in the new theater.

While in Russia, members of the company had noticed that Mr. B. paid particular attention to one girl from the corps—Suzanne Farrell. At first, he seemed only courteous and helpful, and 17-year-old Farrell was in awe of him. She quickly emerged from the corps to solo roles. Other dancers said that she was an excellent young dancer, but still they wondered at her rapid progress.

One of Balanchine's first large-scale ballets in Lincoln Center was 1965's *Don Quixote* to music by Nicolas Nabokov. The ballet tells about the adventures of an old Spanish knight, Don Quixote, who imagines his ideal woman. She comes to him in many forms, some ordinary and some glorified. In the end, she begs for his protection. When he fights a giant windmill that he thinks is a giant, he is captured and taken home to die. His ideal woman becomes a servant who blesses him at his death.

Balanchine saw Don Quixote as "an old man, . . . but young in feeling and vigorous in movement." Perhaps this was how he saw himself. He created the role of Don Quixote for Richard Rapp, but at the charity premiere, Balanchine danced the role himself. The part was mostly pantomimed, so he managed it easily. He liked to perform now and then, but he wouldn't let the public know in advance. On the night of a performance, a voice would announce, "Ladies and Gentlemen, in

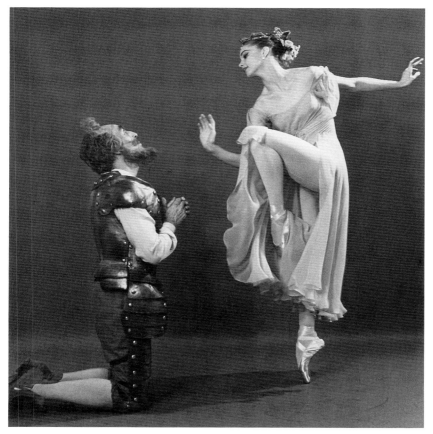

George, as Don Quixote, performs with his Dulcinea, Suzanne Farrell.

this evening's performance, the role of Don Quixote will be danced by Mr. George Balanchine." The applause would roll out even before the curtain rose.

Balanchine created the role of Dulcinea, Don Quixote's ideal woman, for Suzanne Farrell. By now, everyone in the company knew she was Balanchine's new muse. She had strength, fearlessness, and femininity, as well as the perfect body for his style. Her pretty face and wonderful memory were also assets.

Ballet critic Arlene Croce wrote, "We think of Farrell ... as the supreme classicist of our time. She could do anything Balanchine asked of her—and do it on a grander scale, at greater speed, and with a silkier recovery and sense of control than anyone else."

George courted Suzanne, though he was 61 and she was 19. He may have realized that he couldn't marry another young dancer without being severely criticized, but he wanted Suzanne's full concentration and devotion. He won her loyalty by lavishing attention on her and helping her become the perfect Balanchine dancer.

George educated Suzanne the way Diaghilev had educated him. He taught her how to look at art, how to listen to music, and how to view the world the way he did. Like many young dancers, Suzanne hadn't finished high school. Her life had consisted of ballet classes, rehearsals, performances, and sleep, until George added "talking about life and art" to her schedule. They would spend long evenings together in delicatessens and doughnut shops. On tour, they would explore each city.

In July 1966, the state of New York opened a new indoor-outdoor theater for the NYC Ballet at Saratoga Springs. Balanchine and the company now spent part of each summer there. He and Tanny shared a small house where they indulged their love of animals and kept many cats and dogs. George, relaxed and sociable, cooked wonderful meals for friends.

For the 1966 fall season at Lincoln Center, Balanchine assembled one of his most popular ballets, *Jewels*. He designed it in three sections. Each could be shown separately, but when

"Emeralds," "Rubies," and "Diamonds" were shown together, *Jewels* made an exciting full-length program. "Emeralds" had a French feeling, with music by the French composer Gabriel Fauré. "Rubies," danced to Stravinsky's music, had a deliberately witty, jazzy feel. "Diamonds," to music by Tchaikovsky, recalled Russia in the days of the tsars.

Balanchine choreographed "Diamonds" for Suzanne. Like a lover's gift of a diamond ring, this dance was George's gift to her and a showcase for her talent. "Diamonds" was supposed to be the high point of the evening, yet most critics agreed that the "Rubies" section shone brighter and more interestingly.

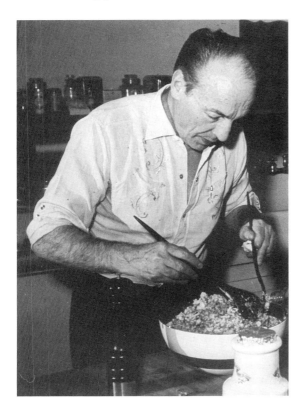

While on tour or at home, George enjoyed cooking for his friends.

For a tour of Scotland in 1967, the NYC Ballet had no male dancer tall enough to partner Suzanne. So Balanchine sent for a young Danish dancer, Peter Martins. Later that year, Balanchine invited Martins to New York to dance in *The Nutcracker.* Soon Martins was shuttling between New York and the Royal Danish Ballet in Copenhagen.

Some excellent dancers left the NYC Ballet during the next few years. They felt they couldn't progress because Balanchine was so obsessed with Suzanne. No one liked it when he refused to teach jumps in class because Suzanne had a sore knee. No one appreciated that he didn't stay in the theater to watch a whole program unless Suzanne danced that night.

By this time, Tanny realized that she couldn't depend on George. She had to rebuild her own life. She developed a method of teaching dance that didn't require demonstration and joined the faculty of Arthur Mitchell's Dance Theatre of Harlem. This position helped her to feel capable and independent.

Tanny knew what everyone in the ballet community knew about George and Suzanne. She kept her pride and agreed to a separation.

Suzanne was going through her own agony at this time. She loved George sincerely but felt their relationship was hopeless. She was a religious Roman Catholic. Even if George proposed, she couldn't give up her religion to marry a divorced man. The age and educational differences formed a broad gulf between them as well. Suzanne was discovering what Brigitta learned years ago: Life as a goddess was tiring.

Paul Mejia, a dancer and potential choreographer, invited Suzanne to take adagio classes with him at S.A.B. In adagio class, the work focuses on partnering. Men learn to lift, turn, and support women, and women learn to help and trust their partners during elaborate or dangerous lifts.

From adagio class, Paul and Suzanne built a friendship, and late in 1968, Paul told her he was in love with her. Suzanne loved Paul but worried about how this would affect George and her position in the company. George heard of his competition and instantly proposed marriage. He suggested they have a child—something he had never wanted for himself or for any of his dancers. Suzanne knew she couldn't marry George.

George thought she refused him because he was married. He had lawyers arrange a permanent income for Tanny. Then he flew to Mexico. On February 5, he was granted a divorce. He couldn't return to New York though, because he'd promised to stage a ballet in Germany. Suzanne and Paul were married on February 21, 1969, without having to face George.

When George heard of the marriage, he gave in to anger and despair. He vowed he would never return to the United States. He had wild ideas. He would go to Iran. He would go to Moscow and teach the Bolshoi Ballet his repertoire. In the end, he returned to New York.

George tried to behave as if nothing had happened, but he couldn't stand to be around Paul. He allowed Paul to take class and collect a salary, but he wouldn't let Paul perform. Finally, Paul told Suzanne he had to go someplace where he could dance. Thinking she could help, Suzanne sent a message to George, saying that if Paul didn't dance that night, they both would leave the company.

George did not like ultimatums. He did not ask Paul to dance. Suzanne packed her personal items and left the New York City Ballet.

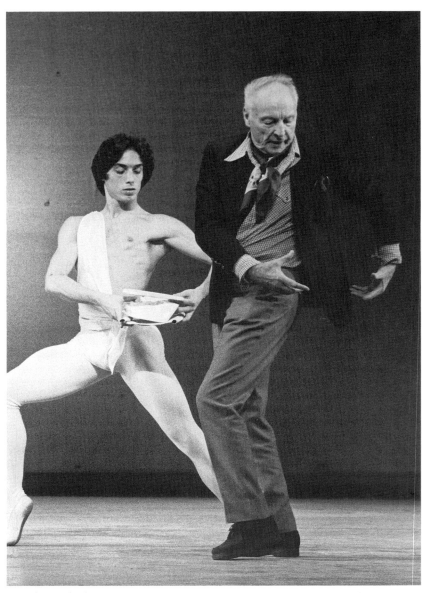

Through the years, George taught his famous choreography to many young Apollos, this time to Jean-Pierre Frohlich.

TWELVE
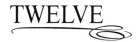

Curtain Call

1969–1983

*A*fter Paul and Suzanne left the NYC Ballet in 1969, Balanchine seemed apathetic and disinterested in his own company. He restaged an old ballet and then found work in Germany and Switzerland.

While he was gone, S.A.B. moved into spacious quarters at the Julliard School in Lincoln Center. This move linked S.A.B. and the NYC Ballet even closer.

When S.A.B. students joined the company, Balanchine liked to tell them they learned ballet steps at S.A.B. At the NYC Ballet, they must learn to perform. When their dancing was awkward or amateurish, he'd tease them by asking, "Where did you learn *that*? S.A.B.? Ah, that's what they teach you. S.A.B. is the worst!"

As S.A.B. produced more and more excellent dancers, Balanchine began to see them as interchangeable. When his ballet mistress asked about casting a certain dancer, he'd answer, "Just put anybody, because they're so good—anybody."

Lincoln Kirstein was still the active administrator of S.A.B., which he had run since 1934. He was also chief fundraiser for the board of directors of the NYC Ballet. If Kirstein could find money for a new ballet, it got produced.

If he couldn't, Balanchine would have to do something else. Kirstein's impeccable taste, the result of his knowledge of art, often influenced Balanchine's decisions about the look of a ballet.

Danish dancer Peter Martins joined the NYC Ballet in 1970, but Balanchine didn't seem pleased with Martins' dancing. Martins didn't have the speed and musicality needed for Balanchine's ballets. After months of struggling, Martins finally asked Balanchine what was wrong. Balanchine replied, "You see, dear, you don't seem to be interested . . . . When people show interest, I use them. If they don't, I leave them alone." As soon as Martins asked for help, he got it.

Sometimes when Balanchine left dancers alone, he did so because he knew instinctively that they didn't need special attention. "You never cared about me," Karin von Aroldingen accused him. He answered, "No, dear, I knew you could do it on your own."

Just as Balanchine varied his encouragement of dancers, he also varied their training. He was not consistent. If dancers compared what he told each of them privately, they would find conflicting instructions. One day he would say, "Don't listen to the music, just count." The next day, he might say, "Don't count, just follow the music."

New York ballet audiences wondered if their resident company would ever give them an exciting new ballet again. Finally in 1970, Balanchine produced *Who Cares?,* a ballet to famous songs by George Gershwin. When Balanchine chose the song "Who Cares?" as the title of the piece, dancers thought it was a message to Suzanne Farrell.

Balanchine had definite ideas about his future relationships with women. "I'm free. I am an old man. And nobody is going to get me any more."

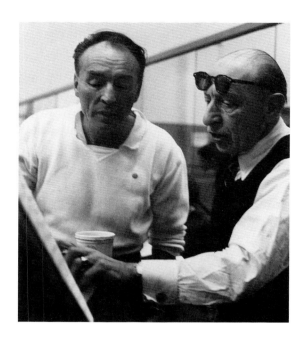

Balanchine and Stravinsky, a memorable creative team

In 1971 Balanchine's great friend Igor Stravinsky died. This sad event seemed to rekindle Balanchine's creative powers. Two months after Stravinsky's death, Balanchine announced "Next year, Stravinsky Festival." He assembled this program with his usual imagination, energy, and skill.

He insisted that the festival open on the day that would have been Stravinsky's 90th birthday, June 18, 1972. The company would give performances every night for a week, plus two matinees. No two programs would be alike. He had one year to prepare, during which the company still had to present its regular programs. Balanchine required a quarter of a million dollars to produce this festival and demanded that the theater be closed for the week before the festival. That demand cost Lincoln Center $130,000 in lost ticket sales. Balanchine didn't care. He needed the theater for rehearsals.

He called former NYC Ballet dancers to Lincoln Center from all over the United States. He needed their memories to rebuild old Stravinsky ballets. For new works, Balanchine couldn't or didn't want to choreograph them all himself. He invited six other choreographers to create new dances for the program.

The Stravinsky Festival presented 31 ballets with only 10 restorations of old ballets. Excitement about the festival spread all over the United States. Balanchine was more famous than ever, but few of the dances became part of NYC Ballet's permanent repertoire.

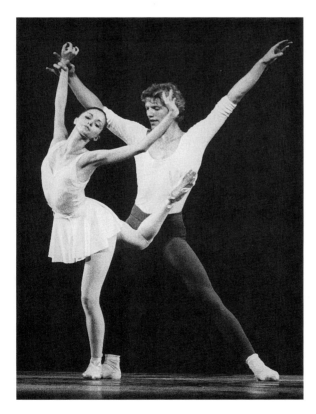

Kay Mazzo and Peter Martins dance in Duo Concertante, *which George choreographed for the 1972 Stravinsky Festival.*

In 1973 and 1976 Balanchine had to deal with strikes by the orchestra and the dancers. The dancers complained that everyone in the company—administrators, musicians, stage-hands—earned more than the dancers. The company and the state of New York lost over a million dollars because the shows did not go on.

Balanchine was not very sympathetic to his striking dancers. When they complained that dancers earned less than garbage collectors, he explained that "garbage stinks." If there was no settlement, he said, "We'll close the theater, and everyone will go home. The girls will marry; the boys will go and drive taxicabs."

This was a cold attitude. If the company disbanded, Balanchine could work anywhere and command high fees. But most dancers couldn't do anything but dance. Without his company, Balanchine implied, they were worth very little.

During these years, Suzanne Farrell and her husband Paul danced in Belgium. In the summer of 1974, they came back to visit and bought tickets to see NYC Ballet perform in Saratoga Springs. They did not try to take class or make themselves conspicuous.

Later that year, Suzanne wrote a short note to ask Balanchine if she could rejoin the company. To her amazement, he said yes. Not only did he welcome her back, he welcomed her as his personal friend once more.

But Balanchine still couldn't accept Paul. At first, Paul worked wherever he could in New York. Then he went to Guatemala for a year. Eventually Balanchine helped him get work with the Chicago Lyric Ballet, where Maria Tallchief was the director. Paul worked in Chicago for eight years. Each summer he and Suzanne met in the Adirondack Mountains, where they ran a ballet camp.

Balanchine's greatest inspiration may have been Suzanne, but Karin von Aroldingen became more important to him as he grew older. Karin had started with the company in the corps de ballet in 1962 and became a soloist in 1967. During her time in the corps, she married and had a child, but she didn't let anything interfere with her first priority— to become the best Balanchine dancer she could be.

Once Balanchine was sure that Karin put her career before her marriage, he behaved like a father to her and a grandfather to her little girl. He bought a condominium on Long Island next door to Karin's family. Karin and George shared a love of cooking and spent hours making everyday meals into feasts. Before Russian Easter each year, they spent two weeks cooking a traditional holiday meal to serve to everyone they knew.

In 1978 Balanchine had a mild heart attack. He was 74. Karin arranged for his care and saw him through rehabilitation. George hadn't had a serious physical problem since his early days in the United States. If his bad knee was sore, he never spoke of it. If he was short of breath because he had only one usable lung, he could still demonstrate steps and technique. But the heart attack reminded George that he was mortal.

George made a will. In it, he left the rights to 80 ballets to Tanny and distributed another 20 ballets among other dancers and administrators of the NYC Ballet. His will completed, Balanchine went back to work and toured with the company.

Late that year, he suffered alarming attacks of angina, a condition in which pain radiates from the heart to the left side and affects the jaw, shoulder, and arm. A low-fat diet helps prevent angina, but Balanchine was used to high-fat food and wasn't willing to change his habits. He broke his

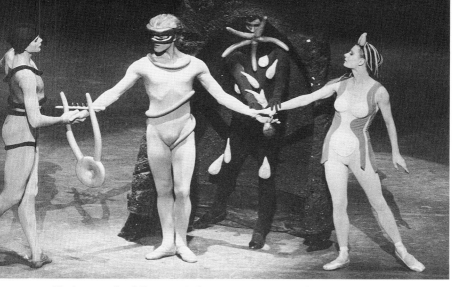

Karin von Aroldingen, right, was a favorite dancer and close personal friend to George. She performs here in Orpheus *with Adam Lüders, left, and Peter Martins, center.*

own rule against allowing surgeons to cut into his body and chose bypass heart surgery to replace blocked arteries with healthy arteries. After the surgery, George had more energy.

In 1981 Balanchine choreographed a ballet with religious themes called *Adagio Lamentoso (Slow Lament)* to music by Tchaikovsky. Dancers were mourners, angels with immense wings, hooded figures in purple, and monks who prostrated themselves in the shape of a cross. A child entered with a candle and on the final chord of the symphony, blew it out, plunging the theater into darkness. The audience was so shocked they could not applaud. It looked too much like Balanchine was staging his own public funeral.

Balanchine began to weaken. First his vision faltered,

and though he had cataracts removed from both eyes, he still could not see well. He had trouble with his hearing. Worst of all, George's sense of balance deteriorated, and he fell often. He heard noises in his head that interfered with his conversation and his enjoyment of music. Yet when he vacationed in Saratoga Springs in the summer of 1982, he composed song after song, writing both music and lyrics. He joked that he needed a change of career.

He persuaded Brigitta to narrate a role in *Persephone,* a dance drama by Stravinsky, while Karin danced the role. But George wasn't up to his task of choreographing, and Karin had to help him. She suggested positions and steps and asked George what he wanted. She had to draw the choreography out of him.

Finally he could not work at all. Every day was a struggle. He broke bones when he fell. A nurse came daily, and his personal assistant, Barbara Horgan, and Karin tried to be with him as much as possible. George knew he was becoming a problem to people who loved him. He decided to check into New York's Roosevelt Hospital on November 4, 1982.

For five months, George Balanchine lay in a hospital bed. Doctors had no idea what was making him so ill. There was nothing they could do to ease his symptoms. On good days, he recognized everyone and could laugh and joke with visitors. On bad days, he could not function.

Friends, dancers, and students visited regularly. People brought food to tempt him, gave parties for him, and tried to behave as though George would recover. Gifts of radios and taped music arrived for George, but he preferred the music he heard in his head. To that music, he watched dancing that only he could see.

His turquoise bracelet hung loosely on his sticklike wrist.

In February 1983, President Ronald Reagan chose Balanchine to receive the Medal of Freedom, the highest award the U.S. government gives to honor a citizen. When someone told him the president was honoring him, he joked, "Of what country?"

Of course, Balanchine could not go to Washington, D.C., so Lincoln Kirstein, Barbara Horgan, and Suzanne Farrell accepted the honor for him. Suzanne wondered why the government had waited so long to make the award. Clearly it would give George no pleasure now.

On April 30, 1983, George Balanchine died.

Since medicine had been useless to ease Balanchine's symptoms or keep him alive, doctors wondered why he had died. They performed an autopsy but found nothing obvious. Tissue samples later revealed the cause of death to be Creutzfeldt-Jakob disease, an infection of a slow-acting virus that attacks the nervous system.

The day Balanchine died, the NYC Ballet and the S.A.B. had three performances scheduled. Before each curtain went up, Lincoln Kirstein made a short emotional speech to the audience, telling them that Balanchine had just joined his friends Mozart, Tchaikovsky, and Stravinsky.

For three days before the funeral, memorial services were held at a Russian Orthodox cathedral in New York. At these services, Tamara Geva, Choura Danilova, Tanny LeClercq, and Maria Tallchief could be seen near the casket. Brigitta was in Europe when he died.

Balanchine was buried on May 3, 1983, at Sag Harbor, Long Island. At the funeral, Lincoln Kirstein stood on the steps of the church and quaked with sobs. His friend of 50 years, the man who had made his dream of an American ballet come true, was gone.

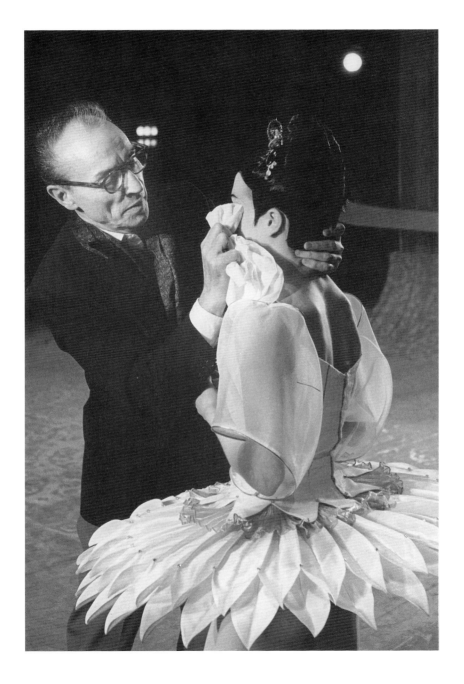

EPILOGUE

$\mathscr{B}$alanchine's work lives in the memories of his students, who are now the teachers of a new generation of dancers. His ballets are still performed regularly. In 1993 the NYC Ballet produced a Balanchine Celebration to revive or reproduce many of his ballets. Once again, Balanchine's former students and colleagues participated in restoring the repertoire. They used films of performances in which they had danced many years earlier to help them remember the choreography.

Someone owns the rights to every Balanchine ballet. An organization called the Balanchine Trust guards the legal rights to all the ballets. Whenever a company anywhere in the world performs a Balanchine ballet, the owner of the ballet or a representative of the trust supervises the production and receives royalties. Suzanne Farrell owns *Don Quixote*. Lincoln Kirstein owns *Concerto Barocco* and *Orpheus*. Karin von Aroldingen owns six other Balanchine ballets.

Balanchine was sure his ballets would change after he died. He said, "Somebody will rehearse them different and it will all be a little different, with different approach, different intensity. So a few years go by... [they] will be my ballets, but will look different."

Some people now claim that the ballets look *too* different. They say that no one teaches the Balanchine technique any longer, that the stress on dancing the music is gone.

They may be right. Some people find it difficult to devote their lives to someone else's vision. Others can dedicate themselves to doing just that. If a dancer wants to learn the Balanchine style now, he or she must find a teacher devoted to that style.

Balanchine ran the NYC Ballet the way the tsars ruled Russia. His word was law. "People don't realize," Lincoln Kirstein said, "the specific way in which George ran the company.... There was nothing except what he wished, and that's why it's very difficult now—because there isn't that kind of single purpose or tyrannical behavior. It's much harder to run a company now, without him...."

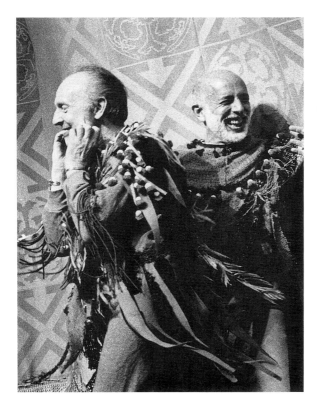

Jerome Robbins, right, *takes a bow with George.*

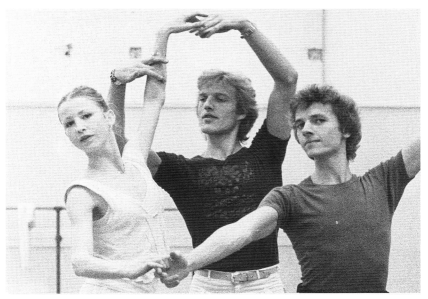

Peter Martins, center, *carried on as teacher and director of NYC Ballet.*

Before Balanchine died, everyone wondered who would follow him as director of the NYC Ballet. Balanchine said he didn't care who followed him. "Nothing is forever. There will be another kind of dancing. . . . Would you want Washington to be president today? Or Lincoln? . . . They were very great men, but they were in their times, not ours. I only live now. That is the only forever: right now."

Jerome Robbins was the obvious choice to head the company and carry on the standards of Balanchine. But he was over 60 years old and didn't want the responsibilities Balanchine had carried into his old age. The board of directors offered joint leadership roles to Robbins and Peter Martins. Later, Martins took over every aspect of the enterprise. He even took on the fundraising job from Lincoln Kirstein.

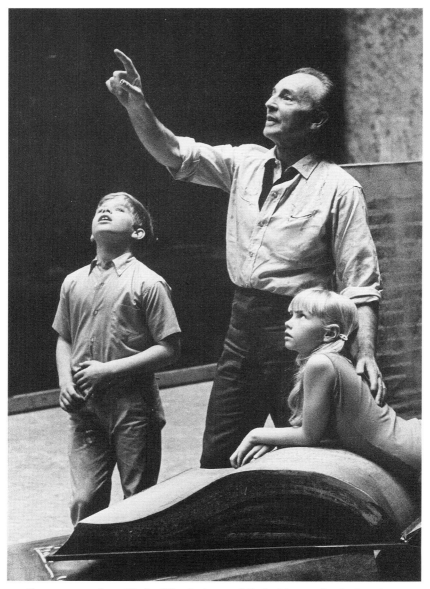

George coaches Chris d'Amboise and Judy Fugate in their roles for Don Quixote.

Scholars have written that the musical genius Mozart heard his compositions, complete, in his head. He copied down the music as if he were remembering it rather than inventing it. Balanchine's creativity operated in much the same way. He used to say that he didn't *create* ballet. "Only God creates; I assemble."

He seemed to listen to an inner music when he assembled dances. One dancer described how easily Balanchine heard that inner music. "He'd just take us by the hand and start to choreograph. . . . He'd do a few nose twitches, lead you to the center, the music would start, and he would show you the steps. It would all come out and just flow."

The company's doctor once asked Balanchine, "How do you do all this stuff?" The answer: "Oh, it's really very easy. I hear music, and I see people doing things, and I just go in the studio and I have them do what I see them do in my mind." Then Balanchine pointed to the sky and said, "He tells me."

Sources

p.17   Bernard Taper, *Balanchine: A Biography* (Berkeley, California: University of California Press, 1987), 43.

p.26   Ibid., 69–70.

p.28   Alexandra Danilova, *Choura: The Memoirs of Alexandra Danilova* (New York: Alfred A. Knopf, Inc., 1986), 66.

p.30   Moira Shearer, *Ballet Master: A Dancer's View of George Balanchine* (London: Sidgwick & Jackson, 1986), 49.

p.34   Taper, *Balanchine,* 91.

p.36   George Balanchine and Francis Mason, *Balanchine's Complete Stories of the Great Ballets* (Garden City, New York: Doubleday & Company, Inc., 1977), 28.

p.37   Edwin Denby, "The Power of Poetry," *New York Herald Tribune,* 23 October 1945.

p.39   Taper, *Balanchine,* 110.

p.42   Ibid., 125.

p.43   Lili Cockerille Livingston, "Inside Interview with Mr. B.," *Dance Magazine,* July 1983, 49.

pp.49–50   Taper, *Balanchine,* 149.

p.50   W. McNeil Lowry, "Profile: Conversations with Balanchine," *The New Yorker,* 12 September 1983, 54.

p.50   Richard Buckle, *George Balanchine: Ballet Master* (New York: Random House, 1988), 68.

p.51   Edward M. M. Warburg, "Fifty Years Ago: The Beginning of the School of American Ballet," *Playbill,* NYC Ballet Winter Season 1983–1984.

p.52   Lowry, "Profile: Conversations with Balanchine," 54.

p.53   Francis Mason, *I Remember Balanchine: Recollections of the Ballet Master by Those Who Knew Him* (New York: Doubleday, 1991), 124.

p.57   Ibid., 125.

p.59   Taper, *Balanchine,* 163.

p.60   Ibid., 164.

p.61   Ibid., 165.

p.61   Ibid., 166.

p.62   Ibid., 175.

p.63   Shearer, *Ballet Master,* 114.

p.63   Mason, *I Remember Balanchine,* 129.

pp.64–65   Vera Zorina, *Zorina* (New York: Farrar, Straus & Giroux, Inc., 1986), 171. Reprinted by permission.

p.70   Taper, *Balanchine,* 196.

pp.72–73   Ibid., 177–78.

p.73   Mason, *I Remember Balanchine,* 225.

p.77   Taper, *Balanchine,* 212.

p.79   Ibid., 226.

p.79   Anatole Chujoy, *The New York City Ballet* (New York: Alfred A. Knopf, Inc., 1953), 202–203. Reprinted by permission.

p.79   Taper, *Balanchine,* 227.

p.84   Zorina, *Zorina,* 202.

p.85   Taper, *Balanchine,* 213.

p.87   Mason, *I Remember Balanchine,* 343.

p.89   Taper, *Balanchine,* 244.

pp.90–91   Mason, *I Remember Balanchine,* 351.

p.92   Barbara Newman, *Striking a Balance: Dancers Talk About Dancing* (Boston: Houghton Mifflin Company, 1982), 107.

p.92   Edward Villella, *Prodigal Son* (New York: Simon & Schuster, 1992), 141–142.

p.92   Buckle, *George Balanchine,* 238.

p.94   John Gruen, *The Private World of Ballet* (New York: The Viking Press, 1975), 282.

p.94   Taper, *Balanchine,* 293.

pp.97–98   Ibid., 275–276.

p.100   Buckle, *George Balanchine,* 249.

p.101   Suzanne Farrell, *Holding on to the Air* (New York: Simon & Schuster, 1990), 127.

p.101   Arlene Croce, "Books: Angel," *The New Yorker,* 15 October 1990, 124.

p.102   Farrell, *Holding on to the Air,* 98.

p.107   Jennifer Dunning, *But First a School* (New York: Elizabeth Sifton Books for Viking, 1985), 145.

p.108   Buckle, *George Balanchine,* 264.

p.108   Mason, *I Remember Balanchine,* 491.

p.108   Ibid., 259.

p.108   Joseph H. Mazo, *Dance Is a Contact Sport* (New York: E. P. Dutton & Co., 1974), 253.

p.109   Buckle, *George Balanchine,* 296.

p.111   Ibid., 295.

p.115   Farrell, *Holding on to the Air,* 264.

p.117   Arlene Croce, "The Balanchine Show," *The New Yorker,* 7 June 1993, 103.

p.118   W. McNeil Lowry, "Profile: Conversations with Kirstein," *The New Yorker,* 15 December 1986, 44.

p.119   Mazo, *Dance Is a Contact Sport,* 294–295.

p.121   Taper, *Balanchine,* 257.

p.121   Mason, *I Remember Balanchine,* 319.

p.121   Ibid., 581.

Bibliography

Balanchine, George and Francis Mason. *Balanchine's Complete Stories of the Great Ballets*. Garden City, New York: Doubleday & Company, Inc., 1977.

Buckle, Richard. *George Balanchine: Ballet Master*. New York: Harper & Row, 1982.

Danilova, Alexandra. *Choura: The Memoirs of Alexandra Danilova*. New York: Alfred A. Knopf, Inc., 1986.

Dunning, Jennifer. *But First a School*. New York: Elizabeth Sifton Books for Viking, 1985.

Farrell, Suzanne. *Holding on to the Air*. New York: Simon & Schuster, 1990.

Geva, Tamara. *Split Seconds*. New York: Harper & Row, 1972.

Gruen, John. *The Private World of Ballet*. New York: The Viking Press, 1975.

Kirstein, Lincoln. *Portrait of Mr. B*. New York: Viking Press, 1984.

Mason, Francis. *I Remember Balanchine: Recollections of the Ballet Master by Those Who Knew Him*. New York: Doubleday, 1992.

Mazo, Joseph H. *Dance Is a Contact Sport*. New York: E. P. Dutton & Company, 1974.

McDonagh, Don. *George Balanchine*. Boston: G. K. Hall & Company, 1984.

Newman, Barbara. *Striking a Balance: Dancers Talk About Dancing*. Boston: Houghton Mifflin Company, 1982.

Shearer, Moira. *Ballet Master: A Dancer's View of George Balanchine*. London: Sidgwick & Jackson, 1986.

Stravinsky, Igor. *An Autobiography*. New York: Simon & Schuster, 1936.

Taper, Bernard. *Balanchine: A Biography*. Berkeley, California: University of California Press, 1996.

Tracy, Robert and Sharon DeLano. *Balanchine's Ballerinas: Conversations with the Muses*. New York: Simon & Schuster, 1984.

Villella, Edward. *Prodigal Son*. New York: Simon & Schuster, 1992.

Zorina, Vera. *Zorina*. New York: Farrar, Straus & Giroux, Inc., 1986.

Index

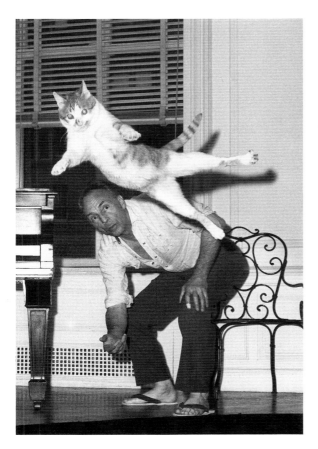

George helps Mourka dance.

127

Photo Acknowledgments

Front cover: George Balanchine rehearses a dance sequence for the 1937 movie *The Goldwyn Follies.* Vera Zorina stands in the center.

Back cover: Balanchine instructs a Ringling Brothers elephant for Stravinsky's *Circus Polka.*

Page 1: Balanchine poses with the stars of his ballet *Jewels: (from left)* Violette Verdy, Mimi Paul, Suzanne Farrell, and Patricia McBride.